Intellectual

Giftedness

in

Disabled Persons

Contributors

Shirin Antia
Anne L. Corn
Joanna Gartner
Patrick M. Ghezzi
Gladys Knott
S.J. Obringer

John Robertson
Sandra Ruconich
Anne Udall
Martha Lentz Walker
Nancy Wingenbach
Doris Senor Woltman

Intellectual

Giftedness

in

Disabled Persons

Joanne Rand Whitmore
Kent State University

C. June Maker
University of Arizona—Tucson

AN ASPEN PUBLICATION®
Aspen Systems Corporation

1985

Rockville, Maryland
Royal Tunbridge Wells

Library of Congress Cataloging in Publication Data
Whitmore, Joanne Rand, 1938
Intellectual giftedness in disabled persons.

Bibliography: p.
Includes index.
1. Gifted children—Education—United States. 2. Learning
disabilities—United States. 3. Handicapped children—Education—
United States. I. Maker, C. June. II. Title [DNLM: 1. Child,
Gifted—education. 2. Education, Special. 3. Handicapped. LC 3993
W616i]
LC3993.9.W45   1985   371.95   85-15039
ISBN: 0-87189-236-7

Editorial Services: Martha Sasser

Library of Congress Catalog Card Number: 85-15039
ISBN: 0-87189-236-7

Printed in the United States of America

1 2 3 4 5

This book is dedicated to
CURT WHITESEL

who invited and guided our development as authors while providing just the right balance between freedom and direction; whose giftedness as an editor will long be remembered; and whose perseverance and adaptation to becoming disabled in a losing battle with cancer lives on in our memories to inspire our work.

Table of Contents

Preface

This book, *Intellectual Giftedness in Disabled Persons*, is somewhat unique in that its purpose is to give impetus to the development of a new field of inquiry that will improve professional practices and community responses related to disabled children and adults. We have been motivated by a strong desire to acquaint others with some of the remarkable disabled individuals who have achieved significantly despite handicapping conditions and have profoundly shaped our thinking, and to consequently create a provocative dialogue about prevailing attitudes, beliefs, and practices.

The content of this text is a product of our collective and complementary experiences of inquiry and discovery over a period of approximately 15 years. Those experiences have included assisting gifted adults in seeking appropriate employment and sharing the frustration associated with rejection; working with children and teachers to prepare them for the "mainstreaming" of handicapped students; participating in the process of evaluating students with specific disabilities for admission to or continuation in teacher education programs; consulting with highly skilled educators in schools puzzled by the identification of intellectual giftedness in a disabled student; assisting in the development of pilot or experimental programs to serve gifted students with special needs; interviewing successful disabled professionals; serving on committees and councils, such as the National Council for the Accreditation of Teacher Education (NCATE), to develop accreditation standards to require every teacher to be prepared to work effectively with disabled and gifted students; struggling to establish a healthy concern about gifted handicapped students through a committee of the Council for Exceptional Children; and participating in efforts to increase integration and collaboration among teacher educators preparing professionals in various programs and departments. We hope the synthesis of our experiences, analyzed from theoretical perspectives, will heighten the awareness of our readers and encourage them to join us in this line of inquiry.

We wish to acknowledge our extreme indebtedness to the subjects of the case studies presented in this book who have so effectively taught and inspired us and who have so generously responded to our questions with gifts of time, candor, perceptiveness, and caring. A special thanks goes to John Robertson, who endured the tedious process of writing more than 60 pages of manuscript for the chapter entitled Gifted Adults Incurring Severe Disabilities. His personal story and insightful analysis were a most significant contribution to our effort. We are deeply grateful also for Gladys Knott's co-authorship of Chapter 6 and the expertise regarding learning disabilities that she contributed.

Since our book was conceptualized to create dialogue, the willingness of colleagues to initiate discourse over the in-depth case studies by writing brief reactions to Chapters 2 to 6 also was a vital contribution. We wish to express our appreciation to the writers of these chapter reactions, who significantly enriched the content of the text: Shirin Antia, Ph.D.; Doris Senor Woltman; Sandra Ruconich, Ed.D.; Anne L. Corn, Ed.D.; S.J. Obringer, Ed.D.; Patrick M. Ghezzi, Ph.D.; Martha Lentz Walker, Ed.D., C.R.C.; Joanna Gartner, C.F.C.; Anne Udall; and Nancy Wingenbach, Ph.D.

As all authors know, the quality of available secretarial support in the production of a manuscript is a critical factor in the ease or difficulty of completing the task. We are grateful for all assistance provided at both of our institutions, but particularly for the special talents of Janie Knight at Kent State University, who produced the final manuscript. Her exceptional skills—from typing on the word processor, to identification of the occasional need for editing, to careful consideration of format and content, all at the highest level of professionalism and cooperation—made our task much more simple, efficient, and pleasant.

We have identified that it has been our intent to create a dialogue. Therefore, as our readers collect new information or find evidence to confirm or refute our hypotheses and theories, we encourage them to communicate with us. We intend to continue our inquiry and to participate fully in the professional discourse that we hope will ensue with heightened curiosity and vigorous commitment!

Joanne Rand Whitmore
C. June Maker

Part I

Introduction

Chapter 1

The Emerging Field: Education of Gifted Handicapped Students

Most people do not consider the possibility that an obviously handicapped person may also be mentally gifted. Although the public has admired and enjoyed the life stories of persons who overpowered severe handicapping conditions to evince exceptional courage and achievement (e.g., *The Story of Helen Keller* by L. Hickok, 1958; *Biographical Sagas of Willpower* by H. Baker, 1970), such persons have been viewed as remarkable exceptions. In general, expectations for achievements by handicapped individuals, particularly those regarded as severely disabled, have excluded accomplishments of significant social value. Even when handicapped children have been identified as intellectually gifted, the lack of appropriate educational programs has severely limited the development of such children's potential for exceptional achievement.

The last decades of the twentieth century offer some exciting challenges to the professional leaders in psychology and education in relation to this specific population of persons who possess both superior intellectual abilities and specific disabilities. Current research on the nature of intelligence or cognitive functioning, on the educational implications of neurological and psychological characteristics of the brain, and on the relative effects of various educational treatments for specific groups of learners promises an emerging body of knowledge and educational technology that will enable all children to receive a truly appropriate education allowing full development of their abilities. Accordingly, this text is intended to arouse awareness and concern and to stimulate questions and dialogue about professional activity that may lead to the pursuit of the knowledge and technology needed to serve more appropriately the important subpopulation of gifted disabled individuals.

This chapter provides a definition of the emerging field in historical perspective; a description of current understanding of the phenomenon called "gifted handicapped" (intellectual giftedness in a person with a specific disability), and related problems and concerns; and an overview of the content of this book.

3

DEFINITION OF THE FIELD

The History of the Current Movement

Through the 1950s, research in education and psychology tended to be dominated by a desire to establish norms of human behavior, with exceptional patterns considered only as deviations from the norms. Consequently, texts and courses on child development and education focused on normative characteristics of children at given ages and directed little attention to the recognition or accommodation of individual differences and special needs. In fact, the early efforts of Binet and others to measure intelligence were directed at identifying mentally handicapped children who could justifiably be excluded from schools because of an inability to benefit from educational opportunities. It was in the course of developing such a measure of intelligence that Lewis Terman became intrigued by the performance of individuals who excelled on the tests. Subsequently, he spurred the growth of interest in "gifted" children by his classical, longitudinal study of 1500 mentally gifted children, then called "geniuses."

In the late 1950s, the attention of United States educators turned dramatically to the identification and special education of mentally gifted and academically talented students, particularly in science and mathematics. The sociopolitical nature of this interest in gifted children and their special educational needs has been well documented elsewhere (Newland, 1976; Whitmore, 1980; Tannenbaum, 1983). The post-Sputnik era illustrated this phenomenon as Americans became obsessed with a desire to develop more scientific leaders in order to maintain world power and leadership in competition with Russia. Consequently, efforts were directed toward the identification and full intellectual challenge of actual and potential high achievers, particularly in mathematics and science. Mass identification procedures employed in early elementary school years generally included group-administered aptitude tests, standardized achievement tests, and teacher referral based on high academic achievement. While special programs for gifted students, often with segregated classes, were evolving, this preoccupation with the need to develop a greater number of scientific leaders affected all children, because more challenging courses in mathematics and science were introduced into the general curriculum of the elementary school.

By the middle of the 1960s, professional discourse about individual differences and the need to individualize instruction had intensified and permeated the literature. However, attention to the needs of gifted students waned as new concerns about the culturally different, the educationally disadvantaged, and racial minority students emerged as a significant part of the Civil Rights Movement. During the 1960s many innovative programs were funded by the federal government in an attempt to ensure equality of educational opportunity. Concurrently, steadily increasing amounts of federal subsidy were allocated in support of research and the development of special education, in particular for the handicapped. The field of special education received substantial support to do research, to train teachers, and to implement experimental programs. A technology for diagnostic-prescriptive instruction and educational materials for highly individualized instruction rapidly became available to classroom teachers. Especially skillful in this more sophisticated methodology for enhancing learning by handicapped children were the newly trained special educators, who generally taught small groups of children with similar educational needs in segregated classrooms for all or part of the school day. The majority of severely handicapped children were placed in such self-contained, segregated classes.

In 1969, Congress decided to ask the Commissioner of Education to conduct a study on the status of gifted education or, more specifically, what was happening to gifted students educationally in America's schools less than ten years after the intense post-Sputnik developmental period. The Marland Report, published in 1971, indicated that fewer than 4 percent of the children in the gifted population were receiving any special educational services.

As the Marland Report was stirring renewed concern about the neglect of gifted students, the Civil Rights Movement and the court cases won in behalf of excluded or inappropriately educated handicapped students resulted in what has been commonly called the "mainstreaming movement." What could be described as growth in moral consciousness produced investigation into the damaging effects of labeling and segregating handicapped children (Hobbs, 1975; Reynolds & Birch, 1977). The outcome was Public Law 94–142, The Education for All Handicapped Children Act (1977)—legislation requiring the protection of every handicapped child's right to a free, appropriate education in the least restrictive environment. The law basically required an annual review for each child, in which careful diagnostic assessment was the basis of an individual educational plan developed by a multidisciplinary team (M–Team) of professionals working with the parents. Refinement of the assessment procedures and efforts to identify handicapped children at an early age resulted in the identification of a surprising number of young children who were classifiable as both disabled and mentally gifted.

The new field of education for gifted handicapped students is emerging as a result of the intersection of special education for handicapped and for gifted students. The intersection of these two fields occurred largely as a by-product of the process by which Public Law 94–142 was implemented. In addition to the occasional identification of superior intelligence during the diagnostic process, some disabled students were recognized as intellectually superior after they were "mainstreamed"—transferred from segregated classrooms for handicapped learners into regular classrooms. In the less restrictive setting of the regular classroom, which included a more stimulating or challenging curriculum and more "normal" models, gifted students with specific disabilities evinced their exceptional potential for learning and exhibited rapid intellectual development and achievement that exceeded teacher expectations.

Mary Meeker, Merle Karnes, and Anne Sanford were among the first educators of the gifted to investigate the nature of this subpopulation. As a result of their leadership, there has been some development of special programs in recent years. Descriptions of those programs were provided in the first publication focused on this subject, *Providing Programs for the Gifted Handicapped* (Maker, 1977). Those programs generally have been funded through the Federal Office of Special Education in grants to universities. Therefore, most systematic activity in program development has occurred outside the public school systems, though individual teachers have reported cases in which children have been identified as both intellectually gifted and disabled and appropriately modified programs have been developed.

In the early 1970s The Association for the Gifted (TAG), a division of the Council for Exceptional Children (CEC), established a national committee comprising professionals interested in the development of the field of gifted handicapped education. National conferences on the topic were held in 1976 and 1977, but the difficulty of gaining a sufficient number of participants became obvious as available travel monies decreased. As a result, the plan for annual national conferences on gifted handicapped was dropped. Members of that original national committee have continued to seek ways to create greater interface between various "handicapped" divisions of CEC and TAG. In 1977 the category of "gifted handicapped" was added to the indices of the Educational Resources Information Center (ERIC), but the number of existing publications referenced remains very small. However, the continuous receipt of inquiries by the authors on this subject suggests that interest is growing, and a significant increase in research, program development and subsequent publications over the next ten years can be expected.

In summary, the field of education for gifted handicapped students is emerging within the context of moral concern for the civil right of all children to have an appropriate public school education that will help them fully develop their potential for life satisfaction and contribution to society. The field is developing as a product of the intersection of the two special fields focusing on the educational needs of the disabled and the gifted. Most systematic programming for gifted students with specific disabilities has occurred in university research settings with special programs subsidized by federal grants. The next decade offers unlimited opportunities for special educators from both fields (education of the handicapped and the gifted) to continue the effort to establish a body of knowledge and programming technology critically needed to appropriately serve this significant subpopulation of American children.

Definitions and Concepts

Before operationally defining the gifted handicapped population, one must define independently both the terms "gifted" and "handicapped." These definitions also will serve to define the parameters of the focus of this book. Although there are handicapped persons with special talents (Maker, 1977), the authors have chosen to address only intellectual giftedness because of its direct implications for the nature of instructional programs and the preparation of teachers. This more narrow focus does not deny the importance of recognizing and nurturing special talents, such as in art, psychomotor skills, and music.

Giftedness

For too many years intellectual giftedness was equated with a "high" intelligence quotient (IQ), the score on an aptitude test (usually over 130). Placement in gifted programs, however, typically required high scores (usually seventh stanine or higher in all subjects) on standardized achievement tests, consistently superior grades, and a positive recommendation from the classroom teacher(s). Generally this practice continues to be the method of identification and selection for program participation, with many districts using only group-administered IQ tests as the least costly measure of aptitude. The resulting operational definition of intellectual giftedness—high academic achievement, with emphasis on verbal and test-taking skills—has obvious limitations.

Intellectual giftedness, as established by Terman and others, has been defined as superior aptitude for learning and achievement on cognitive or academic tasks. Individuals classifiable as intellectually gifted manifest superior cognitive abilities in their ease, speed, and quality of processing information. The gifted child or adult assimilates and accommodates new ideas with greater facility than others; produces new insights and constructs of notable quality; and readily perceives relationships and their implications across categories of thought and events. The mind of a gifted person processes and produces information with distinctive facility and qualitative results.

Cognitive characteristics that reliably discriminate gifted from nongifted individuals, when accurate observations or measurements are used, cluster around four key abilities: (a) communication of ideas, (b) problem-solving skills, (c) creative production or thought, and (d) retention and use of knowledge. Frequently children are recognized as gifted because of their fluent and advanced use of language, superior quality of self-expression, and complex language structure. In problem-solving tasks they are remarkably analytical, drawing from a wide range of knowledge and relevant experience to select a viable alternative solution to be tested. They evidence superior evaluative skills as they judge each step of the problem-solving process.

Gifted persons also evidence the potential of inventing new methods or solutions, creating new ideas or experiences, and engaging in exceptional divergent thinking. These traits foster expectations that gifted persons will become distinguished inventors, creative writers, and innovators. They seem most motivated to communicate, to solve problems, and to be creative. Another primary indicator of intellectual giftedness, however, is exceptional retention and use of knowledge. The gifted individual evidences not only remarkable memory but also superior facility in organizing information for storage, retrieving it as needed, and perceiving appropriate relationships among bodies of knowledge.

The purpose of aptitude tests has been to provide an objective and efficient assessment of potential for intellectual achievement, thereby predicting school performance. The IQ score actually is a means of sampling some principal cognitive abilities and describing intellectual functioning in relation to chronological age. Performance on the intelligence test originally was translated into a ratio of mental age (M.A.), the age of most children producing that score, to the child's actual chronological age (C.A.), which is then multiplied by 100. A child with a C.A. of 6 and a M.A. of 9 has been described as having an IQ of 150—indicating a performance comparable to that of most children with a C.A. of 9. Although this formula is no longer used, the IQ score being calculated now to reflect deviation from the norm (average performance), the fundamental concept of a ratio between mental and chronological age seems to remain valuable in explaining the nature of intellectual giftedness.

Intelligence tests were intended to assess ability independent of educational opportunity. In reality, group aptitude tests produce results very similar to achievement tests because of the necessary design and content for mass administration. Most significant, perhaps, is the fact that the Stanford-Binet Intelligence Scale and Wechsler Intelligence Scale for Children–Revised (WISC–R)—the two standardized tests that have been regarded as the most reliable and valid indicators of potential academic ability—are administered in a one-to-one relationship, with the administering psychologist reading all instructions and items so that the child is not required to read or write. In spite of their limitations and weaknesses, such as cultural bias and narrow scope of content, the Stanford-Binet and WISC–R scales have been very useful in establishing the giftedness of disabled learners or underachievers (Whitmore, 1980).

Individual intelligence tests, the Stanford-Binet and WISC–R scales have been commonly used to identify gifted learners. Therefore, an accurate understanding of the nature and meaning of such tests is critical to proper use and interpretation in the identification of gifted and/or handicapped individuals. Giftedness can be defined simply as the capability or potential for exceptional achievement and contributions in a specific area of human ability. It is assumed that the gifted person will surpass 95 to 98 percent of the total population in competitive performance. Thus, in order to identify gifted individuals in an area of ability, or to assess how an individual compares with others on a specific set of skills, a measure must be designed to sample that kind of ability. If standard procedures are followed to test reliability and validity, the content of the test can be assumed to be a fair sample of what is required in the area of ability—that is, if the test were administered to the total human population, performance would be distributed in a normal curve, with the majority scoring in the middle range. It is important to note, however, that generally norms used to interpret scores have been derived from population samples of nonhandicapped individuals. Thus, accurate interpretation of the score of a disabled person remains a problematic issue in the field of education.

As previously discussed, an awareness of the inherent limitations of IQ tests is important. Too seldom are educators reminded, in texts or courses, of the meaning of a score that is implicit in the design of the instrument. In effect, a particular IQ test score is merely a statement of probability that, given an appropriate educational program, a child with that score will excel in intellectual tasks similar to those measured by the test—that is, vocabulary, comprehension, memory, logical problem solving, and so on. The most widely used individual intelligence tests contain a heavy emphasis on verbal skills, but that is a reasonable factor given its high degree of accuracy in predicting success in school, which is a highly verbal enterprise.

Two major challenges confront researchers and test developers concerned with increasing accuracy in identifying giftedness. First of all, more accurate means of estimating intellectual ability as innate potential, rather than ability dependent on school experiences or other educational opportunities, must be developed. Second, there is a need to broaden the current thinking regarding giftedness, and to develop tests that examine more accurately a wider range of mental abilities than those represented on the Stanford-Binet or WISC–R scales, which measure primarily verbal skills with some measure of logic and perceptual-motor performance. Guilford's hypothesized 120 to 150 specific mental abilities have helped to eliminate the assumption that an individual exceptionally capable in one area of cognitive functioning will have similar ability in all other areas. The Structure of Intellect (SOI) test battery has been designed to assess many specific intellectual abilities, and norms are being developed, along with characteristic profiles, for subpopulations of exceptional or atypical individuals. Similarly, the new Kaufman Assessment Battery for Children (KABC) has been designed to yield measures of aptitude and achievement as well as a precise analysis of the relationship among abilities and performance, in an attempt to measure thinking "processes" as well as "products." Although this promising new test battery has not yet gained widespread popularity, children from minority groups as well as the handicapped and gifted were included in the normative samples. Certainly many mental abilities associated with scientific inquiry, including mathematical reasoning, are not assessed accurately by the currently most popular aptitude tests. The development of more verbal-free measures involving a wider range of cognitive abilities obviously would help many gifted children to evidence their special mental abilities.

In summary, giftedness may be defined as exceptional potential for learning. Since intelligence tests sample primarily the verbal skills that have proved to be predictive of success in school, a score in the top 3 to 5 percent—perhaps in the top 10 to 20 percent—of the tested population suggests an exceptional potential for learning and the probability of high academic success. Individuals gifted in less verbal areas of cognition may have to be identified by other measures—for example, achievement tests and observed behavior. It is most accurate to say that a mentally gifted child is one who has exhibited exceptional potential for (a) learning, (b) achieving academic excellence in one or more subject areas, and (c) manifesting superior abilities through language, problem solving, and creative production.

Handicapped

Children are considered handicapped when their normal learning and development are impaired by one or more specific conditions, so that special educational programming and related services are required in order to develop their abilities. A child may be disabled in one, several, or all areas of development and performance: intellectual, physical, social, and emotional. Not only may a child be handicapped in one developmental area (e.g., physical) and be normal or gifted in other areas of ability (e.g., intellectual), but within a specific developmental domain, a child may be both gifted and disabled. Examples of the latter condition include an individual who is physically impaired in the area of gross and fine motor coordination yet exceptionally skilled in the use of auditory senses, and a child who is disabled in the intellectual domain requiring verbal performance but excels in the use of cognitive skills involving the manipulation of spatial relations.

Many intellectually gifted disabled adults with whom the authors have spoken have objected to the practice of calling persons "handicapped." During a panel discussion on the subject at the 1978 meeting of CEC, one blind scientist stated passionately, "I do not regard myself as handicapped, but I do regard as handicapped those 'normal' people around me who are handicapped when it comes to knowing how to deal with my differentness!" With respect for this view and the intense feeling accompanying it, the authors recommend the use of the term "specific disability." Even with that term, we are aware that there are individuals who philosophically oppose the *concept* of handicap or disability. They argue that an absence of a specific ability (e.g., to have normal vision, to have average motor coordination, to be able to hear) is *a disability or handicap only to the extent that it limits or prevents* an individual from pursuing a career or hobby of personal value. For example, a blind person cannot choose to become an airline pilot; an orthopedically handicapped person cannot aspire to become a professional baseball player. But it is only a matter of perspective as to whether such limitations are in fact handicaps or disabilities. Readers should pause to reflect on their own strengths and abilities: in any one person, the possession of abilities necessary to pursue every possible career or hobby of special interest is highly unlikely! Adolescents may express a strong desire to succeed in many roles—for instance, to be a successful professional musician, athlete, artist, scientist, and astronaut; they must engage in serious self-study to determine which careers best combine their special abilities and personal interests. To the extent that a woman always has aspired to be a popular singer of romantic love songs, she is handicapped if she cannot carry a tune and lacks a fine quality of voice—but, many would argue, she is not otherwise in any way disabled!

In spite of the philosophical debate, funding agencies—most notably, governmental agencies—continue to define a variety of "handicaps" with intended precision for identifying qualified recipients of special services. For the purposes of this book, the authors have selected the following categories of impairment for the study of gifted persons with specific disabilities: learning disabled, hearing impaired, visually impaired, neurologically impaired, and orthopedically or motor impaired. Another major category of special education, emotionally disturbed or "behavior disordered," is not included, owing to the difficulty in gaining access to appropriate cases and research data. The authors decided to discuss characteristics of emotional disturbance or behavior disorders only as secondary characteristics associated with other handicapping conditions, rather than to attempt to address the special characteristics and needs of the mentally ill or psychiatrically disordered. As the reader will see in Chapters 2 to 6, the characteristics attributed to members of a specific category of disability are delineated in the chapter treating that particular category.

Gifted Handicapped

Children classifiable as gifted and handicapped require special educational programming both to accommodate one or more disabling conditions and to develop fully their potential for exceptional achievement in one or more areas in which they may be gifted or talented. Such children possess two sets of exceptional characteristics, giftedness and disability, that must be the basis for educational programming.

It seems accurate to state that virtually all gifted persons with specific disabilities were first described and treated medically and educationally in terms of their handicapping condition. Therefore, many disabled persons have not had the opportunity to evidence or to develop their superior mental abilities in ways recognized by others as giftedness. Although there is no accurate statistic for the incidence rate of gifted persons with specific disabilities, a reasonable and perhaps quite conservative estimate is that 2 percent of the handicapped children could be classified as mentally gifted. By this estimate, of the 6 to 9 million handicapped children identified in 1976, a minimum of 120,000 to 180,000 were intellectually gifted (Gearheart & Weishahn, 1976). Increasing the estimate to 5 percent would suggest a gifted disabled population of 300,000 to 540,000 in 1976. It is obvious that appropriate educational programming for these children could release a very significant amount of creative productivity of great value to society and would also reduce the possibility of economic dependence in adult years, as is often the case when suitable employment cannot be obtained.

It should be quickly noted that many gifted adults with disabilities, including those described in subsequent chapters, have distinguished themselves in prestigious careers. As the reader will later discover, they claim their accomplishments generally have been secured in spite of inadequate and frustrating educational opportunities. Nevertheless, the reader should not conclude that no help is needed for this subpopulation: the common misconception that gifted students can ''make it on their own'' in realizing their full potential is as inaccurate for the disabled as for the nonhandicapped! Rather, the reader must contemplate the unrecognized potential in many others about whom chapters also could be written. The authors have shared the anguish of numerous gifted college students with mild to moderate handicaps who were unable to secure or sustain employment in such roles as teachers, child caregivers, librarians, engineers, or counselors in community agencies because of slow movement, minor physical limitations, or the appearance of a person perceived as handicapped and weak—a high risk employee. It is our hope that information presented in this book will help to dispel fears about employing handicapped persons otherwise qualified for positions.

In summary, the emerging field of education of gifted handicapped students requires the reintegration of educational responsibility and expertise. Specifically, regular classroom teachers must become more aware of the characteristics and needs of both students who are disabled and gifted, and become more skillful in observing those characteristics for identification and referral, if necessary, for special services. Special education teachers who work with handicapped students must also become more informed about the characteristics and educational needs of intellectually gifted students, and they must develop the habit of teaching to stimulate and nurture exceptional cognitive potential that may be present in each child. Teachers of gifted students must recognize that mental as well as physical disabilities can impair the learning and achievement of their students in specific areas. In all schools there should be more collaborative teamwork among professionals and parents in the identification of special needs, the planning of appropriate programs, and the evaluation of pupil progress.

The field of education of gifted handicapped students is emerging in an educational context in which there are obvious conflicting trends in philosophy and practice. On the positive side, in the judgment of these authors, is the ''mainstreaming movement'' which over the last decade has raised our collective moral conscience regarding the need to (a) guarantee the right of every child to a free, appropriate public school education in the least restrictive (or most enabling) environment; (b) function as interdisciplinary teams of professionals in consultation with parents to plan and evaluate each child's individual educational plan; and (c) integrate handicapped and gifted education programs, special and regular education programs, and community and school agencies, in order to provide appropriate educational services needed and deserved.

The "mainstreaming movement" has produced appeals within the profession for (a) cooperative efforts to help the field of education mature as a profession; (b) a renegotiation of professional roles and an increase in the number of alternatives made available to children; (c) a genuine respect for and accommodation of individuality in classrooms to maximize opportunities for academic and social success for all children; and (d) continuous evaluation and responsive flexible programming in order to avoid ''locking'' a child into a program less than optimal for his/her development. Much of the resulting dialogue and collaboration between special educators of the handicapped and of the gifted that has occurred, though very limited, has clarified the extent to which those professional groups share a common ground of (a) concern for individuals and their maximum growth, (b) technology for individualizing instruction in a diagnostic-prescriptive mode for basic skill development, and (c) commitment to the principles of providing appropriate individual educational plans.

On the negative side, from the authors' perspective, is the "back to basics movement," with an accompanying conservative philosophy that stresses "firm discipline"; highly structured classrooms with strong teacher control and little or no student choice; opposition to "individualization," which is equated with permissiveness; and a return to a more simplistic, singular mode of instruction often called "direct teaching." Although there is wide variability among the attitudes of the conservative public, beginning in the 1980s there has been a definite movement toward increased local control of schools and a reduction— elimination where possible—of federal control through subsidized programming. It appears that in many communities, both desegregation and special education either for the handicapped or for the gifted within the community's public schools will receive little support in the near future. This movement significantly colors the context in which the field of education of gifted handicapped students is seeking to emerge and develop.

PRINCIPAL GOALS OF THE NEW FIELD

The movement among professionals seeking to establish the field of education of gifted handicapped students seems to be directed toward five principal goals that encompass numerous related concerns. The first goal is, predictably, that of increasing the accuracy of the diagnostic process so that more children are accurately identified as mentally gifted when they are also disabled in some way. The second goal is that of increasing the amount of research and development activity directed toward expanding the body of knowledge and instructional technology necessary to equip professionals to address competently the needs of gifted students with specific disabilities. The third goal is implementation of the necessary major changes in the preparation of medical and human services personnel as well as of preservice and inservice teachers. The fourth goal is that of increasing the sense of shared responsibility for the total development of gifted children with specific disabilities—shared among professionals in the schools and in the community with the parents. The fifth and last major goal pertains to preparing the gifted individual with a specific disability for lifelong satisfaction in a career and in various self-selected avocational pursuits that allow full development of potential for exceptional achievement.

Goal 1: Identifying Gifted Students with Specific Disabilities

Two specific objectives are involved in addressing the goal of identification of disabled children as intellectually gifted: (a) removing obstacles to their formal identification as gifted, and (b) developing systematic methods of increasing the probability that characteristics of intellectual giftedness will be elicited and recognized in disabled children. Before suggesting how the second objective might be pursued, it will be helpful to consider some of the major reasons that gifted disabled children in the past generally have been overlooked in terms of their giftedness and treated only in terms of the disabling condition.

Obstacles to Identification

In addition to clearly defining the terms "gifted" and "handicapped" or "disabled," in order to increase the probability of accurate identification being made, it is helpful to examine reasons these individuals might not be recognized as gifted and consequently provided more appropriate educational programs. Four major categories of obstacles to identification of disabled individuals as mentally gifted contribute to the formulation of more productive identification procedures.

Obstacle 1: Stereotypic Expectations. Fundamental to the successful search for anything is the ability to recognize it once it has been found. Therefore, an accurate expectation of identifiable characteristics must first be formulated. Terman's classic work helped parents and teachers to realize that gifted children were not always weak ectomorphs with thick horn-rimmed glasses, but that such children more often appeared to be normal or above average in physical size, appearance, and health. Terman established the fact that gifted children are normal youngsters with some exceptional characteristics or abilities in specific areas, so he was successful in correcting certain misinformation about giftedness. However, over time, the public and the education profession developed from Terman's work somewhat erroneous stereotypic expectations regarding the characteristics of gifted children that today pervade schools and communities: (a) the gifted child excels or exceeds the norms in all areas of development; (b) gifted students always are high achievers with high motivation to excel in school; (c) the best single indicator of intellectual ability is language—advanced, appropriate, fluent; and (d) the gifted child is a mature, independent, self-directed student.

Although these expectations will not impede the accurate identification of a large portion of the gifted population, a significant percentage will be excluded. Namely, giftedness will go unrecognized when handicapping conditions limit verbal ability (reading, writing, and/or speaking), independence, opportunity for leadership, or academic achievement. Furthermore, the stereotypic expectations described have produced the popular belief that, because a gifted student excels in the regular program and is so capable in all areas, no special education or assistance is needed. The common comment from educators and citizens alike is, "Perhaps it would be nice to provide special programs for gifted students, but with severe limitations on our financial resources it is impossible to do everything. Therefore, it makes no sense to expend resources to provide more to those students who possess more to begin with and can achieve well in regular educational programs."

The probability of overlooking giftedness in an individual who is disabled is increased by the stereotypic expectations held for persons with disabling conditions. A major thrust of the "mainstreaming movement" has been the awareness, cultivated by leaders such as Nicholas Hobbs in *The Futures of Children* (1975), that labeling and segregating children for prescriptive treatment have some serious negative effects. With attempts to set reasonable expectations and to plan appropriate programs for exceptional children came *new* sets of stereotypic characteristics as the "norm" for each classification. A natural consequence, then, was a tendency on the part of the medical and educational professionals to prescribe treatments that limited the development of the child's abilities because of the expectancies associated with the cluster of characteristics defining that labeled condition or syndrome. In fact, the presence of a few primary traits led to the inference that other characteristics judged to be related were also present. The danger in the use of labels, descriptive categories, and illustrative case studies (as in this book!) is the human tendency to generalize to other individual cases. But in each case, judgment should be suspended until a thorough examination has been completed and until prescriptive treatment, resulting from an analysis of all information, has been subjected to reevaluation for appropriateness by ongoing assessment of the individual's needs and responses to treatment.

Examples of negative effects of the stereotypic expectations of others for persons who are gifted and disabled can be provided easily. The authors have seen the unfortunate results of such negative expectations in gifted children with the condition called cerebral palsy.

Kim was classified at birth as "profoundly handicapped," owing to cerebral palsy of severe degree. Early treatment began with a physical therapist and a language development specialist, but at 7 years of age, Kim still had extremely limited motor control and no expressive language. Confined to a wheelchair, she slumped considerably and had difficulty holding her head erect. Her droopy posture, continual drooling, and lack of language skills led professionals to design educational experiences for her that were identical to those provided for mentally retarded children. She was placed in a public school for the profoundly and multiply handicapped, in which development of basic self-help skills comprised the principal educational goals.

Kim's parents, who were teachers, had observed through the years her increased effort to communicate with her eyes and began to believe there was more intellect within that severely limited body than they had assumed. They stimulated her with questions and problems to solve while providing her with a relatively simple means of indicating responses. When a group of students from the school for multiply handicapped were scheduled to be mainstreamed into an open-space elementary school, they insisted that Kim be included. After two months of stimulation in a normal classroom setting, the provision of an adapted communicator she could manage, and participation in a more normal instructional program, Kim evidenced remarkable development. She exhibited a capacity to learn quickly and to remember exceptionally well; superior problem-solving and reasoning skills; and a keen interest in learning. Within four months she was reading on grade level (second) despite missing two years of appropriate reading instruction in school. An adapted form of the Stanford-Binet was administered, and her performance qualified her as mentally gifted.

Since beginning to study this area, the authors have come across an impressive number of similarly dramatic examples of severely disabled children who are intellectually gifted. The stereotypic expectations that impede identification of intellectual superiority in disabled children are related to (a) the absence of language, as used in questioning, explaining, sharing knowledge, and so forth; (b) the lack of physically active investigation that is typical of many gifted youngsters; and (c) the assumption that gifted children "look bright." The physical appearance of severely disabled children, such as Kim, seems to lead even physicians to assume the child is mentally handicapped also. If the image presented bodily by the child is one associated with intellectual dullness (e.g., drooling, slumping, dull eyes staring), mental retardation often is assumed. In fact, it was only one small deviation in the pattern that led to the discovery of Kim's intellectual potential—her bright, communicating eyes. She possessed the eyes of a gifted child!

Obstacle 2: Developmental Delays. Specific handicaps delay the development of some abilities that facilitate the recognition of intellectual giftedness (Maker, 1977). These delays are critical factors in the assessment of abilities by measures based on norms for the chronological age (C.A.). Although the skills will be acquired later, the delay in early years causes the handicapped child to score below the norm for the appropriate C.A. group, obscuring the exceptional potential to excel intellectually that is associated with accelerated, advanced development from birth. Accurate estimates of intellectual potential in such children may not be obtained until later childhood or adolescence. Aptitude test scores of young disabled children may require compensatory adjustments to produce more reliable estimates of potential.

Cognitive development and intellectual performance are delayed when characteristics of the handicapping condition limit the child's ability to receive and respond to cognitive stimulation and to manifest cognitive abilities through self-expression and problem solving (Maker, 1976, 1977). Visually impaired children show some developmental delay in abstract thinking that seems related to the absence of visual images. Language-disabled children (e.g., who are hearing-impaired or have cerebral palsy) seem to experience some delay in cognitive development, although the cognitive characteristics are difficult to assess accurately because of the absence or immature level of oral language. Similarly, severely limited motor ability (e.g., as with orthopedic or neurological impairment) curtails the child's interaction with the environment, consequently reducing the stimulation that normally fosters cognitive growth. In spite of exceptional potential for learning and intellectual achievement, impairments that limit cognitive stimulation or the ability to enjoy discourse with the world of people and things can be expected to delay the development of mental abilities and the demonstration of intellectual superiority. Therefore, for purposes of evaluation, the abilities of a disabled child should be compared also with those of others having similar handicaps.

The well-known story of the life of Helen Keller provides an extreme example of the obstacle presented by developmental delays. With limited mobility and stimulation as a result of her lack of vision, confounded by an accompanying lack of hearing that presented normal language development, Helen Keller undoubtedly suffered significant delay in the development of her superior cognitive abilities. When the breakthrough in language finally occurred, and she discovered how to formulate and communicate concepts, her cognitive growth was rapid, and she became capable of demonstrating her exceptional intellectual powers. The potential for exceptional learning and intellectual achievement was present in her mind from birth, but the severe handicaps impeded its development because basic understandings of her world were missing. The intense frustration she experienced as a young child, manifested in violent temper tantrums, was undoubtedly a function in part of that exceptional intellect trapped in a severely limited body that required living with acute sensory deprivation and isolation from others.

The likelihood of significant delay in the cognitive development of young disabled children should warn professionals that premature judgments regarding mental abilities can lead to treatment decisions and conditions that limit such children's opportunities to fully develop those superior characteristics. Early identification of handicapping conditions is very important to reduce the negative effects of disabilities, to facilitate growth in all areas of development, to guide the acquisition of constructive skills for coping and adapting, and to assist the parents in their critical role. However, judgments about cognitive ability should be made only tentatively, subject to modification according to observed responses to intellectual stimulation; such responses more accurately indicate the potential for learning as it develops and becomes more evident through the childhood years.

Medical and educational professionals must be trained to communicate accurately to parents the possible range within which the child can be expected to perform intellectually in later years—that is, if there is no certainty of damage to the brain impairing cognitive processing, memory, or reasoning, then the entire range of possibilities remains open, and it is reasonable to assume the child's performance will be within the normal range. Few physical disabilities are inevitably accompanied by a general cognitive disability. No ceiling should be placed prematurely on expectations for the cognitive growth of a child with a specific disability. Parents and teachers should seek the most effective means for stimulating the child's cognitive abilities and for developing an ability present to communicate and to interact with the world of ideas, people, and things.

Obstacle 3: Incomplete Information about the Child. All professionals dealing with the disabled child tend to have a narrow view of problems and possibilities because of a limited amount of information provided through observations, tests, and parent reports. Educators seldom are provided with specific information explaining medical diagnoses and the characteristics of the conditions that should be considered in the design of an appropriate educational plan. Similarly, physicians seldom receive complete information about the child's performance in school, such as precise descriptions of behavior that might be helpful in medical diagnosis or treatment. Counselors and parents also have limited information regarding the child's assessed capabilities and behavioral responses in other settings, such as the school and doctor's office.

Incomplete information can lead to inaccurate assessments and inappropriate educational programming. For example, physicians frequently advise parents on educational programming or placement without consulting with educational professionals. Similarly, educators frequently prescribe educational programs without medical information that might be significant in determining the appropriateness of the plan—for example, the amount of physical exercise or stress that can be beneficial; the nature of physical therapy received elsewhere and the appropriateness of the exercises or services provided at school; or the possible effects of various medications or medical treatments. The following case study (Whitmore, 1980) provides a simple example of this problem area.

Nancy was a chubby girl somewhat large for her age. She appeared very lethargic and, to her teachers, uninterested in learning activities and intellectually dull. Her eyes revealed no spark of interest or enthusiasm in school, and by second grade she was almost totally noncommunicative. She did not attempt to answer any items on tests administered by the classroom teacher. She stared into space instead of completing any learning assignments. The seeming lack of response to sensory stimulation, her glassy eyes, and the consistent failure to attempt learning tasks suggested mental retardation as an explanation of her behavior in the classroom. These observations during Nancy's first three years of school led to teacher referrals for testing, with the expectation that she would qualify for placement in a program for the mentally retarded.

However, when tested privately by a sensitive school psychologist who carefully developed rapport with her, Nancy scored 130 on the Stanford-Binet test. It was the psychologist's knowledge of a gifted sibling in Nancy's family, his suspicion about her physical and emotional health, and his gentle persistence that allowed him to gain this insight into her potential as a learner. She certainly did not belong in a class for mentally retarded children! Thorough medical examination indicated a metabolic problem probably related to diabetic tendencies in the family, discomfort created by a constricted colon in response to tension, and poor mental health. The appropriate educational placement for Nancy was in a special class for gifted children failing in school because of mildly handicapping conditions or developmental delays.

Obviously, a lack of complete information about the child's health, home, extraschool activities, and performance in school can result in misdiagnosis and inappropriate educational placement or programming. Acknowledgment of this fact accounts for the required multidisciplinary team (M–Team) under Public Law 94–142 regulations. All persons with significant knowledge about the child should be participants in the design and evaluation of an appropriate educational plan.

Obstacle 4: No Opportunity to Evidence Superior Mental Abilities. As has been suggested, it is extremely difficult to recognize superior potential for learning and intellectual accomplishment in a child who has no expressive language. In such cases, identification occurs as a result of highly perceptive and skilled parents and professionals who accurately observe nonverbal manifestations of intellectual giftedness. However, a large segment of the gifted population is overlooked because of a lack of opportunity to develop and demonstrate exceptional intellectual abilities in social settings, including the classroom to which they are assigned. This obstacle is especially apt to occur with children who are placed in special classes for the handicapped—such as Kim, the gifted child with cerebral palsy.

Special education programs have tended to focus on the development and remediation of self-help and basic skills (reading, writing, and arithmetic) because the field of special education was created in response to that recognized need. The primary focus of such classes has tended to be directed toward the child's mastery of basic skills through educational strategies of (a) reinforcement to condition responses and (b) memorization and practice exercises for mastery of basic facts. Special education programs typically include very little content in the sciences (Schnur & Stefanich, 1979); if instruction in science and social studies is included, it usually is taught with methods similar to those employed in the basic skills subjects (i.e., memorization, direct teaching of factual information), with little attempt to engage the students in active problem solving, discussions, and actual use of information. Exceptional mental abilities can be discovered easily in science education, which offers opportunities for inquiry. The child can then develop and reveal skills in analysis, synthesis, evaluation, utility of knowledge, and creative and critical thinking. Similarly, special education programs typically include little curriculum in the arts, which stimulate creativity (Hokanson, 1976). Creative self-expression is another primary mode by which the disabled child can evidence exceptional intellectual abilities.

Without appropriate gifted education in the sciences and the arts, opportunities to observe gifted behavior are infrequent in most classrooms; consequently, giftedness is not revealed. This lack of opportunity to evidence superior ability is illustrated in the following case study.

Kitty was born blind. Her parents were advised by the family doctor to place Kitty in a residential school for the blind as soon as she could be admitted, which they did. In her early years at home, the parents did not know how to help Kitty develop and essentially tried to meet her physical needs to keep her content; normal stimulation by parents, other relatives, and friends through conversation and engaging activities did not occur. Kitty found some intellectual stimulation in the state school, but over the years she was provided with only an educational program of vocational training. In her classes there was no expectation that students might pursue a college education, and her intellectual development was not sufficiently stimulated.

The astute observations of a counselor during the high school years, however, led to Kitty's decision to attend college to prepare to become a teacher. Without the support of her parents, who were confused by the decision, Kitty enrolled in a small, private college; there she slowly restructured her self-concept. As she became more independent and developed confidence in her intellectual abilities,

Kitty became an honors student in teacher education and completed rigorous programs for certification in elementary and special education for the visually impaired. Kitty graduated with a commitment to helping visually impaired children receive appropriate education in regular classrooms of the public schools—a much more common practice today.

Methods of Accurate Identification

The previous discussion of the obstacles to identification of giftedness in disabled persons suggests the procedures needed for more accurate identification. To begin with, persons working with parents and training professionals must help them to recognize and eliminate inappropriate stereotypic expectations and to examine ways of penetrating the disabling condition to assess the child's potential for developing superior qualities of thought—analytical and creative problem solving, organization and use of stored knowledge, perception of relationships and events, formulation of principles and generalizations through transfer across settings or events, social sensitivity and insight into people, and creativity. The challenge is to find ways to stimulate the expression of such potential. With disabled children, alternative modes of expression must be found where the common modes of expressive language, problem solving, and creative production are blocked by the disabilities.

In order for giftedness to be identified in disabled young children, professionals must be trained to stimulate productive and creative thought and to observe the manifestation of those traits in atypical forms. Whereas traditional methods of identifying gifted children have relied on oral and written language to indicate the need for further testing, when children are impaired in those modes of expression, techniques of evaluation must rely more on direct assessment of mental abilities through tasks requiring problem solving, memory, critical thinking, and creativity. Parents can be skillful observers whose records of the child's behavior can suggest the possibility of gifted abilities. Exhibit 8–3 and Table 8–2 in Chapter 8 outline reliable indicators of intellectual giftedness that can facilitate accurate identification of cognitive giftedness despite impeding characteristics of handicapping conditions.

Two factors are critical to the successful identification of giftedness in children with handicapping conditions. First, opportunities must be provided that will elicit indicators of mental giftedness. The most accurate information is obtained when a child is placed in an environment that stimulates such performance and when mental abilities are assessed by means of tasks not requiring performance skills impeded by the handicapping condition. Tests of mental ability must be appropriately adapted and scores adjusted for severe disabilities where there is reason to believe cognitive functioning exceeds performance capabilities on that measure. Second, the most accurate picture of a child's abilities and characteristics is composed of the pooled information gathered by a team of professionals and the parents. The M–Team approach to diagnosis of educational needs and to the design of an appropriate educational plan is critical to meeting the needs of the gifted and disabled child. With accurate early identification, appropriate educational programming can be instituted immediately to develop the child's intellectual giftedness.

Goal 2: Research and Development

There is serious need for research and development (R&D) activities that are directed toward expanding the body of knowledge about gifted persons with handicapping conditions and providing the instructional technology necessary to optimal programming for these students. Three areas requiring R&D activity are particularly important: identification and diagnosis, effective programming, and resources for teaching.

Identification and Diagnosis

Research needs to be conducted that builds on the pioneering work of Merle Karnes at the University of Illinois (1979). Because of the difficulties encountered by those attempting to identify giftedness in young handicapped children, most of the limited body of research has involved adult subjects who, by virtue of their accomplishments, became recognized as gifted persons with handicapping conditions (Maker, Redden, Tonelson, & Howell, 1978). However, with the use of more precise methods of identifying handicapping conditions in young children, the characteristics of intellectual giftedness can be discovered more often. Systematic research on the effects of early identification of disabled children who begin to evidence intellectual giftedness in early childhood years should become a priority for the same reason that Terman's work was a major contribution after years of post hoc analyses of the recalled life experiences of gifted adults.

Research is therefore needed to continue to define and describe the subpopulation of gifted individuals who possess specific disabilities. As more complete information about their characteristics is obtained, more accurate methods of identification can be devised. A related need is to develop diagnostic instruments that will more accurately assess the specific educational needs of the child. With accurate diagnostic information, parents and professionals can formulate more appropriate expectations for the achievement of the child so that optimal educational programming can be provided.

The Effects of Alternative Programs

As in all areas of education, more research is needed to determine the relative effects of various alternative programs for different groups of students identified as gifted and having specific disabilities. At present there are insufficient data to guide the M–Team in predicting the outcomes of certain program decisions for specific kinds of learners—in particular, the gifted and disabled. The M–Team could make more accurate decisions about programming if data were available regarding outcomes of past decisions for similarly diagnosed learning needs. A major research question pertains to the effects on severely disabled children of a decision to place them in a regular mainstream program with supportive assistance from special education resource teachers. An evaluation of the social, instructional, and curricular characteristics of the most effective programs for mentally gifted children who are handicapped in varying degrees of severity is needed to guide the prescriptive process.

Resources for Teachers

In order for appropriate programming to occur, teachers must be equipped with curriculum resources. For example, technological devices, when appropriate, must be available to enable the disabled student to function with minimal impairment. A prime need is the development of a larger variety of electronic communicators that enable the severely motor-impaired child without oral language, like Kim, to be self-expressive and responsive to others. Adaptive use of computers perhaps is the most promising single aid to improving instruction of disabled students.

There are more technological resources to accommodate handicapping conditions than there are materials for the gifted child who cannot read or has a language deficit. The problem is one of motivation when the interests of the gifted child are similar to those of older students but the content of curriculum materials requiring low reading-language skills is based on characteristics of young children. More curriculum materials must be developed for handicapped children that contain the highly challenging cognitive content essential to appropriate programming for gifted students. As mentioned earlier, especially lacking are resources in the sciences and the arts. A related need for visually impaired students is to avoid long delays between the request for specific reading materials and the provision of the text in braille or on tape by Community Services for the Blind. Library research is extremely difficult for blind students. The recently developed Optacon offers much greater accessibility to reading resources for those who can use it to read the printed word through their fingers. Also the Kurzweil Reader has made library research and general reading more feasible for visually impaired persons.

Dissemination of Information

A fourth related need in R&D is for the development of a communication network through which pertinent information can be disseminated. Although ERIC provides this service, additional networks may be needed to assist in problem solving and decision making by all those who work with gifted disabled students. Dissemination must go beyond circulation among researchers to include practicing professionals, and beyond professionals to reach parents and citizens. Networks of dissemination among disabled persons are needed also, such as *The Blind Teacher*, a newsletter published through the National Association of Blind Teachers.

Goal 3: The Preparation of Professionals

One of the major purposes of this book is to bring about immediate revisions in the preparation of professionals in the fields of human services including medicine, counseling, psychology, and education. Those persons who may comprise a team evaluating a handicapped child must be prepared to investigate the cognitive potential of the child and to explore numerous alternatives for early and continued educational treatment. The curricula of most medical schools include almost no attention to the educational needs accompanying various child characteristics, nor are physicians informed of the need to allow a special educator or educational diagnostician access to medical diagnostic information. Nonetheless, when a handicapped child is born, it is the physician and the nurses with whom the family has close interaction who typically influence the parents' decision—whether to provide care at home or to place the infant in a residential facility. In the initial discussions with the parents, the family doctor tends to set expectations regarding the extent to which the child may achieve a normal life. Seldom, if ever, is it mentioned to the parents of a severely impaired infant that the physical handicaps do not rule out the possibility of exceptional cognitive ability and potential for learning. Nor is the development of cognitive abilities closely monitored to guide appropriate stimulation and, ultimately, educational programming.

Similarly, a family may rely on the advice of a counselor, minister, or social worker to decide how to provide for the disabled child. Persons in these influential roles must be trained to withhold judgments regarding intellectual potential and to encourage normal stimulation and careful observation to determine how the infant's abilities are developing. The effects of the handicapping condition on cognitive development should be explained to the parents so that some developmental delay is expected and stimulation is continued. Information about the alternative programs available to handicapped children in the early years is important also. Consulting professionals should be well informed about local resources in order to guide families in the procurement of assistance.

Certainly educators need to be prepared differently also. In many schools, teachers and administrators know very little about handicapping conditions and giftedness, having been prepared for ''regular'' teaching. Public Law 94-142 has led to the funding of projects directed toward the revision of teacher preparation programs at the preservice college level and toward the provision of inservice training of teachers in regular classrooms (and sometimes administrators) to provide better understanding of the characteristics and educational needs of handicapped children. Teacher education has definitely moved toward the reintegration of special education and regular teacher preparation programs (Reynolds & Birch, 1977; Whitmore, 1983).

Unfortunately, most special education programs include only token attention to gifted children in an introductory course on characteristics of exceptional children. To date, a small percentage of colleges and universities have required all future teachers to have substantial information about gifted learners, and in only a small percentage have special programs been developed to prepare teachers of the gifted. Furthermore, programs to prepare teachers of gifted students often have emerged from a department of educational psychology or curriculum that has little interaction with a department of special education.

At the inservice level there are continuous and rather intensive efforts to inform teachers about gifted students and their needs in specific school systems around the nation. Generally the inservice information has focused on gifted students who need special programming because of their exceptionally high achievement, however, and generally no attention has been given to underachievers or handicapped students who also qualify as gifted. Therefore, institutions of higher education and school systems must begin to integrate accurate information about giftedness as well as handicaps so that all teachers are better prepared to identify those students and recommend appropriate educational programming. Certainly all special educators should be both knowledgeable about and skilled in identifying and planning for gifted children with handicapping conditions.

An additional need is for professionals to determine how services could be extended into the adult years for gifted persons with severe impairments, so that they are able to live normal lives within the community. This need is discussed further in the next two goals.

Goal 4: Increasing the Sharing of Responsibility

An indisputable and well-known fact is that parents of newborn and infant children with disabling conditions need supportive help in understanding how to provide for the child and in coping with the emotional impact on their lives. Especially when parents discover their child is severely disabled, extensive support is needed. It is always the medical profession that has the first opportunity to provide helpful guidance and assistance. Referrals are usually made to appropriate human services agencies for counseling of the parents of the disabled child. In the early years, social workers and therapists or nurses may also become involved with the child and family.

From the birth or identification of a disabled child, the medical and human services professionals in contact with the family should consult with appropriate educational agencies in the community to obtain the earliest possible educational diagnosis and assistance with educational planning. Many of the mechanisms for shared responsibility and collaborative planning are used in providing for the needs of disabled children in some communities. These same mechanisms need to be extended to the gifted student who later is identified as having a mild handicap or who acquires severe impairment, as in the loss of sight or hearing. More extensive use of those mechanisms needs to occur in most communities. Often it is left to the parents to piece together information from each source, never gaining the participation of all professionals in a conference to synthesize information about the child and to share responsibility with the parents for making critical decisions regarding the child's care and education. If the team of professionals functions only to provide fragmented pieces of information to the parents, the evaluative process is violated, and its purpose of providing more complete knowledge and understanding is not achieved. True collaboration to synthesize a picture of the whole child must occur.

Within the education profession alone, there is much room for significant growth in collaboration among special education (for the handicapped) resource teachers, teachers of the gifted, regular classroom teachers, and administrators. The busy schedules of each professional group do make M–Team meetings difficult to arrange, but schools may need to be restructured to accommodate that need. Certainly, the number of gifted children with disabilities is low enough to allow the desired collaboration to occur. Through such collaboration—and documentation of the findings—the body of knowledge about these children can be expanded while professionals become more cognizant of the problem and alternatives. School administrators particularly need to assume responsibility for contributing to the development of an appropriate plan for the disabled child and for creating a school climate that enables each student to feel accepted, valued, and capable of success socially and academically. In attending to the special needs of the exceptional students in a school, the administrator will improve the learning environment for all students.

Goal 5: Preparation of the Student for Adult Living

As the reader will discover from the case studies in this book, most disabled adults with successful careers feel as though they achieved success despite the educational system and often without the encouragement of medical or human services professionals. A common error has been in the tendency to program disabled students for vocational training and to deter them from interest in careers requiring advanced education or skills regarded as unsuitable because of the handicapping condition. Even when such students have been enrolled in regular educational programs, there has been a tendency to limit career alternatives and to discourage college attendance.

This goal is directed toward early counseling of gifted and disabled students to develop their skills of self-evaluation, assessing personal strengths and weaknesses as well as natural interests, and also to explore career alternatives. Even when a particular career seems out of the question because of physical limitations, technological devices may be available that will functionally eliminate the impediment. For example, there are phones to accommodate the quadriplegic or person with a weak voice; the Optacon has been developed to enable a blind person to read the printed page; prosthetic limbs may allow movement. Students should be helped to recognize their special abilities and to accept the limitations created by their disabilities. Limitations include the social handicap that may be imposed by the discomfort of others dealing with the disabling condition. Students deserve assistance in the development of constructive ways of coping with the stress created by degrees of social rejection, especially when seeking employment. Special agencies to assist disabled persons in securing employment and group housing should be available in every community of significant size.

Most important is the development of a healthy self-concept and sense of worth in every gifted person with a disability. Inclusion of career exploration in the curriculum can contribute to the identification of special abilities, the recognition of career potential, and the development of the expectation that life as a socially accepted, relatively independent adult is possible. Adult living for the disabled person should also include hobbies and cultural interests developed during the years of education as a child and youth—for example, music, art, or games. The development of the field of education for gifted disabled students can contribute to a fuller realization of the intellectual and social potential of gifted persons with handicapping conditions through making accessible to them a broader and more appropriate curriculum. The authors assume that the case studies to follow will clarify those specific educational opportunities necessary to the full development of the potential of gifted persons with disabling conditions.

OVERVIEW OF THE BOOK

As has been stated, the purpose of this book is to facilitate the establishment of the field of education for gifted disabled students as an area for focused R&D, professional preparation, and educational planning. Since the field is embryonic, the authors cannot present confirmed results obtained from a large body of literature, but they hope to stimulate thinking and investigation through the raising of questions, the definition of issues, and the telling of stories—the life stories of some successful gifted adults with disabling conditions. A critical need is to increase dialogue within and among professions that will lead to the production of knowledge and resources through R&D. To stimulate that dialogue, professional colleagues have been invited to react to the authors' presentation and discussion of each case study. It is hoped the reader will find the discourse provocative and helpful in the direction of thought.

Chapter 1 has described the emerging field of education of gifted handicapped students. Part II, which follows, presents case studies, followed by discussions and reactions, of gifted persons who are sensory-impaired, motor-impaired, severely physically disabled from birth or by accident in adulthood, or learning disabled. Part III examines implications and recommendations for improved practices to facilitate affective and cognitive development, and the achievement motivation of disabled persons through experiences at home, at school, and in the community.

Part II
Case Studies

Chapter 2

Hearing-Impaired Gifted Persons

A CASE STUDY: MYRON

> I was motivated to read at an early age . . . . When I was very young, every night my parents would come in and turn the lights out and say goodnight. I had a flashlight under my bed. When they closed the door I would pull the covers over my head and take out a book, and I'd read six, eight, ten books a week!

This statement by Myron, the subject of the following case study, suggests why he has achieved a higher level of success in his career than that achieved by most other individuals with a comparable degree of congenital hearing loss or even normal hearing. He attributes much of his success in school to his enormous desire to read, and his success in his career and personal life to a similar degree of motivation.

In his late 40s, Myron is a physician in charge of a specialized center for research in hypertension at a large university's medical school. His educational background includes an undergraduate major in zoology, English, and history with minors in physics, chemistry, and psychology; a medical degree; internship and residency in internal medicine; and, finally, a research fellowship at Stanford University. After this training, he became an assistant professor and physician in internal medicine at another university, where he rapidly moved through the ranks and became a full professor within seven years. The center he directs has received millions of dollars in research support and is known for its major breakthroughs in hypertension.

Myron's congenital hearing loss of 80 to 90 decibels classifies him as legally deaf. He was evidently deaf from birth because his loss is sensorineural. However, no one knew he was deaf until he was 6 or 7 years old! He learned to read lips at an early age, learned to read before going to school, and attended regular public

31

schools with no assistance other than a powerful hearing aid. Currently, the only electronic aids he uses are a hearing aid, a telephone amplifier, and an electronic amplifying stethoscope. He has never used manual communication and very seldom receives the services of oral interpreters for the deaf.

Myron is one of two children in a Jewish family, with a mother who graduated from high school and a father who completed eighth grade. His mother is not employed outside the home, and his father is a businessman. The other child in the family, a younger sister, also has a hearing loss. Myron is married and has three children of his own.

Personal View of Self

Myron has only recently viewed himself as handicapped, having resisted the notion even to the extent of refusing to associate with other handicapped people or to become involved with advocacy groups for the handicapped. He talks at length about his belief, shared with many other individuals with handicaps, that a person with a disability cannot admit to related limitations until success on that person's own terms has been achieved. According to Myron,

> . . . I think you have to achieve a certain amount of success before you can admit that you have a problem. There has to be a large amount of denial in order to cope. Until you feel you've reached a level of success which is acceptable to you as an individual without a handicap, then you can admit you have a handicap.

He does feel, now, that he has achieved success on his own terms and is willing to affiliate with advocacy groups and to identify himself as a deaf person.

Generally, Myron sees himself as one with high intellectual ability, an excellent memory, and very good lipreading skills. However, he attributes most of his success to his motivation. When discussing motivation, he often uses the term "perverse" and continues with an explanation of both the positive and negative effects of such determination to succeed. It seems that his motivation and desire on his part enabled him to maintain a perception of himself as capable of high achievement regardless of the negative views of others around him. In fact, because of this self-confidence and determination, when others told him he could not succeed at something, he became even more determined to be successful. He had to "show them"—to prove them wrong. Because he was determined to succeed, he was persistent in asking questions until a concept was understood, he was unwilling to quit applying when first denied admission to medical school, and he spent a great deal of time reading when he was young.

With respect to the negative aspects of this "perverse" motivation, Myron discusses a quest to prove his mother wrong in her belief in her son's ability to succeed despite his deafness.

> . . . she overcompensated by convincing me there was nothing I couldn't do. She set a goal for me. And so I began to set my own goals. Then as a result of that, I spent about 15 years trying to find out what I couldn't do . . . . There was a protective environment, taking care of our own kind, as well as a shelter from hurt by saying you can do everything. I was filled with so much disbelief that I felt compelled to find out what I could not do. And I found I couldn't play musical instruments, I couldn't hear a flute, a whole series of other things . . . it was sort of like she lied.

This determination to prove others wrong even carried over into his participation in medical school. When he was initially turned down, Myron decided to apply again to show the admissions committee that he was determined. After his admission, when he was deciding on a specialty area, he was encouraged to go into areas where communication and hearing ability would not be a concern. He was determined to go into patient care in internal medicine, which he did, and when told he should not pursue cardiology because of his deafness, he became determined to pursue that specialty as well.

Another aspect of Myron's success is his ability and willingness to use nontraditional ways of getting information. Even though he uses an electronic stethoscope, for example, to magnify the sounds made by the heart and lungs, there are times he cannot hear these murmurs because they are too high-pitched. He has learned to detect certain types of heart murmur through feeling the patient's chest, and to detect clues through an individual's pulse in the arm and leg.

An obvious weakness he sees in himself is difficulty in communicating on the telephone and in other situations in which lipreading is not possible, such as in conversation with a person whose back is turned. As a physician who deals with people, Myron feels he must use the telephone. As he indicates,

> Communication is a vital problem. For a long time I would not use the telephone, and I would rely heavily on other people to take messages or to talk for me. Several of the people associated with me at the time offered to do that, but it got to the place that I resented the self-image that was being generated by those sorts of activities. I simply forced myself to learn to use the telephone.

When asked how he overcomes problems in communication, Myron indicated that he first finds out who is calling, since that often gives him an initial clue as to the purpose of the call. He then must concentrate intensely on trying to pick up one or two words out of every five or ten and then try to formulate in his own mind what the person is saying. He then reformulates the idea as a question, asks the question, and hopes that he can get a "yes" or "no" response. If the response is "no," he must formulate another question. It is interesting to note his description of talking on the telephone.

> I have a certain pattern. First I need to know who it is. Once I know who it is I can make out a vowel, some sort of sound, [and can infer] what it might be regarding. Then it's a searching operation to try to find out what's going on. It's almost amusing when people call me because I have a well-established reputation now, and people call me who don't know me, but they know of me. They'll be talking awhile, asking for information, and I say, "Who is this? Repeat your name please, I'm having trouble hearing," then I'm alert to them saying, "We must have a bad connection, I'll call back." Then I'll say, "No, there's nothing wrong with the connection, I have a hearing problem, and bear with me and repeat what you said, then we'll go from there." Then there's a long silence and they they start talking again, slowly, very loudly, sometimes, which makes it worse. When they shout into the phone, everything gets obliterated.

Rather than emphasizing Myron's difficulties in talking on the telephone and labeling this disability as a weakness, many individuals consider his methods of coping as a sign of his strengths. Very few individuals possess his level of ability to discern the content of a conversation with so very few clues. His skill in determining the reason for a call, formulating a question isolating the "essence" or meaning of a section of conversation seems remarkable. Such skills can be useful to him in many other situations as well, and could be the reason for his success in group meetings or similar situations in which he cannot follow an entire conversation using speechreading skills.

Another characteristic that could contribute to his ability to communicate and to fill in missing information is Myron's knowledge and understanding of a variety of subjects. While in college, he majored in zoology, English, and history, and minored in physics, chemistry, and psychology. He also enjoyed sports, especially football. Because he has had experience and has knowledge in each of these areas, Myron is more likely to be able to "fill in the gaps" in conversations resulting from his inability to hear than would someone who knows very little about such topics.

Myron describes his needs related to self-concept and acceptance as a "need to be superior to other people in order to be accepted." He gives the following example:

When I played football I weighed 220, and in the ninth and tenth grade in high school, I was pretty tough. It was not very difficult for me to be an effective football player, but I had to do better; it wasn't just making the football team, I had to be on the first string, and even then that wasn't enough, because what happened was; because I couldn't wear my hearing aid (they were afraid I would rupture my middle ear), I had to watch the center move the ball, and as soon as it left his hands I moved while others were listening for the hike signal, so I would always be the first one across. The referees would call an offside penalty an average of 4 times a game, and my teammates would yell; it would cost 5 yards, and another 5 yards, so I had to be better to overcome that penalty. I had to be more aggressive than anyone else on the team.

As many academically-oriented adolescents often do, Myron went through a period in which he felt that he had to make a concentrated effort to avoid being labeled a "brain." He deliberately did poorly in school and spent most of his free time playing football, drinking, and "running around." Although he recognizes that such behavior is more or less typical, he feels that in his case the behavior was more flagrant and perhaps more pronounced than usual.

Myron also describes his need in a similar context with his motivation. For example, he felt a strong need to test himself and the system to see what he was really capable of doing. As discussed earlier, there was a big discrepancy between his mother's view of his capabilities and the expectations, both overt and covert, held by others. His mother led him to believe there was nothing he could not do, whereas others told him repeatedly there were many things he could not do because of his handicap. He explains as follows:

I had to test the system to see really what I was capable of doing. Everyone, when they realize what their problems are, their handicap or whatever, spends a certain amount of time being very depressed, saying "Why me?" and "Why can't I be like everyone else?" But eventually you pick yourself up and say, "Well, that's the way it is and what do I do now?"

He eventually decided that it is more important to satisfy himself; his own perceptions of his capabilities were more important than those of others around him.

Personal View of Perceptions and Treatment by Others

Facilitators

Clearly, Myron's mother was the most important facilitator in his life. She provided a protective environment, in a way, because she was convinced that there was nothing he could not do, and she set a goal for him—he would be successful. Along with her "protection," however, his mother provided every opportunity she could for his growth. Her reading to him greatly facilitated his learning to read: "I can remember her reading to me. She didn't really teach me to read, she just read. And that stimulated me to read because she wasn't always there when I wanted to be read to." When his hearing loss was discovered (in the second or third grade he believes), his mother immediately began to explore the possibilities for instruction in lipreading skills. She found that there was a school for the deaf and that the public schools provided a class in which lipreading skills were taught. Even though the class was quite a distance from his home, Myron's mother made arrangements for him to attend. Interestingly enough, he went to the class for one day, and when the class was over, the teacher sent him home with a note saying that there was nothing she could teach him. He had already learned it all on his own!

In addition to the specific influence of his mother, Myron attributes much of his motivation and success to the whole home environment with its "emphasis on success, in a fairly identifiable form, with intellectual growth being the primary one; . . . my parents always, as most Jewish parents do, placed physicians on pedestals, [as] the epitome of success." Even though he does not specifically address the influence of his father, it seems that the whole home environment placed an emphasis on his ability and need to be successful. Myron has also noted that he believes the fact that he was the firstborn son made a great deal of difference in the way he was treated. Even though his sister was provided with many opportunities, she did not show the same motivation to succeed academically, and Myron is not certain whether her lesser degree of motivation stemmed from some inherent difference between them or from subtle differences in the way the two children were treated.

It also is interesting to note the influence of Myron's wife. In discussing the issue of identifying with advocacy groups for the handicapped, he notes his wife's surprise when he agreed to testify before a congressional committee about education for the handicapped. His wife asked why he wanted to do this and wanted to know if he had not felt uncomfortable. When recounting the incident, he reflects,

> She has never been able to admit that I have a handicap. She was very uncomfortable; she doesn't see me as a handicapped person. Somehow she finds it demeaning that I would consider myself handicapped because I've never been around handicapped people.

Thus, the home environment emphasis on high expectations as well as a certain denial of the existence of a handicap has continued into his adult life.

Obstructors

The major obstructors or inhibitors in Myron's life tended to be educators who wanted to discourage him from going into medicine. He vividly remembers a high school biology teacher who tried to encourage him to go into biology. The man, whom Myron considered a very interesting teacher, took an interest in the students and spent a lot of time with them. He considered Myron a very good student and one day asked what career he was considering. When Myron answered "I want to be a doctor," the man said, "There's no way; you can't make it with your handicap. You ought to consider biology [because] you're very good at it, but you've got to be realistic. You can't spend years [trying] to do something you can't do." According to Myron, this man was the first of a whole series of people who constantly reminded him of his supposed limitations.

It is interesting to note, however, that the overall effect of these obstructors in Myron's life was to increase his motivation and effort rather than to decrease it. When remembering the incident, Myron reflects on his reactions: "All of a sudden I started crying and turned away from him. And then I said, 'We'll see about that.' I said, 'Okay, I'll show you!'" Afterwards he was even more determined to become a physician. Most of the people he encountered were not as forceful in saying "you can't," but they tried to discourage him by telling him how difficult his chosen course would be. Myron's reaction was "so what's new about that?" Throughout medical school, there were individuals who attempted to discourage him from pursuing clinical medicine, and to encourage him to go into radiology or another area not requiring much communication at the personal level. As previously, however, the comments of these people served only to increase his determination to pursue a specialty that was supposed to be the most difficult for someone with his handicap.

The first real barrier for Myron was being denied admission to medical school the first time he applied—in his junior year of college. When this occurred, for the first time Myron realized that he might not be able to reach his goal: " . . . all of a sudden the end had come. I had to ask myself, well maybe I'm not going to make it, what am I going to do?" Because of his wide range of interests and his ability, he saw that there were many options, including creative writing, so he continued in college for another year while further exploring his career options. At the end of his senior year in college, Myron applied again to medical school; this time he was accepted. His reflections on the events are interesting to note:

> Even though I cannot get anyone to admit it, I think the concerns were whether I was motivated enough to do whatever I had to do to get through medical school. They felt that if they turned me down the first time, and if I wasn't sufficiently motivated, then I wouldn't come back.

But if I did apply again, they'd give me a chance. That's essentially what happened.

Statement of Specific Needs

Myron very clearly believes that determination and self-motivation must stem from the home environment. There must be an emphasis on success as well as high expectations for what can be accomplished. By providing an environment that emphasized goal orientation and achievement, was rich in experiences and resources, and had many role models for success, his family encouraged the development of high motivation and specific goals. He also notes the importance of his mother's willingness to read to him and to provide those resources. His family was helpful in getting him reading material after he learned to read. Even though the public library had a policy that children could only check out two books each week, this rule was waived for him—he could take as many books as he wanted so long as he took them back on time. There was, to a certain degree, also an element of denial on his parents' part that any handicap existed. In effect, his parents treated him as a normal, nonhandicapped person, and his wife continued the same treatment in his adult life.

With respect to the school environment, Myron recalls interesting events that occurred before his hearing loss was discovered. One of his most vivid memories is of his difficulties in the reading groups:

> In the first grade of school (we had a very traditional, structured school system), they had reading groups of six or eight children in a circle. The teacher would call on different people to read, and I couldn't lipread and follow the book at the same time. I'd learned lipreading by then by myself, but not ever having heard I didn't know what it was to hear, so I couldn't watch people and read at the same time, so I just read. Then she would call on me and frequently she would have to come and tap me on the shoulder and I'd start reading where I was and I was eight or ten pages ahead of everyone else. On the report card it said for reading: he does fine, but he doesn't pay attention in class. So my parents gave me hell, and they emphasized the business of paying attention.

As one who did not attend special schools or special classes, Myron emphasizes the importance of mainstreaming because "segregation of people with similar disabilities breeds very low self-image." According to him, the situation causes development of a common image and lowers expectations for academic performance. There are very few role models for success. Since everyone is deaf, no one tries to communicate in any form other than what can be understood by everyone else. When asked what effect going to a regular public school had on his life or achievement, Myron replied:

> Well, it enabled me to see myself as a normal individual long enough to get the ego reinforcement I needed in order to say okay, I'm handicapped. Being in a deaf school would have forced me to communicate in sign language . . . . I would have quickly found out there was no chance for a job, and I would have lowered my aspirations, figured my mother was dead wrong, and I would have simply stopped. I see [being mainstreamed] as a very integral component in motivation.

To make the mainstreaming experience successful, Myron believes that teachers must be selected who are amenable to the concept; that students need the support of the environment both at home and at school; and that the students must have motivation and potential. With regard to this last point, Myron believes that students who are above average or gifted intellectually will be more likely to succeed in a mainstream setting than those without the same level of ability. Ability is not enough to assure success, however. Students must also possess a high degree of motivation to learn and achieve at a high level. Teachers must recognize that students with handicaps can and do have academic potential.

Myron also feels strongly about oral communication. He believes that the biggest deficiency of "sign language" is that it tends to cause people to think only in concrete terms, so that the development of abstract concepts is difficult or impossible. Interestingly enough, Myron recommends that schools concentrate on teaching deaf children to read early, rather than on teaching them manual communication. He believes that this would enable the children to concentrate on how to think and write more precisely, for example, rather than on learning vocabulary. Reading can enable gifted deaf children to pick up the meaning of many words through contextual clues.

Medical school presented the biggest educational challenge to Myron. He says that " . . . for the first time in my life I had to study and I didn't know how . . . ." He notes that many of his lectures in medical school were in darkened rooms because of the need to show slides. Such settings made lipreading and notetaking impossible. To gain needed information, he had to rely on notes taken by others or on reading textbooks and other resources.

Since he must continue to communicate in academic settings, Myron often requests the assistance of colleagues and others. He asks to have people with whom he must communicate within lipreading distance. He also asks that the lighting on people's faces be increased, and that they take care to make their faces and lips more visible. He also requests that colleagues take notes for him at scientific meetings.

DISCUSSION

Traditional Views of Deafness and Hearing Impairment

Deafness and hearing impairment are often viewed as the most debilitating in the academic setting as well as the most limiting to the choice of careers. Because the development of early language and intellectual skills depends on being able to hear, and because early school success depends on language, vocabulary, and reading, children with severe hearing impairments are at a distinct disadvantage.

Classification of an individual as deaf or hearing-impaired results from consideration of the degree of loss and the effect of that loss on the individual's speech and language development, educational adjustment, and psychological adjustment (Myklebust, 1964; Newby, 1972). The most recent classification was developed by the Ad Hoc Committee to Define Deaf and Hard of Hearing (1975), which recognizes two categories—deaf and hard of hearing. A deaf person is one whose disability precludes successful understanding of language through the ear alone, whether or not a hearing aid is used, and a hard of hearing person is one who has residual hearing that enables the processing of linguistic information through audition, usually through the use of a hearing aid.

The intensity of sound is measured in decibels (dB). Zero dB indicates the intensity of the softest sound that can be heard by a normal young adult. At the other extreme, 140 dB represents the intensity of sound measured 80 feet from the tail of a jet airplane at takeoff; this level is so loud it is painful.

The extent of hearing loss is often categorized as mild (20–40 dB), moderate (40–60 dB), severe (60–80 dB), or profound (80–100 dB) (Green, 1981). Individuals with a mild loss cannot hear such things as a whisper at 5 feet, the rustle of leaves, or noises in a quiet office or residential area at night. Those with a moderate loss have difficulty hearing conversational speech at 5 feet, the noise made by a washing machine, or the noises usually heard in an office. People whose losses are considered severe are not able to hear a quiet typewriter, an automobile at 65 miles per hour, or the noises in an average "quiet" factory. Persons with a profound loss cannot hear a loud shout at 5 feet, a noisy factory, or a chain saw (Green 1981). These are, of course, only general indicators of sound intensity, and what an individual can hear or understand also depends on the type of loss and the frequencies of detectable sounds. Generally, however, the degree of loss gives an indicator of the level of difficulty an individual will have in communicating and in understanding the environment.

There are four usual types of hearing loss resulting from a number of factors, conditions, and illnesses (Green, 1981): conductive, sensorineural, mixed, and central. A conductive loss results from problems with the structures in the ear, usually through blockage in the mechanical conduction of sound. Most conductive losses can be successfully treated with medicine or surgery. A sensorineural loss results from damage to the cochlea or the auditory nerve and is usually greater in degree than losses caused by conductive disorders. Sensorineural losses are not medically or surgically treatable. A mixed loss is caused by both sensorineural and conductive problems; thus some aspects are treatable while others are not. Central auditory losses are caused by lesions or damage to the central nervous system and result in no measurable peripheral hearing loss. Most hearing losses are caused by conductive, sensorineural, or mixed disorders.

A fifth type of hearing loss, called functional, is not due to any organic problem. Functional losses may be conscious, or intentional (to gain attention, explain poor performance, or avoid a responsibility), or unconscious—that is, unintentional. Unintentional losses usually result from emotional stress or psychological problems.

Generally, the effects of a hearing loss vary, depending on four major factors (Green, 1981; Moores, 1982; Quigley & Kretschmer, 1982): the severity of the loss; the age at which the loss occurred; unilaterality versus bilaterality (that is, whether one or both ears are affected); and the hearing-impaired person's determination to adapt. Those whose learning is most affected are individuals who have a profound loss that occurred at or soon after birth. A person who cannot hear normal speech sounds does not usually develop normal speech and language. When first attempting to make speech sounds, young children listen to these sounds, compare them to the sounds made by parents or others, and repeat a sound that more closely approximates the sounds made by others. By listening to others, children expand the range of sounds they can produce while developing an understanding of the meaning of these sounds.

If the hearing loss is unilateral, the problems will be less noticeable than if it is bilateral. When average hearing in the good ear is in the normal range, for example, the hearing impairment is not generally viewed as a disability because the major problems encountered will be in determining the direction of sounds.

Generally, it is believed that a child born with a mild to moderate loss will develop speech and language skills slowly but eventually learns to use language normally and to speak effectively when therapy is combined with amplification from a hearing aid (Holm & Kunze, 1969; Quigley, 1970). On the other hand, a child born with a severe or profound loss generally grows up with a severe language and speech disorder, usually having no intelligible speech or a "deaf-like" speech and voice (Carhart, 1970). Even a brief exposure to speech and language can give a child a foundation upon which to build later language. Helen Keller, who became deaf and blind at the age of 2 years, is a classic example of one who developed excellent communication abilities even though she could not hear for most of her developmental years. It should be noted, however, that she did have exposure to speech and language during her first two years of life.

Lenneberg (1967, 1970) has suggested that there is a critical stage for development of language, and that if certain skills are not acquired during this critical period, later attempts to learn language will be very difficult. Since this critical stage is the first two years of life, early detection and intervention are extremely important. However, accurate diagnosis of a hearing impairment is difficult during infancy and the first three years of life. The child not only must be able to discriminate differences in intensity and tone but must be able to communicate these differences to the examiner. Testing the hearing of infants has in the past relied on the observation of head and eye movements; more recently, the monitoring of physiological responses such as respiration and movement has also been instituted (Northern & Downs, 1974).

The relationship of deafness to intelligence has been a major concern to educators. For many years, deaf children were often mislabeled as retarded intellectually as well as educationally. Their educational lag was considered to be due both to mental inferiority and to language handicaps. As testing techniques, with more appropriate nonverbal tests, have become more sophisticated, results show that there are very small differences between average levels of measured intelligence of deaf children and those who can hear (Lenneberg, 1967; McConnell, 1973; Vernon & Brown, 1964).

There is a definite difference, however, between the reading skills of deaf and hearing impaired children and those of hearing children. Reported deficits in reading attributed to hearing impairment include the following: (a) reading achievement in the hearing impaired is between three and eight years below the average for children without a hearing impairment (Jensema, 1975; Wrightstone, Aranow, & Moskowitz, 1963); (b) hearing impaired high school seniors have reading vocabularies at the level of 9-year-olds (Myklebust, 1964; Frybus & Karchmer, 1977); and (c) of deaf students over 16 years old in the United States, 60 percent read below grade level, and 30 percent are functionally illiterate (Williams & Vernon, 1970).

The most outstanding problem of children with severe and profound hearing losses is language (Suppes, 1975). Children have difficulty producing sounds, articulating properly, making tone discriminations, and developing voice quality. They also have problems in the content and structure of language. For example, hard of hearing children use fewer adverbs, pronouns, and auxiliaries than those noted in the speech of children who hear, and totally deaf children use fewer adverbs, pronouns, prepositions, and modifiers than those used by hard of hearing children (Brannon, 1968; Brannon & Murray, 1966). Clearly, language should not be used as a basis for assessing either the intelligence or the achievement of a deaf child unless it is compared with that used by children with a similar hearing loss.

However, the influence of language deficits on concept formation and achievement should not be ignored. Language indirectly affects thinking because it either inhibits or facilitates patterns of cognitive stimulation and interaction with other people. These effects are apparently cumulative since the differences between concept attainment abilities in deaf and hearing children have been noted to increase as they grow older (Meadow, 1980).

Social and emotional adjustment also are problems for individuals who are deaf (Meadow, 1980). Perhaps the most difficult problem is coping with feelings of isolation. Communication is always difficult, especially with those who can hear. Interaction is therefore also difficult, and many people who can hear do not take the time and make the effort to communicate with deaf people. For this reason as well as the difficulties in communicating their own feelings of inadequacy, deaf people often interact almost exclusively with others who have the same handicap.

Career choices are limited because of others' perceptions of the deaf person's capabilities as well as specific difficulties in communicating (Schein & Delk, 1974; Lerman & Guilfoyle, 1970). Jobs that require very little verbal interaction through personal or telephone contact often are considered the most appropriate career choices. Manual labor and other unskilled occupations are often the only choices because of the deaf person's lack of reading and other academic skills.

Educational Programs

A range of services usually is available for children with hearing impairments. These services may be provided in residential schools, day schools, or self-contained classes in regular elementary or secondary schools. Regular schools may have part-time or integrated programs, in which children spend part of the day with hearing children in regular classrooms and a part in resource rooms with hearing impaired peers; alternatively, itinerant services may be provided for hearing impaired children placed in regular classrooms. The degree and type of loss, as well as the age at which the loss occurred, are the major factors usually considered in determining placement.

Children with severe or profound hearing losses are usually placed in residential or day schools for the deaf, whereas those with mild or moderate losses are usually educated in special classes or in a mainstream setting in public or private schools. Because of their extensive needs for language development, auditory training, instruction in speechreading and/or manual communication, and development of academic skills, a special school with constant instruction is usually considered the best for those with severe or profound losses. Some educators believe that being in a community of deaf people is essential for those whose hearing loss is severe or profound. Those whose hearing loss allows them to develop normal speech and language are considered more able to function in a regular classroom or school setting.

For many years, there has been a continuing controversy about whether to teach deaf children "oral" or "manual" communication techniques. Oral communication methods focus on specific speech production, using the residual hearing to the greatest extent possible, using environmental cues in conversation, sharpening the ability to discriminate among sounds and words, and the development of skills in speechreading. Manual communication methods include the use of sign language—usually either American Sign Language or Manual English (Quigley & Kretschmer, 1982). Children are taught many of the techniques used in oral communication, but the major means of communication is through signs.

Those who advocate the use of manual communication emphasize the difficulty deaf persons have in understanding a speaker using oral methods. Only 30 to 40 percent of the sounds in language can be associated with visible lip movements, so the hearing impaired individual must fill in many gaps in information. Speechreading requires a great deal of concentration, excellent attention skills, and good visual acuity. Certain characteristics of the speaker and the environment also influence a deaf person's ability to read speech. For example, the deaf person must be able to see the speaker's entire face from the front and at close range and must be able to see body gestures as well. If the speechreader is familiar with the speaker, the task is easier.

Other advantages of manual communication include the fact that signs are clearer, larger, and more easily made visible than lip movements, and that children's skills in oral communication vary greatly. Signs are easier to learn. According to the advocates of manual communication, use of sign language allows the deaf person to understand all the information being transmitted; thus, the problem of social isolation does not occur, and communication skills are developed more easily.

Although the "oralists" recognize that speechreading is difficult and that much information is lost or must be inferred, they have emphasized certain disadvantages of manual communication. First, it is more difficult to communicate with those who hear because most hearing people do not know sign language. Second, signing immediately labels the individual as hearing impaired or deaf. Third, not all forms of manual communication use the same signs. Last, some forms of manual communication do not contain all the words and phrases used in normal language. Manual methods usually include both finger-spelling (using finger positions to represent letters of the alphabet) and American Sign Language (a system based on ideas and concepts with a structure very different from English). Oralists call attention to several problems related to the actual signs (Larson & Miller, 1978): (a) lack of a one-to-one correspondence between sign language and English, (b) differences in meaning between the signed word and its English equivalent, (c) differences in structure between American Sign Language and English, (d) the lack of relationship between reading and signing since reading is based on English, and (e) confusion associated with the use of several systems. Oralists also call attention to the fact that most hearing-impaired people speechread to a certain extent without having been taught and without really being aware that they are doing so (Berger, 1972). Oral communication is seen by these advocates as a necessity if the deaf person is to function in a world of people who can hear. Manual communication is seen as limiting personal interactions to those who can understand and use sign language—usually those who are also deaf.

In the past, one or the other of these approaches was advocated very strongly, although manual communication was emphasized for those with severe and profound losses, whereas those with mild or moderate hearing losses were educated in oral methods to supplement their hearing. Often, however, the controversy extended to the preferred method for those with severe and profound losses. Strict oralists would not allow the use of any sign language at all because of the belief that the deaf person would rely so heavily on signs that speechreading skills would never be developed. Advocates of manual communication were not as strict, however, and taught students many of the techniques used in oral communication.

Research comparing the two approaches is limited and inconclusive but the following findings support some of the assumptions of those who advocate the use of manual communication: first, children taught manual methods tended to demonstrate better achievement than those taught speechreading (Stevenson, 1964; Vernon & Koh, 1970, 1971); second, use of sign language does not interfere with the development of good oral techniques (Montgomery, 1966; Moore, 1976); and last, young deaf children born of deaf parents who use manual communication are superior in academic achievement and socialization to deaf children born of deaf parents who do not use it (Meadow, 1968; Vernon & Koh, 1971; Brasel & Quigley, 1975). Many researchers have concluded that this last finding shows the value of early and intensive use of manual communication in the homes of these children.

Currently, the debate over oral versus manual communication is becoming much less heated, and most educators are recommending "total communication." This philosophy advocates the use of every possible method to increase the deaf person's ability to communicate and to develop a basis for further learning of language. Techniques included in both oral and manual approaches are taught to hearing impaired children. Such a philosophy also recognizes that no single method is appropriate for all children, and that it is more realistic to teach a variety of skills, thereby allowing students to choose, and use, the techniques that work best for them. Research seems to favor use of simultaneous techniques involving both manual and oral methods rather than either method used alone (Moore, 1976; Towne, 1979). However, three specific problems associated with this approach have been identified: sentence structure and syntax in speechreading and in American Sign Language are different, posing obvious problems when the methods are used simultaneously; many individuals have difficulty processing two different visual stimuli at the same time; and residual hearing is not always being trained.

It seems that the most effective approach may depend on individual characteristics and attitudes. Another important consideration is the goal of the instruction. Academic achievement may be facilitated more by use of sign language, whereas social interaction with hearing individuals may be facilitated more by use of oral techniques. However, interaction with hearing individuals may not be considered important. Certainly, the needs of individuals and the preferences of families should be considered in decisions about which methods to employ.

Since children with mild losses may not be identified in early school years, they may be inappropriately labeled as slow learners, learning-disabled, behavior problems, stubborn, or lazy. Early detection of hearing losses is thus important so that the appropriate services can be provided. Parents should be alert for such signs as a lack of functional speech by the age of 2 years, failure to pay attention when spoken to, and behavior problems. In a school setting, some indicators of hearing impairments are the following: behavior problems, failure to articulate certain speech sounds correctly, omission of consonant sounds, failure to discriminate between words with similar vowels but different consonants, frequent need to have words or sentences repeated, and frequent earaches, "runny" ears, colds, allergies, and upper respiratory tract infections (Duffy, 1967).

Children with mild, moderate, or even severe and profound losses should be fitted with a hearing aid if it is determined that they can benefit from amplification. Such decisions should be made by professionals, and when an aid is provided, auditory training should be included. It is important to remember that amplification causes all sounds to be intensified and distorted to a certain extent. Auditory training can help to overcome some of these problems by assisting the child to recognize common sounds, to discriminate speech from other sounds, and to use contextual cues.

Educational intervention for children with mild or moderate losses may include only the auditory training necessary to help them use their residual hearing and/or minimal changes such as seating them close to the teacher. Other techniques that can assist in the learning process include the use of visual materials to supplement verbal instructions or explanations, provision of extensive written materials, and instruction on an individual basis. Children also should be encouraged and allowed to maintain visual contact with those who are speaking. Speakers should keep their hands away from their mouths and should make certain that objects do not obstruct vision. Students can be given reading assignments or new vocabulary words in advance so that they can gain maximum benefit from instruction.

Indicators of Intellectual Giftedness

In numerous ways, Myron does not fit the traditional view of a deaf person with a similar type and degree of hearing loss. His loss of 80 to 90 dB is classified as profound. It seems most likely that he was deaf from birth because his parents cannot recall any illnesses or trauma that could have caused it. Because of his sister's deafness, Myron believes that the problem is hereditary, and because his loss is of the sensorineural type and has not progressively worsened over the years, he must have had a profound hearing loss at birth. The development of normal speech is extremely rare in an individual with a profound hearing loss, and almost unheard of in someone with a profound loss present from birth.

Nevertheless, Myron's speech is normal, with almost no hint of any abnormality. During initial telephone contact to arrange an interview for this case study, it was difficult to believe that he had any hearing impairment at all. His lipreading skills are excellent, and he functions well in small groups.

A review of Myron's developmental history will reveal many early and continuing indicators of superior intellectual ability. The most obvious of these is the fact that his deafness was not discovered until he had been in school for a year or two. He must have had fairly normal speech and language development or his family, pediatrician, and others would have suspected there was a problem. He apparently developed excellent speechreading skills without formal instruction and learned to read without being taught. As a youngster, he enjoyed reading and did so extensively and well. In two of the incidents he describes, this early interest and skill are apparent. Before going to school, he read as many as ten books a week and devised interesting ways to spend time reading. In school he obviously read well and rapidly, since he was given good reports on his reading ability, but he was chided for his lack of attention because he would be several pages ahead of the group when called upon to read aloud.

Other typical indicators of intellectual ability seen in Myron include excellent memory, ability to function well in a regular classroom and school situation, superior performance in school, and a wide range of interests. As Myron indicates, many people believed that he had a photographic memory. He attended regular classes in the public schools and did not receive extra assistance from special education programs or itinerant teachers. Yet he consistently performed at or near the top of his classes in elementary and high school. In high school he also played football. He maintained a B average in his undergraduate program while majoring in zoology, English, and history and minoring in physics, chemistry, and psychology. In medical school he also had a B average.

The authors have evaluated Stan, another individual profoundly deaf from birth, who showed unusual development in different ways. As a child, he was always interested in taking apart his mechanical toys to see how they worked. His constant interest in "knowing what was happening" in school was translated into doing science experiments and reading, and later through his employment as a research chemist. Such mechanical interest and ability could certainly be identified in a child with limited verbal skills.

Interestingly enough, Stan's case presents a direct contrast to that of Myron. Born to deaf parents, he had no difficulty in learning language, primarily through manual communication, and performed extremely well in school. He attended a special school for the deaf throughout elementary and high school and experienced no social or academic difficulties. In fact, he performed at the top of all his classes and progressed through school very rapidly. After high school, he went to Gallaudet College, majored in chemistry, and became employed immediately as a research chemist. While in college, he enjoyed the challenge of being in school with others who were "just as smart." He was involved in student government and spent a great deal of out-of-class time in intellectual discussions with classmates. Thus, in comparison to others with hearing impairments, he could have been identified as gifted since his achievement and development were highly advanced over others with a similar disability.

Identification of Giftedness

Many of the methods typically used to identify gifted students are inappropriate for use with those who are deaf. Most intelligence tests require verbal responses, and almost all rely on verbal instructions. Thus, a deaf individual is at a disadvantage in many ways. Because of their slower language development, deaf children may lack both the vocabulary to express their thoughts and an understanding of the abstract concepts usually learned through language. Since they cannot hear their instructions, they may misunderstand the directions for a task. Tests of abstract reasoning, critical thinking, and achievement have limitations similar to those identified for intelligence tests.

Tests of intelligence used with deaf and hearing impaired individuals should rely most heavily or even exclusively on nonverbal tasks—those not requiring a verbal response or verbal instructions. Usually these tests are called "performance" tests and include many visual and manipulative tasks. Instructions are given in a variety of ways, including demonstration, pantomime, and manual communication. Only one test has been developed exclusively for measuring the intelligence of deaf individuals: *the Leiter International Performance Scale*. This test uses pantomimed instructions and only visual materials. It has been criticized, however, because only one type of item is included. The most commonly used test of intelligence for the deaf is the performance section of the *Wechsler Intelligence Scale for Children–Revised*. This section includes several different tasks such as assembling objects, replicating designs with blocks, and noticing missing parts of pictures. Instructions are verbal, however, and no normative data exist for individuals with hearing impairments. The *Ravens Progressive Matrices* also can be used with the deaf. Although no norms exist for the performance of deaf individuals the task is easily understood and extensive instructions are not necessary. However, it has the same lack as that criticized in the Leiter: there is only one type of item. Nonverbal tests of creativity such as the figural form of the *Torrance Tests of Creative Thinking*, visual analogies, and tasks measuring rate of visual learning are also helpful in identifying intellectual ability.

Myron is quite different from many deaf individuals, and his language development far exceeded that of most children with his degree and type of deafness. Thus, he may have been easily identifiable as gifted—especially because of his high reading ability. However, in general, the most accurate assessment of intellectual ability in deaf individuals will come from nonverbal tests. Verbal tasks may be given as supplementary measures to provide further information, but decisions about whether or not a deaf child is gifted or about the specific level of intelligence should be based on performance on nonverbal tests.

Other methods that are becoming more common can be used in the identification process. Interviews with parents may reveal an early interest in reading, early ability to read, and the range of interests. Similarly, the examiner can gather data about mechanical aptitude, scientific interests, and exceptional ability to communicate manually. Interviews with teachers produce information about current reading ability, success in school, interests, and language. In addition, written products can be examined to determine their sophistication and to monitor achievement in school.

The level of success Myron attained in school without special classes or special assistance also indicates his high levels of intellectual ability, as does the achievement of the man who attended schools for the deaf. Therefore, an interview with the subject of the evaluation may produce valuable insights into motivation, self-confidence, and the skills developed for coping with the disability.

Potential Interaction Between Giftedness and Hearing Impairment

One view of the interaction of giftedness and a handicapping condition suggests that a handicapped person succeeds in spite of a disability and because of other abilities that allow compensation for the loss. An opposite view suggests that many abilities, such as attention to visual cues in the deaf or auditory memory in the blind, are developed or sharpened because of a disability and that the individual's determination and motivation to achieve are increased, thereby increasing chances for success. Certainly, both these viewpoints offer insights into the possible interaction between abilities and disabilities. One of the characteristics most frequently attributed to the gifted handicapped children identified in a preschool project (Leonard, 1978, p. 88) was an extraordinary ''ability to learn or develop alternate ways of doing tasks to compensate for handicaps.''

Myron exhibited to a high degree an ability to develop alternative ways of doing tasks. He was developmentally advanced in reading ability despite a handicap that generally retards learning to read. His language development and speech were not noticeably delayed or abnormal as these skills usually are in deaf persons. Other indications of Myron's ability to cope with his disability or to develop alternative ways of doing tasks include learning speechreading and observation skills without formal training; his methods of participating in oral reading groups in school (following the process by reading rather than trying to lipread and follow the book at the same time); his methods for using the telephone; and, at the professional level, his ability to detect certain heart murmurs through the patient's pulse.

Myron obviously possesses certain abilities, however, that increased his chances for academic and career success. His memory, described by some as "photographic," may well have been sharpened by his reliance on it to compensate for gaps in receiving information. However, it is most likely that high ability was present at an early age. Myron has another important ability, good visual acuity, which when combined with his excellent powers of concentration enabled him to gather clues from his environment, to read lips, and then to interpret these clues and the gestures made by speakers. Ability to make visual discriminations, combined with these skills, made him a good reader, thereby allowing the gathering of information that he could not pick up through listening.

With regard to characteristics developed because of the handicap, Myron very clearly believes that his motivation and determination to be successful were due to his deafness and the reactions of others (particularly his mother) to this disability. His mother essentially denied the existence of any handicap and told him there was nothing he could not do. She led him to believe that not only was he as good as everyone else, but that he was *better*. Myron received different messages, however, from other people in his life: teachers told him to be more realistic in his expectations, and peers were not willing to accept him as an equal. As a result of these dual messages, Myron developed what he calls a "perverse" determination or motivation to succeed. On the one hand, he felt his mother had "lied" to him by telling him there was nothing he could not do and by leading him to believe he was better than anyone else. For this reason, he felt he had to search for things he could not do as a way to prove her wrong. On the other hand, she had fostered in him a belief that he was a capable individual, so when other people told him he could not do something, or that he should not try because it was too difficult, he felt he had to prove these people wrong also, by showing them that he could far exceed their highest expectations. With regard to peer acceptance, Myron believed he had to be better than others in order to be accepted by them since he was at a disadvantage because of his handicap. In effect, it seems that he was constantly searching for some realistic evaluation of his potential and his limitations. He was not willing to accept either of the extremes—his mother's positive evaluations or other people's negative evaluations. He developed a strong determination to have this realistic perception accepted by others.

Although much of his determination and motivation can be attributed to the presence of a disability and the development of a desire to overcome it, one must not ignore the cultural and environmental conditions that may have contributed to the development of high achievement motivation regardless of a handicapping condition. As Myron indicates, he believes that being the firstborn son in a Jewish family was significant. In most Jewish families, there is an emphasis on success, cultural enrichment, and intellectual growth. Children are given a great deal of encouragement and are provided with many opportunities for intellectual development at an early age. Many studies of the backgrounds of gifted children (Gallagher, 1966) show that there is a higher percentage of children from Jewish families than might be predicted from the percentage of Jewish persons in the general population. Thus, Myron's case is similar to those of many gifted individuals who are not disabled. Furthermore, studies of giftedness in general show that in a significant proportion of cases the gifted child is the oldest child in the family (Gallagher, 1966).

Obviously, there were negative effects of this extreme motivation and determination, which Myron alludes to when he uses the term "perverse" to describe his motivation. He seemed to be constantly in need of proving himself and could not relax or let down his guard for a moment. If he was not trying to prove himself academically, he was trying to prove that he was a "good guy" by impressing his peers with his social skills or athletic ability.

This desire for success and determination to prove himself also led to a certain denial that a handicap existed. As Myron indicates, he needed to achieve a certain amount of success—his own definition of success, and on his own terms—before he could admit that he is handicapped. He believes that a certain amount of denial is necessary in order to cope. There was no identification with groups of deaf individuals, and he often made extensive attempts to cover up the fact that he is deaf. Interestingly enough, even though Myron has gained a great deal of perspective and has worked out many of his problems, he still does not want many of his colleagues or professional associates to know the extent of his impairment.

SPECIFIC GUIDELINES

The insights gained from careful examination of Myron's background and experiences suggest several recommendations for dealing with deaf or hearing-impaired children and adults who are also bright or intellectually gifted. It is important, however, that these recommendations take into account differences in abilities, interests, and other characteristics possessed by the gifted handicapped individual. To help the reader go beyond Myron's case, information from interviews with other bright deaf or hearing-impaired individuals (Maker, Redden, Tonelson, & Howell, 1978) is integrated into the following discussion. If research exists to support certain recommendations, such information is also included.

Parents, Siblings, Neighbors, and Friends

Perhaps the most important recommendation for families is to establish some means of communicating with the child as early as possible. Whether this is achieved by oral, manual, or a combination of oral and manual methods depends on the child's hearing and other characteristics. This means that if the child can best use manual communication, all members of the family should learn it as well, so that they can teach the youngster new words. Deaf children need to learn some kind of language as a means of expressing themselves and of interacting with the family. If the child can benefit from amplification, use of a properly fitted hearing aid should begin as soon as a hearing problem has been identified. If, as some researchers believe, the first two years are critical for the development of language, a means of communication is crucial for later development as well as for normal daily interaction with the family.

All those who will be interacting on a long-term basis with persons who are deaf or hard of hearing should constantly strive to improve their ability to communicate with the hearing impaired. If the individual uses manual communication, advanced vocabulary should be practiced and used by all members of the family. If speechreading is used, the family, friends, and neighbors should learn ways to make their speech more ''readable.'' When total communication is the philosophy practiced and advocated in school, family, friends, and neighbors should learn about and practice these techniques.

Another important recommendation for parents and siblings is to develop an environment in which intellectual achievement is valued, encouraged, and expected. This includes providing a variety of experiences as early as possible, securing resources such as books whenever needed, reading to the child, and encouraging the development of reading skills. When reading aloud, the parents or siblings should make certain the child can see their lips; simultaneous manual communication may also be used. Parents can arrange contacts between the deaf child and successful adults who are deaf or have hearing problems. Perhaps even more important than providing resources and arranging experiences is the family's expectations for the handicapped child's level of achievement. Myron emphasized the importance of having a mother who did not seem to believe that his disability would put him at any disadvantage at all. Other deaf individuals, as well as Myron, suggest that the total denial of a handicap (illustrated by the attitudes of Myron's mother) is not the best strategy to use, nor is the extreme opposite: belief that the disability places major limitations on potential. A more realistic attitude and expectation is that a disability such as deafness will place limits on some of the individual's activities but will not interfere with or limit others. The most important aspect of these perceptions is that with a hearing disability, neither intelligence nor possibility for success in a challenging, rewarding occupation is impaired.

As a companion to these high expectations and positive attitudes, families, friends, and neighbors should adopt a creative, problem-solving approach when interacting with a gifted deaf individual. This guideline can have different meanings in different settings, but generally there should be an emphasis on assisting the person to develop alternative plans for reaching goals when a barrier is encountered, rather than suggesting that the goals be changed. If a family member or friend believes that a deaf person's goals are unrealistic, discussing this belief is important, but the emphasis should be on assisting the individual in developing or identifying ways to make the necessary tasks easier. Support and assistance are necessary, as is an honest expression of reservations about the goal a deaf individual has selected.

Another aspect of a problem-solving approach is the development of coping skills (e.g., strategies for minimizing the effect of a disability, techniques for increasing ability to learn, strategies for making everyday tasks easier). Successful adults who are deaf or hard of hearing are rich sources of information about coping strategies that can be taught to or developed in younger individuals. In addition, certain strategies have been reported by other individuals interviewed by the authors (Maker et al., 1978). Some of the strategies involved family members and friends. One man, for example, asked his children and wife to point out any errors he made in pronunciation or grammar. Another asked his family and friends to act as an audience for him to practice speech and presentations. A deaf woman asked her family to help her develop answers for potential employers who wanted to know how she would do certain tasks requiring communication. She wanted to go into a job interview with prepared answers to possible questions.

A third area of importance, especially for parents, is cooperation and coordination with the school or educational program. This includes not only assisting in completing homework and monitoring progress in school but also working closely with educators to identify areas in which enrichment or extension activities could be provided. The purpose of these extension activities is to enhance the learning of the deaf individual and to minimize restrictions in the process of information gathering due to the hearing disability. For example, parents can ask teachers for a list of the specific topics being studied in school. Then they can assist the student in finding books at a public library on these topics, or they can arrange trips to museums or other places where the student can have concrete experiences that will supplement reading or other means of getting information.

Community Services and Agencies

The major component of any program or service for a gifted person who is deaf is high expectations for success. It is important to resist developing stereotyped images of what an individual with a certain handicap should be expected to accomplish. Individual capabilities are different, so parents and professionals alike must keep an open mind about the appropriateness of their expectations.

Although Myron's case did not illustrate a need for transition from the "deaf world" to the "hearing world" (because he was never a part of the deaf world), such a transition is important for many profoundly deaf individuals. The story of

Stan, the research chemist introduced earlier, may provide some insights. Born profoundly deaf to deaf parents and educated entirely in schools for the deaf, his only contact with those who could hear was with certain teachers or others proficient in manual communication. He had always been comfortable participating in group activities and had never experienced the social isolation many deaf individuals encounter at a very early age. However, when he left school and began working in the chemistry laboratory, he had, in his words, quite a "culture shock." He was not really prepared for the fact that he was the only deaf person in his work environment. People were very considerate, and many of them eventually learned sign language, but interaction was difficult for quite some time. The shock of realizing that there were many situations in which he would be totally left out of the conversation was something he was totally unprepared to face.

The need to prepare adequately for a transition from the deaf world to the hearing world suggests two major recommendations for agencies and groups. The first is that activities be arranged in which deaf and hard of hearing children participate with children who do hear, and that professional groups encourage the participation of hearing impaired graduate students or young professionals so that they can begin early on to develop skills for participating in the hearing world. Perhaps even more important, such programs encourage hearing individuals to develop skills for communicating with hearing impaired individuals, to gain an understanding of their problems, and to overcome their fear of these people who communicate differently.

A second recommendation is that employers of people who are hearing impaired attend to the social needs of their employees. Many individuals who are deaf are not as lucky as Stan. His co-workers were warm and friendly, and because they were interested in learning sign language, they eventually learned how to communicate with him. Other deaf persons have described very painful emotional situations in the work environment: co-workers turn their heads the other way when walking by the hearing impaired person, and the only method of communication with others is through writing notes. Co-workers as well as the employer need to learn techniques of communication. The employer can facilitate this by providing instruction on site or allowing time off from work for taking classes.

Since this discussion is directed toward a variety of agencies and groups, not all guidelines will apply in all cases. The following list provides some brief suggestions:

1. Provide scholarships for bright deaf students, and encourage them to compete with nonhandicapped students.
2. Arrange for interpreters at meetings or activities in which deaf people are involved.
3. Select counselors, social workers, or case workers who are familiar with the concerns of bright people with hearing problems.

4. Provide inservice training for staff members that addresses the special concerns of gifted hearing-impaired persons.
5. Hire capable deaf people.
6. Organize groups of parents who have gifted handicapped children and facilitate their communication and cooperative development of creative solutions to common problems.
7. Organize "big brother" or "big sister" or other mentorship programs in which older people with a similar degree or type of hearing loss are paired with a younger person. These mentors must be at least somewhat older so that they can give advice based on their perspective, but optimally the child should have contact with those of a variety of ages.
8. In any advertisements or literature from the agency, make certain that the abilities of deaf individuals are shown in a positive light.
9. Whenever conferences or meetings are planned, arrange a number of "poster sessions" or others with a visually oriented format. In such sessions, the focus is on discussing the project, research, or ideas in a small group or individually.

Educational Professionals

As for other groups, the most significant guideline for education professionals is development and communication of realistically high expectations for accomplishments. A child's deafness may make learning more difficult, may place some limits on career choices, and may restrict certain activities. However, it is important to communicate to the child that being deaf or hard of hearing does not limit the basic capacity to learn. Furthermore, even though educators are familiar with the limits on career choices or learning difficulties usually caused by deafness, they must remain open-minded about the possibilities for achievement in individual cases, especially when a child is gifted. Myron provides a perfect example of someone who is an exception to almost every rule about deafness.

It is very important that educators avoid making judgments about intellectual capacity based on a deaf child's language skills. Generally, the first clues to giftedness are an extensive vocabulary, appropriate use of words, and use of more complex statements than expected for the chronological age. Slower language development and use of less sophisticated language are normal characteristics of children who are deaf or hard of hearing and should not be taken as an indication of lower intelligence.

Development of a problem-solving approach is important for educators. Rather than discouraging, for example, choice of career or specialty because of deafness (as in Myron's case), the educator should share concerns about possible problems and then assist in identifying ways to overcome these problems. It would also be appropriate to assist the student in identifying alternative career goals of interest in areas in which the possibility of advancement or success is less affected by any limitation imposed by a particular disability.

As an integral component of a problem-solving approach, counseling should be provided on a regular basis. Counseling of gifted handicapped individuals is essential for several reasons: (a) to close the gap that typically exists between the handicapped individual's expectations for performance and the actual ability to perform a task; (b) to aid in developing a healthy self-concept and a realistic perception of capabilities and limitations; and (c) to aid in resolving differences between personal perceptions of capabilities and perceptions held by others. Counseling can be provided on an individual basis but may be more effective when conducted with a small group of students with similar concerns. If there are not enough bright deaf or hard of hearing students to constitute a group, bright children with other disabilities could be included.

To complement a problem-solving approach, educators also should teach students the coping strategies that have been successful for other deaf individuals. This can be done through having successful deaf adults talk with students or through simple sharing of information. Some of the coping and learning strategies used by successful deaf and hard of hearing adults are the following (Maker et al., 1978):

1. Read extensively on topics covered in classes to supplement classroom learning.
2. Ask questions until concepts are clear.
3. When reading, attempt to grasp the author's style and method of expression.
4. Make an effort to connect abstract concepts (such as those in calculus) with concrete ideas more easily represented visually (such as those in chemistry and physics).
5. Ask teachers and professors to set up a weekly or daily individual student conference to discuss assignments and topics presented in class.
6. Sit in on college classes the semester before taking them for credit so that information is familiar and there has been an opportunity to do outside reading. An alternative strategy was developed by one man who was not allowed to sit in on classes: he signed up for the class for credit and then withdrew on the last possible date; the following semester, he again signed up for the course and completed it!
7. Observe other members of the class for the first few days, and notice how conscientiously they take notes. Ask the two best note-takers for a copy of their notes in return for extra paper and carbon paper.
8. Take classes with friends, or develop friendships with classmates who are willing to discuss classes and help fill in information gaps.

9. Whenever possible, substitute independent study, independent reading, or internships on a one-to-one basis for lecture classes or classes with large groups of students.

In early education programs and in elementary schools, there needs to be a dual focus on language and cognitive development. Even though language is important in cognitive development, very often so much time is spent teaching deaf children communication skills that the development of other intellectual skills is totally neglected. Gifted students, especially, need to develop their capabilities for abstract reasoning and to be involved in intellectually challenging experiences. This neglect of thinking and reasoning skills may be a major factor contributing to the slower academic progress of deaf students. There are numerous guides for providing nonverbal reasoning or thinking tasks (see Guilford, 1967 and Meeker, 1973). The Midwest Publications Company, for instance, produces numerous workbooks and teachers' guides for the development of nonverbal critical thinking abilities.

Young deaf and hard of hearing students should be encouraged to participate in many activities that involve language skills including reading, spelling, grammar, and composition. Creative writing and story-telling are excellent complements to recreational reading as ways to challenge these children while allowing them to develop and refine skills of self-expression.

At higher levels of education, particularly in high school and college where many teachers lecture to large groups of students, several methods have been identified as helpful to those who have hearing impairments. Teachers need to be willing to spend extra time on an individual basis, explaining assignments, answering questions, and asking questions to make certain that hearing impaired students have the correct information or have not missed important concepts or ideas. One easy way to help such students is to provide a copy of the lecture notes to read before class. This provides students with some "advance organizers" that can help them understand better what is being said. The classroom also should be arranged to facilitate good speechreading, and interpreters should be provided when needed. If no interpreters are available, the teacher can ask other students to provide assistance, such as through taking notes or spending time explaining assignments, to those who cannot hear well.

Teachers and administrators also need to be willing to substitute individual reading courses, independent study, and internships for formal classes when possible and when needed by students. Often, these students can be more successful and learn much more when they interact on a one-to-one or small-group basis with the teacher. Since advanced classes and special programs for the gifted often have smaller numbers of students, these may be more attractive placements for gifted students who are deaf than are regular classrooms. In place of a course in research methodology, for example, a program of apprenticeship to one or several professionals involved in different types of research could be instituted. Gifted students profit from methods that allow them to learn at their own pace, so these individualized methods accommodate both their strengths and weaknesses.

Myron has recommended that gifted deaf and hard of hearing children be educated in a mainstream setting and has emphasized the advantages, including higher expectations from teachers and peers, an atmosphere conducive to success and high achievement, and an environment that more closely approximates the "real" world. He feels that he would not have had such high motivation if he had been in a special school or class for the deaf. Most hearing impaired persons who were interviewed agreed with him. However, several who are profoundly deaf did not; they emphasized the difficulties they had in getting information and in communicating with peers. These individuals believed strongly in the importance of developing language and communication skills as early as possible to enable them to take in more information. However, gifted students can usually learn language and communication skills more quickly than normally expected, and they can be moved into a mainstream setting as soon as their communication skills enable them to participate. Assessment is necessary first. Educators must not make assumptions about the effect of a disability. As in Myron's case, there is always a possibility that some severe or profoundly deaf individuals will not need a special class or school placement. Such individuals may have learned language and communication skills on their own.

Regardless of the type of setting in which gifted hearing impaired students are educated, teachers and other students should learn to communicate with them as effectively as possible. Teachers and students should learn advanced techniques in manual communication, lipreading, or other techniques for use in communicating with gifted deaf students.

Learning to communicate with students who are deaf and encouraging other students to acquire these skills can go a long way toward preventing one of the most significant problems deaf students face: isolation. Deaf students who are also gifted may have a greater tendency to become isolated than those who are not gifted. Many highly gifted individuals often feel isolated because there are no "intellectual peers" who understand and relate to them. Others tend to isolate themselves because they are interested in pursuing their individual projects. Because of the combined tendencies toward isolation, teachers should make an even greater effort to develop an atmosphere in which all students feel a responsibility to learn how to communicate more effectively with a deaf person in their classes.

Two other suggestions for educators include the hiring of capable teachers who are deaf or hard of hearing, so that children, both handicapped and nonhandicapped, have role models of success in the face of disability, and making arrangements for hearing impaired students to have contact with adults who have a similar degree or type of hearing loss. Another important program component is a strong cooperative relationship with parents. If such a program is developed, school projects can continue at home, concrete field experiences can supplement the abstract learning occurring at home, and clear educational goals can be established for the student.

CONCLUSION

Although Myron's case is in some ways a unique one, many insights into the needs of gifted students who are deaf can be gained through analysis of his development and concerns. According to him, the most important needs that can be met by both educators and families are high expectations for success and an environment that facilitates achievement. Both negative stereotypes and positive encouragement, interestingly enough, can have a similar effect on motivation, as they did in Myron's case. The desire to "prove himself" to those who did not believe he was capable was a strong factor in his success, as was his mother's positive attitude that denied any disability. However, high expectations for the performance of any child, especially one with a severe disability, should be realistic. Critical to the positive response Myron had to his mother's denial was his innate ability to succeed. What if he had not succeeded in meeting his goals? Parents and educators must develop realistic expectations based on a process of continuous assessment, observation, and presentation of challenging experiences in which the child can demonstrate both success and failure. Only then can limits be tested and performance expectations be realistic.

If educators and parents have an underlying belief in the capabilities of people with handicaps, they will be more likely to develop effective methods for working with deaf children. Beyond this belief, however, there are many specific methods that may be employed to facilitate the fuller development of each child's intellectual potential.

Chapter Reaction

Shirin Antia, Ph.D.

Educators of the hearing impaired should make it a practice to read about or to meet successful hearing impaired (HI) individuals at least once a year to realign their expectations of their students and their knowledge of the limitations of the handicap. It must be constantly kept in mind that the research describing the characteristics of the hearing impaired population cannot assist in predicting the abilities of any one individual. Often, successful gifted HI individuals vanish into the mainstream of society and are not included in these studies. As a result, educators are likely to underestimate the learning potential of bright HI children and perhaps focus on their disabilities rather than their abilities.

Both Myron's home background and his personal characteristics would be considered by professionals in the field to be predictors of success. His mother denied the limitations that society imposes on individuals with hearing losses. Both parents had high expectations of Myron and provided him with an environment rich in learning opportunities. Myron's persistence, his ability to find ways and means of achieving his goals, and his constant search for his limits are probably key ingredients to his success.

A significant difference between Myron and many other HI individuals is his ability to discover coping strategies to perform tasks that most people would think of as being difficult, if not impossible, for a person with a severe to profound hearing loss. For example, Myron has developed a successful strategy relying on linguistic closure (reconstructing an incomplete linguistic message using knowledge of linguistic rules) and contextual cues to communicate on the telephone. It may be worthwhile for educators to study the coping strategies of successful HI individuals and apply these to the education of other HI students.

Mention is made of Myron's excellent speech, an unusual achievement for a congenitally and severely or profoundly HI person. The stimulus for speech production is generally considered to be auditory input of speech. As pointed out in the discussion section, the child who does not hear speech cannot learn to use speech. It is not clear whether Myron's speech was intelligible before the discovery of his hearing loss or whether speech intelligibility was acquired after he was fitted with amplification.

A note of caution needs to be interjected here: Myron would probably be considered successful by most hearing people not only because of his professional accomplishments but because of his ability to "pass" in the hearing world (the term "pass" is adopted from Goffman, 1963), because of his excellent oral communication skills. It must be remembered that ability to "pass" by communicating orally should not be the only or even the major goal of a gifted HI person or any other HI person. Oral communication skills certainly enhance vocational and social opportunities for HI individuals. However, oral skills are neither a necessary nor a sufficient condition for success. Gifted HI individuals may be "oral failures" owing to the lack of usable residual hearing but may still achieve success in their chosen field. Parents should not let their child's feelings of self-worth be dependent on the ability to use intelligible speech, to lipread, or to be indistinguishable from a hearing person.

Myron discusses two issues that are controversial in the field of education of the hearing impaired: communication mode and educational setting. The question of which mode of communication, oral or manual, should be used to educate deaf children has plagued workers in the field for over 200 years. The arguments of both "camps" are outlined in the discussion, and only a few additional points need to be made here. The term sign language or manual communication, as used in the field today, refers actually to several different systems, divided by Quigley and Kretschmer (1982) into two broad categories: American Sign Language (ASL) and Manual English. ASL is a language with a vocabulary and syntax derived from its spatial and visual nature. Manual English refers to a number of different sign systems that use the vocabulary of ASL (i.e., the signs for many of the words are the same) but that attempt to follow English rules for word order and word inflections.

ASL has no written form, has not been commonly used to impart instruction, and is primarily used for social communication. As a result, it has been characterized as a "concrete" language incapable of expressing abstract ideas. ASL has a smaller vocabulary than English (Moores, 1982), but as it becomes more acceptable and more widely used, its vocabulary is increasing.

Manually coded English, with the help of finger-spelling, is theoretically capable of conveying any concepts and vocabulary that can be conveyed in English. The use of manual communication in and of itself does not limit abstract thinking or the acquisition of abstract concepts. The problem may be with teachers and parents, whose command of manual communication often is limited and who therefore confine themselves to simple messages, thus depriving the child of the opportunity to learn complex vocabulary and ideas. It should be pointed out that a rudimentary knowledge of any language—ASL or English—will restrict the concepts that can be learned or expressed through that language.

Educational placement is related to communication skills insofar as children with good oral communication skills are more likely to be placed in integrated classrooms. However, even these children may have difficulty following directions given while students are writing, since it is difficult to focus visual attention on two areas at once. They may also have difficulty following group discussion and rapid question-and-answer sessions. Integrated classrooms can be challenging and stimulating environments for many gifted hearing-impaired students, but it should be kept in mind that ideally, educational placement decisions should be based on individual needs, and that no one solution is best for all gifted hearing impaired children. Also, the lack of oral communication skills does not necessarily prevent a child from attending integrated classes, because interpreters (oral and manual) and the alternate learning strategies described in the discussion section can be employed profitably in many situations. Some of the disadvantages of integrated settings can be the lack of successful HI role models, isolation from peers owing to communication difficulties or a sense of being different, and lowered expectations by teachers for a child with a hearing loss.

Finally, educators of the hearing impaired need to learn more about gifted HI individuals: how best to facilitate their learning, how to keep them motivated, and how to provide them with the most appropriate educational environments.

REFERENCES

Goffman, E. (1963). *Stigma*. Englewood Cliffs, NJ: Prentice-Hall.

Moores, D. (1982). *Educating the deaf: Psychology, principles, and practices* (2nd ed.). Boston: Houghton-Mifflin.

Quigley, S., and Kretchmer, R. (1982). *The education of deaf children*. Baltimore: University Park Press.

* * * * *

Shirin Antia, author of this chapter reaction, is Assistant Professor of special education at The University of Arizona, where she is coordinator of the teacher education program in hearing impairment. A former teacher of the hearing impaired, Dr. Antia earned her doctorate from the University of Pittsburgh. Her current interests are in the areas of social interaction, mainstreaming, and communication development in the hearing impaired.

Chapter Reaction

Doris Senor Woltman

As an evaluator/diagnostician working in the field of deafness for the past five years, I have been in contact with a large number of deaf students who have demonstrated a wide variety of skills and abilities. These skills and abilities have ranged from limited mastery of basic concrete concepts to mastery of abstract concepts beyond their age or grade level. This latter group includes those students who are typically identified as gifted. Although they are unique in some of their abilities, they each share characteristics that are common to the majority of those individuals identified as hearing impaired gifted.

Myron demonstrated many of the characteristics common to those identified as hearing impaired gifted. These characteristics, along with his family background, are representative of the hearing impaired gifted individual. Myron comes from a supportive home that was success- and goal-oriented. As the chapter indicates, Myron's home background was rich in experiences and resources. Neither he nor his family viewed his hearing impairment as a handicap but only as a disability. Myron, himself, possesses the self-confidence, determination, and motivation needed for accomplishment. Although the characteristics are not exclusive to the gifted, they are essential for success and achievement. He demonstrated excellent skills in compensating for his hearing impairment. Myron is not afraid to ask for clarification if he does not understand information presented to him and demonstrates excellent closure skills in receptive communication with hearing peers. In addition, Myron demonstrates excellent reasoning and problem-solving ability. This is most easily seen in his approach to complex problems or unique barriers imposed by his hearing impairment. He is quick to develop alternative solutions to the problems at hand.

Although the above characteristics Myron possesses are representative of the gifted, I do not believe Myron is representative of a hearing impaired individual demonstrating a severe/profound sensorineural hearing loss. There are questions, which if answered, could possibly explain Myron's extraordinary abilities although he would still be viewed as a unique case. If Myron's severe/profound hearing loss was present from birth, it is phenomenal that he developed such a commanding control over language. It is equally a feat that Myron demonstrates perfect speech ability without having ever heard a human voice, much less his own voice. Although it is mentioned that Myron received amplification in elementary school, there is no mention of the amount of benefit he received from amplification. The amount of benefit received from amplification is unique to each individual but even with optimal benefit, hearing for all speech sounds is typically not obtained nor is sound ever clear. The final factor that makes Myron unique from other hearing impaired peers with the same degree of loss is his general attitude of denial concerning the existence of his hearing impairment. Although this denial can be commonly found in individuals with mild to moderate hearing losses, it is not typical in individuals with losses as great as Myron's. It is possible that due to Myron's outstanding compensatory abilities, he has not ever had to deal with his hearing impairment except in the area of music. Most individuals with a severe/profound hearing loss since birth have had to deal with their impairment early on and it is only with the help of a supportive family and school that they were able to confront it and move on.

The majority of deaf individuals with whom I work are school age children (3 to 21 years), who demonstrate hearing losses in the severe to profound range. The majority of these students are prelingually deaf. They all attend a state school for the deaf either as day or residential students. Total communication is used that incorporates speech, speechreading, signing, fingerspelling, audition, reading, and writing. This educational background is very different from Myron's and, therefore, offers two different insights and/or suggestions.

Students traditionally served at day/residential schools for the deaf need a comprehensive educational program where language acquisition is the major concern and goal. Presentation of language is carefully controlled in all subject areas. Although there are some students who might be well served by the public school system, their language needs are extensive and are usually greater than the resources of the public school. This incomplete mastery of concepts in language can be seen even in those students identified as gifted. Identification of deaf students as potentially gifted is complicated due to this language issue. It is important for schools to look at the language requirements of a test prior to using it as an identification measure. The limited number of identified gifted handicapped students is partially the result of biased identification procedures. Standardized tests may not be appropriate for specific individuals whose abilities, as tested, are masked by their handicap. Even without the mastery of language, several tests are available which are non-verbal in nature, and may be used appropriately with the deaf. These tests measure areas such as reasoning, problem solving, and creativity.

After gifted hearing-impaired students are identified, our responsibility to provide them an appropriate education that responds to their giftedness has only begun. In the area of special education, remediation is typically the primary concern with limited emphasis on developing strengths and/or special abilities. Special education teachers are typically not familiar with the characteristics or needs of gifted students nor are they familiar with techniques used by teachers of the gifted. In order to provide the most appropriate educational program for the gifted hearing impaired, teachers in special education must be willing to learn more about curriculum and programming for the gifted. This includes curriculum and programming that emphasize building on strengths, encouraging motivation, and developing positive self-concepts.

* * * * *

Doris Senor Woltman is a psychology assistant at the Arizona State School for the Deaf and the Blind. She earned a master's degree in Vocational Evaluation and Rehabilitation Counseling with the Deaf. Doris is also a doctoral student in Special Education Administration at The University of Arizona, Tucson.

Chapter 3

Gifted Persons with Visual Impairment

A CASE STUDY: ABE

The field of study that most interests Abe has always been mathematics, in which he obtained a bachelor's degree. Because he is legally blind, however, he was unable at first to find employment in his field. Therefore, he went back to school and obtained a master's degree in psychology. Nevertheless, he was still unable to find employment related to his education because, in his words, " . . . I guess I graduated during hard times and anyway the age of enlightenment for employing blind people had not yet come upon us." He held a series of odd jobs: sewing pillowcases, loading trucks, collating records, and typing letters for the American Foundation for the Blind. Meanwhile, he took several night school courses in mathematics because he enjoyed them so much, " . . . like going to play poker twice a week or something like that. . . ."

Seeing his discontent, his wife asked, "Wouldn't you rather be an unemployed mathematician than an unemployed psychologist?" She insisted that he go back to school full time to earn a degree in mathematics and she then went to work to support them. While working on this degree, Abe taught mathematics part time at a Catholic school and then for a semester at a nearby college for girls. After receiving his Ph.D., he looked for a permanent job. After sending out 200 letters and applications, he had three offers for interviews. One prospective employer, a university, hired him immediately. He has been at this university ever since, where he is now a full professor in the mathematics department.

Abe is married and has three children and eight grandchildren. He comes from a family of three children; he has a younger brother and a younger sister who is also blind. His mother had an eighth-grade education, and his father quit school after third grade. His parents owned a store, which they operated together, although his mother's activities as a homemaker occupied most of her time. Abe grew up in the days of the Depression, and his family was very poor. However, he remembers this period of his life not as a time of hardship but as a time of "great cooperation and love."

Abe was blind from birth. Although he is legally blind, he does have some light perception. Apparently his blindness and his sister's are not hereditary or linked in any way. Abe describes his visual impairment as a retinal problem and his sister's as a corneal problem.

Abe attended public elementary and secondary schools with resource room services for visually impaired students. Most of the time, these services consisted of one teacher who taught the skill of reading braille and provided needed remedial instruction in academic subjects. Abe had services from an individual who read assignments to him as an undergraduate and during work for his master's degree and then provided transcription services (i.e., translating his braille into English and transcribing books and other materials into braille) during work for his doctorate. His achievement was in the top 40 percent in elementary school and in the top 10 percent in high school, and in college his undergraduate grade-point average ranged from 3.5 to 4.0 (B + to A).

Personal View of Self

Strengths

Abe regards his major strengths to be his keen interest in mathematics, an ability to conceptualize or "to see the overall picture," willingness to think things through until they are learned, and an optimistic nature that includes a belief that he can achieve any goal so long as he is willing to put the needed effort into attaining it. He also considers his attitude toward his handicap and his determination not to get angry as valuable assets. Abe attributes most of his success to his willingness to work hard.

Abe remembers always being very interested in mathematics, even in the early school years. Although he was not a "good" arithmetic student in elementary school, he attributes his lack of success to his teachers' inadequate instructional methods, especially their lack of preparation for teaching mathematics effectively to blind children. Available equipment, Abe suggests, was " . . . invented by the devil. You paid so much attention to handling the equipment that you didn't have any room in your mind left to do the arithmetic." He did have a good teacher in high school, and in three months he acquired the skills in arithmetic he had not mastered during eight years of elementary school! By the ninth grade, his academic achievement in mathematics clearly demonstrated his superior ability—he made an A in algebra. From that time on, he took as much mathematics as possible, both in high school and in college.

Abe was discouraged from taking mathematics courses in college because at the time there was no braille system for mathematics notation. In 1951, immediately after obtaining his master's degree, Abe began serious work on the development of his own system. He had started some notations four years earlier while taking mathematics classes, but while taking graduate courses he realized the acute need for a code allowing a more efficient system of notation. Results were not long in coming once he began, because his ideas had been undergoing "incubation" for many years prior to that time.

The underlying skills Abe needed to develop the code, according to him, happened to be his strengths. First, he had to have "a broad understanding of what I was about to do. . . ." I'm a braille expert, I know the braille system very well . . . and I knew what notations I needed to represent." He then had to pay attention to the details of developing consistency in the symbols, and to resolve any possible conflicts. In developing the code, he followed two basic principles. First, the code must represent all symbols and notations as if they were being read aloud. " . . . For example, if someone would say to me a fraction X + Y over A + B, if I could invent the symbol which means the fraction and another symbol which means over, then [in braille writing] I could get the same effect as [in] listening. . . ." The second principle was that the same symbol had to have the same meaning in every area of mathematics and at all levels, from " . . . first-grade arithmetic to nuclear physics."

The development and subsequent wide use of this notation system, named the Nemeth Code in his honor, made possible a career in mathematics for Abe and many other blind people. The Nemeth Code is now used throughout the United States, particularly in the transcription of mathematics books. One of the strengths of the system is that transcribers do not need to be mathematicians: they need only transcribe what they see.

Development of this system required most of the traits that Abe perceives as personal strengths—ability to see the overall picture, willingness to think things through, and belief in personal ability, in addition to the knowledge of both braille and mathematics. His interest in mathematics and desire to study it at a higher level provided the impetus for spending the time and effort needed to develop and refine the system.

Another characteristic Abe perceives as a strength is his positive attitude in the face of his disability as well as other people's treatment of him. As will be discussed later in more detail, one college professor told Abe he did not expect him to do homework, take exams, or get a grade in the course; Abe's reaction was to do the work anyway, without getting angry, and to invest the effort needed to make the best of the situation. He recalls that " . . . I said to myself, if this is the situation, just apply more effort to make it right than it should take, and set about to make it right." Also, he reports that he "did learn from that experience that there are people who have this attitude toward blind people and that I have to be aware of this situation and cope with it. . . . It wasn't devastating."

In a similar situation, Abe was told he could not take a lab course in physics because he was blind. According to Abe, the most important thing he did was to avoid getting angry. Instead, armed with a "briefcase full" of devices to help him read by sound, slide rules, and other equipment, he went to the head of the physics department and asked to be allowed to demonstrate how as a blind person he could take a lab course in physics. The department head consented, and Abe's demonstration was successful: he was permitted to take the course. "When you become angry, the opposite side becomes defensive, so I just quietly went about to prove that I could do it . . . that worked. A reasoned, quiet approach."

The trait that Abe sees as the most important reason for his success is effort, or willingness to work. Although he sees himself as capable, more capable than most other people disabled or nondisabled, he explains the need for hard work in this way:

> . . . I have to work at what I create; hard effort. . . . I've long since learned that the world judges you by what you achieve and not by how much effort you put into the achievement. Some people are talented, geniuses, and accomplish great things with very little effort; some people accomplish great things only as a result of much perspiration, but the world looks only at the achievement. They don't see how hard one works.

In summary, Abe perceives his major strengths as (a) his long-term interest in mathematics, (b) a well-developed ability to conceptualize, (c) his persistence in working through a problem or situation, (d) his optimism, and (e) a strong belief in himself and his abilities. He attributes most of his success to his willingness to expend extra effort to accomplish his goals, his positive attitude despite his disability, and his determination to avoid getting angry because of other people's treatment of him.

Weaknesses

Abe sees himself as one whose achievements require a great deal of effort. "I have good ability, but I'm not one of these people who can create immediately." He apparently perceives his ability to see the overall picture as not necessarily a strength nor even an interest. If a task is important enough, however, he becomes willing to focus his efforts on working out the details of that overall picture—to put in the work required for success in a particular task.

His blindness causes the biggest weakness—lack of access to the printed word. Abe has always felt that if he could read more freely, he would be able to ". . . grow quicker or faster or in more directions." With easy access to written material, he would not need to rely so much on books that had already been transcribed, to wait for requested materials to be provided, or to depend on others to read material to him or lecture. The ability to read widely would enable him to have more choice in his intellectual pursuits and to do more things well.

Personal View of Perceptions and Treatment by Others

Facilitators

Abe perceives his parents as his first important facilitators. Even though he was blind at birth, they did not overprotect him. They allowed him to "fend for [himself] and take whatever lumps were necessary . . . to learn what the world was about." He remembers his father's taking him by the hand and walking with him through the neighborhood. Instead of just walking, his father was careful to describe what they encountered on their route:

> ". . . this is a bakery, this is a butchershop, this is a grocery store . . .
> the name on the street is [so and so] . . . we are making a right turn . . .
> we are walking west." [He] kept me fully in touch with my environment
> and took me to the same destination by different routes so I would get the
> geography well in my mind.

Since Abe grew up in a "rough" neighborhood, the Lower East Side in New York City, he knew that he had to be successful in coping with the neighborhood, or else he could "wind up in Sing Sing."

Abe's parents allowed and encouraged him to do things for himself. Instead of doing things for him—often an easier course for the family—they encouraged his independence. For example, his father encouraged him to touch things to figure out what they were, rather than telling him. His father often placed a letter in his hand and had him mail it, rather than mailing the letter for him. With reference to another blind person whose parents did not overprotect her, Abe summarized the effect of this kind of treatment: "But if they did not push her toward independence, she would never know what her limitations were."

Another important characteristic of Abe's parents' treatment of him was their high expectations. He always knew that they perceived him as a capable person, and he feels that his disability had absolutely no effect on their expectations for his overall success. They expected him to achieve regardless of his disability because he had other abilities that could compensate: ". . . they didn't see my blindness as a handicap. They didn't excuse me at any time on account of my blindness. They expected the same excellence as they would of their other children." His parents' expectations were clearly communicated both covertly and overtly. Abe remembers being asked, " . . . what's a big boy like you doing sitting around at 2 o'clock in the afternoon listening to the radio?" When Abe did not do very well in arithmetic, his father often talked to the teachers, " . . . promising [them] I would do better next month!"

A second important facilitator was his resource teacher throughout high school. Abe believes that, unlike the other teachers who provided special education services, this man understood how to teach blind children. Under his guidance, Abe was able to learn, within three months, all the arithmetic he should have learned in the preceding eight years. This teacher was very successful in communicating with his student. His method of teaching was directed at conveying a grasp of the underlying principles: once a principle was understood, the details could be filled in. This teacher concentrated on helping his student make a "mental leap" from the principles presented to the conclusion. Later, through concentration and study, Abe found that he could absorb the details.

When asked why this teacher was so important and how he communicated his expectations, Abe emphasized the teacher's attitude rather than the subject matter he taught. This teacher was a mentor and a friend: he often took Abe to the teachers' lunchroom to eat and gave him extra problems to work just to see if he could handle them; in the summertime, he took Abe on hikes or long walks. He made it clear that Abe had, within himself, all the resources necessary to do whatever he wanted to do. Essentially this teacher communicated to Abe that he was not expected to fail in mathematics or anything else—and furthermore, that he was expected to be somebody worthwhile and important.

In response to a question about whether his disability had any effect on this teacher's expectations of him, Abe replied, "I don't know. I think he was able to judge each person as an individual. A person's disability is just one aspect of his total makeup, and his judgment was based on the total makeup." Because he valued this man's judgment, Abe was eager to fulfill the expectations presented; he did not want to disappoint his teacher in any way.

This teacher was the most important facilitator in Abe's educational experience. His encouragement made Abe realize that he had the ability to become a mathematician, and that the obstacles he had to overcome were external rather than internal. Abe took all the mathematics courses he could in high school and then majored in mathematics in college. He still had to face obstacles, however, and often had to decide whether he was willing to put forth the effort required to overcome them. The teacher's encouragement was significant in that it made Abe believe that with hard work, he was capable of overcoming the barriers presented by his disability.

Another important facilitator was his wife. Seeing his frustration from working at unchallenging odd jobs, she encouraged him to expend the effort needed to earn a higher degree in mathematics, the subject he loved. Her attitude was that it seemed silly to try to get a job as a psychologist (he had a master's degree in psychology) when he really wanted to be a mathematician. Since he was working at readily available jobs that required no academic preparation, she believed he should go back to school. She was willing to work to support them while he went to school.

When asked about the effect of his wife's encouragement on his overall development, Abe replied that this event had occurred during his adulthood and that his attitudes were well established by that time. He felt, however, that he had a responsibility to her—to keep a job in order to support her—and that the dream of being a mathematician would have to be forgotten in order to meet that responsibility. However, his wife was willing to work with him and to give him the opportunity to be what he wanted to be. In his words,

> . . . everybody has a dream to do more things than one is able to do, so you have to accept doing one or two of those and keep the others as dreams. She saw the value of encouraging me, she didn't look for the short-run goal of living a quiet life. She was looking forward to the long-term goal of a life of accomplishment, and she was willing to make the short-term sacrifice necessary to achieve the long-term goal.

A physicist who studied at the same university also was a facilitator to Abe's career in that he was instrumental in getting Abe's mathematics notation system published. This man, also blind, asked if Abe had a table of integrals. Abe showed his system to the physicist, who was so impressed that he brought it to the attention of the Joint Uniform Type Committee. Subsequently, the committee invited Abe to write a description of the system for publication. Since the system is easily learned and used by transcribers and allows students access to mathematics books and materials previously unavailable to them, it quickly became an official code of communication for visually impaired persons. Knowledge of the availability of such a system should reduce, if not eliminate, the negative attitudes of professors and others who discourage blind people from going into the field of mathematics.

In summary, Abe perceives his facilitators to have been (a) his parents, who saw him as a capable individual, encouraged him to take care of himself, and taught him about his environment at a very early age; (b) his wife, who encouraged him to pursue a career in mathematics even though his professors discouraged this choice, and who provided the support that enabled him to go to school; and (c) a resource teacher in high school, who understood how to teach him, believed in his intellectual ability, and encouraged Abe to pursue his interest in mathematics. Finally, a blind physicist was instrumental in gaining recognition for Abe's development of a tool for blind persons to use in mathematics courses or careers. What these individuals seemed to have in common was their belief in Abe's capabilities, a willingness to encourage the expression of his ability, and their encouragement of his intense interest in mathematics.

Obstructors

Abe perceives the most important obstructors in his life to have been teachers and professors. In his words, "The educational system did nothing but put obstacles in my way." Most of these obstacles were in the form of attitudes of teachers who did not believe that blind people were capable of learning mathematics or related subjects. As an elementary school student, he felt that the teachers simply did not know how to teach a blind child. They paid more attention to teaching him how to use equipment than to teaching him concepts.

In college, prevailing negative attitudes or stereotypes associated with visual impairment seemed to be even more dominant. All of his professors advised him not to enter the field of mathematics because of the problems he would have: How would he read the material? How would he make notes? How would he do his assignments? Even after he developed his code and it seemed to work well for him, his professors still tried to discourage him. Following their advice, he returned to school for a master's degree in psychology—and still could not get an appropriate professional job!

Abe recalls a very memorable event that provides one example of obstructive professional behavior derived from negative stereotypes of blind students. After he enrolled in a statistics course, his professor told him that, although he would be allowed to remain in the class, he would not be expected to do any homework or to take any tests, and that he would not be given a grade at the end of the term. In response, Abe did all the work and studying necessary to learn the material, even though he did not turn in his work to the professor. At the end of the term, he told the department chairman about the situation. The chairman gave him the examination and was impressed by the fact that he earned an A in the course.

His experience with the statistics course was particularly significant because, in Abe's words, "It occurred to me that if a person that I came upon by chance took such an attitude, how many more people in the world would there be who would take a similar attitude?" Taking that specific course was not particularly important, but he became aware that in other areas and activities, similar negative attitudes and obstructive behavior could present problems. But by successfully handling the situation, he gained the confidence needed to deal with such behavior.

It is interesting that in the context of this event, Abe made a distinction between a disability and a handicap. To him, a disability is a physical impairment, whereas a handicap is more of an effect. A handicap may have nothing to do with a disability. In fact, some people are handicapped who do not have a physical disability at all. Some are handicapped by their attitudes toward themselves, and others are handicapped by others' attitudes toward them.

Another experience in college had a similar effect on Abe. He was told that he could not take a physics lab course because his blindness would prevent him from reading the instruments. He then went to the American Foundation for the Blind and picked up a "briefcase full" of devices. Without disclosing that he had already been denied permission to take the course, he went to the head of the department and said that he would like to demonstrate how, as a blind person, he could take a lab course in physics. Abe wished to establish objectively his ability to participate. After the demonstration was successful, Abe requested permission to take the formerly forbidden class and was allowed to enroll. According to Abe, this "reasoned, quiet approach" to obstructors has worked well for him throughout his life.

Statement of Specific Needs

Abe's discussion of specific needs was in the context of recommendations for others with a similar disability. These recommendations generally fall into three categories: developing a realistic, positive understanding of personal capabilities; developing independence; and learning about the environment and how to get around in it.

Family and Friends

The most important contribution families and friends can make is not to fall into the trap of overprotecting blind children. Parents want to keep their children from getting hurt. Certainly some protection is necessary. However, blind children will not develop the courage or the skill necessary to be independent if they are not encouraged at an early age to do things for themselves. Parents must resist the urge to do things for their children. " . . . If a kid tries to do something for himself, let him do it. Don't say, 'I'll do it for you.'" According to Abe, many parents of blind children "carefully walk them down the middle of the street" so that the children never learn what a fire hydrant, a parking meter, a mailbox, a lamppost, or a door is like. Everyday experiences can be made into learning situations if parents are willing to think in these ways.

Education and Schools

The professionals in the educational system can make a significant contribution through raising their expectations for the performance of blind children, thus encouraging such children to have high expectations for themselves. In Abe's words, "more should be expected of blind students. Too many teachers allow blind children to set their own upper limits. The expectations should be realistic, but there's too much of a tendency to think a child who's blind is really not capable of doing such and such."

Abe believes that going to regular public school rather than a school for the blind was one of his most valuable experiences. This experience taught him that a lot is expected of people who can see; he also learned that even sighted persons have limitations in what they can and cannot do, and he learned to understand individual differences from person to person. Most important, he did not "set [his goal] to the norms for a blind person."

He also recommends that schools provide mobility training at an early age to enable students to gain confidence and to allow them to become familiar with their environment. Schools should provide easier access to braille transcriptions and records of books. Finally, he insists that blind students should not have to expend extra energy and time to get materials and readers in addition to doing their regular studies.

Community

According to Abe, the most important contribution that can be made by other individuals in the community is to

> . . . learn to accept an individual as an individual. There are some disabilities which are apparent, such as blindness, and there are some which are not apparent. Nevertheless, you have to learn to accept the whole individual. You cannot approach the individual with preconceptions.

People also need to watch out for dangerous situations and to be ready to provide assistance in situations in which a blind person obviously will require help. In less obvious situations, assistance should be offered.

DISCUSSION

Traditional View of Blindness

Visually impaired and blind children make up one of the smallest groups of exceptional children. Blindness seems to be one of the most feared handicaps among adults. Many people actively avoid associating with a blind individual, perhaps because such a person reminds them of the frightening possibility that they too could lose their sight. Furthermore, a blind individual's mobility is limited, which increases the social isolation. Thus, it seems that most people know very little about blindness and have had limited contact with those who have severe visual impairments. Individuals who are blind tend to be isolated from the mainstream of society both because of the attitudes of others and because of their lack of mobility.

Generally, visually impaired persons are defined as those who differ from those with normal vision to such an extent that they need special teachers, materials, and aids in order to reach their full potential (Ashcroft, 1963). As with hearing problems, there are two general categories of disability—those who are blind and those who have low vision. Some definitions of these two types are based on visual acuity; and others are based on the educational materials needed.

The legal definition of blindness is based on measurably diminished vision, according to either of two criteria: visual acuity of 20/200 or less in the better eye with the best possible correction or a field of vision restricted to an angle subtending an arc of 20 degrees or less. Partially sighted persons are those whose visual acuity is between 20/200 and 20/70 in the better eye with the best possible correction or those who, in the opinion of an eye specialist, need either temporary or permanent special educational facilities (American Foundation for the Blind, 1961).

With regard to educational needs, the blind student is defined as one whose visual loss requires that she or he be educated primarily through braille and other tactile or auditory materials. The partially seeing student is one who has some vision and can use print or other visual materials (American Foundation for the Blind, 1961).

Of these two sets of definitions, those focusing on educational needs are preferred for educators because they describe characteristics that are helpful in determining appropriate programming. However, definitions based on visual acuity and extent of peripheral vision are appropriate for describing and classifying the characteristics of blind or partially sighted individuals. Some of these characteristics are outlined in the following discussion.

Visual acuity is a way of describing the sharpness and clearness of vision at particular distances. For example, visual acuity of 20/200 means that at a distance of 20 feet, the individual can read what a person with normal vision can read at 200 feet. An index of visual acuity does not describe the visual efficiency of individuals, nor does it relate to the variety of ways in which vision is used in an educational setting. For instance, it does not provide an indication of the ability to read educational materials at a close range. Visual arc provides a measure of the field of vision, which if limited may severely restrict mobility and ability to read. Depending on the effect or type of loss, a limited visual field may make seeing objects that are not directly in front of an individual or reading more than one letter at a time on a page a very difficult task. Thus, a description of visual arc is important in providing information about an individual's vision and its effects on learning.

In addition to different degrees of visual impairment, there are different types and causes of visual problems. Types of disorders are classified as (a) those of the refractive system; (b) those affecting the retinal and optic nerve; and (c) those affecting the muscles. The major causes of blindness and other visual disabilities include diseases, accidents or injuries, poisonings, tumors, and inherited defects.

Disorders affecting refraction, some of the most common in children today (Caton, 1981), are farsightedness, nearsightedness, and astigmatism. Most of these problems can be corrected with eyeglasses or contact lenses. However, the receptive parts of the eye are subject to certain degenerative conditions, sometimes caused by infections and sometimes due to recessive gene traits. Such disorders include degeneration of the retina and the optic nerve and detachment of the retina. These disorders usually cause complete or near-total loss of vision, and there is generally a lack of knowledge about the rate and cause of degeneration. Muscular disorders, another type of problem, can usually be corrected by surgery or other treatment.

Two conditions that were relatively common causes of blindness in the past are retrolental fibroplasia and maternal rubella. Premature infants receiving too much oxygen in the incubator often developed retrolental fibroplasia, but now the oxygen level is regulated more carefully, so fewer children suffer from the disorder. However, sometimes a premature infant's life can be saved only by increasing the oxygen level, thus placing the baby at risk for retrolental fibroplasia. Rubella, or German measles, when contracted by a woman in her first trimester of pregnancy, may cause several disorders in her child, including blindness. Doctors are now more aware of this possibility, so preventive measures are taken.

Glaucoma is a condition that results in pressure on the optic nerve and eventual blindness. This disease can usually be treated and visual loss prevented in adults, but congenital glaucoma may result in visual problems in children.

Before considering some of the characteristics of blind or visually impaired children, it is important to emphasize that there is a disagreement in the field as to the overall effect of the specific disability. Some investigators believe that all mental activities are "distorted" by the lack of sight (Cutsforth, 1951); others (Ashcroft, 1963) believe that visually impaired children are like other children more than they are different from them. There are also many variations in characteristics that cause individual differences, so generalizations are difficult to make. The ability to learn, for example, is influenced not only by the type and degree of visual impairment but also by the age of onset of the problem and by the child's range of experiences, intelligence, and chronological age. The following discussion briefly summarizes information regarding the effect of visual impairment on development in each of the three areas: physical, intellectual, and socioemotional growth.

Although blind or visually impaired children's physical characteristics are usually similar to the physical traits of other children, they often fail to develop specific physical skills. Because of overprotection from parents and the inability to observe the physical activities of others, many visually impaired children do not have adequate opportunity to develop skills. They must be taught many of the skills that others develop without instruction—for example, correct posture, gaits necessary to move through various environments, or basic self-care, such as dressing or bathing.

In visually impaired children, learning is affected by many of the same factors as those identified in nondisabled children (e.g., intelligence, range of educational experience, and age). Other important factors affecting learning in children with vision problems are age of onset of the problem and its degree and type. It is generally agreed that, although some studies have documented lower scores on intelligence tests for the blind and visually impaired (Maker, 1978), such scores probably reflect aspects of the testing procedure or a lack of educational opportunity. Many children tested in the studies were enrolled in segregated or residential schools. Furthermore, the tests were not developed for, or standardized on, children with visual impairments, and some early research did not separate blind people from those with low vision. Finally, many blind children do not have the same opportunities to develop their intellectual potential at an early age because they lack access to the printed word until braille is learned, because their experiences are limited owing to restricted mobility, and because their capabilities are not recognized by those around them.

An IQ score often reflects experience or educational opportunities more than intellectual potential. Accordingly, lower scores for children enrolled in residential schools, who often have multiple handicaps severely limiting the range of experiences, are not surprising. One opinion (Caton, 1981) is that visual impairment does not necessarily lower an individual's intelligence. It may restrict the range of experience and consequently have a detrimental effect on performance on tests that do not take into account the effects of a visual disability. On the other hand, although overall intellectual performance of individuals who are blind or partially sighted may be in the average range, the disability may be associated with certain intellectual deficits in specific areas such as ability to link ideas and objects (Tillman & Osborne, 1969; Kephart, Kephart, & Schwartz, 1974). Whether these deficits can be overcome through the provision of special training and/or experiences is unknown at this time.

There is general agreement that visually impaired children progress through the same developmental stages as those seen in children without visual problems (Caton, 1981), but that they do so at a much slower pace (Maker, 1978; Caton, 1981). A possible cause of slower development is a restricted ability to interact with the environment. In addition, these children lack the ability to learn through imitation. The underlying factor seems to be that they lack the interactive experiences with the environment that are necessary for the development of abstract concepts (e.g., spatial relationships, size, form).

Because of their slower developmental rate and their lack of experiences, as well as other factors, blind and visually impaired children achieve at much lower levels than those expected for age and grade placement (Bateman, 1963; Birch, Tisdall, Peabody, & Sterrett, 1966; Lowenfeld, Abel, & Hatlen, 1969; Caton & Rankin, 1978). Other factors also may contribute to this underachievement (Ashcroft, 1963): they often enter school at a later age; many educational programs are inappropriate; they may miss a lot of school owing to surgery or other treatment; and the use of braille, large-type editions of books, or optical aids may slow ability to gain information.

With regard to social and emotional development, there seems to be little agreement about and little evidence of clear differences between individuals with visual impairments and those without. Children with visual impairments may not be as well adjusted as either the blind or the sighted because of their "marginal status"—that is, neither blind nor sighted (Myerson, 1971). Certainly, blindness causes a child to be isolated from the environment and eliminates the opportunity to communicate through facial expressions or body language. Often the social and emotional problems of children with visual impairments are caused by the attitudes and reactions of others. For example, a typical reaction of sighted people is that all visually impaired individuals are totally blind and dependent. This certainly causes problems in social interactions, as does the fact that many blind and visually impaired persons have mannerisms or personal appearances that do not seem pleasing.

Educational Programs

As with other areas of special education, a range of administrative arrangements for services should be available for children with visual impairments. These include consulting or itinerant teacher services for children placed in the regular classroom, resource rooms for supplementary services, special classes in public schools, and special day or residential schools. An optimal program depends on the extent and type of curriculum modifications needed, as well as the intensity of the services required. Often, for example, children with visual impairments who have associated or multiple handicaps should be placed in special schools because of their need for additional equipment, special instruction appropriate for those with visual disabilities in use of equipment or development of skills such as mobility, or services required by associated disabilities. Children with normal intelligence, no additional handicaps, and a severe visual impairment can receive an appropriate education in the regular classroom if additional programs—such as instruction in academics from a specially trained resource teacher and in reading and writing braille, improving mobility, or using certain equipment—are provided. A child with a less severe visual impairment who is capable of reading regular print with a magnifier, can function successfully in the regular educational program with assistance in instructional techniques or equipment provided to classroom teachers by a consulting teacher.

The most important factors to consider in determining appropriate placement are extent and cause of the loss, age of onset, range of experiences, intelligence, and current age. As a student gets older, educational needs may change, and the program should be altered accordingly. Caton (1981) suggests that students with visual impairments be educated as much as possible in the classes they would be attending if they were not visually impaired. Therefore, gifted students with visual problems should probably be placed in programs for the gifted. Certainly there have been numerous instances in which gifted visually impaired children have done well in educational programs for gifted students.

It is obvious that visually impaired students need the same academic curriculum as that offered to nonimpaired children. In addition, children with visual impairments need to be taught adaptive skills of improved orientation and mobility; daily living skills; braille reading and writing (and print reading, if appropriate); use of tape recorders and other equipment, such as the Optacon, to facilitate learning; and use of unimpaired senses, such as listening, to facilitate adaptation. Orientation training develops the students' ability to understand and recognize aspects of the environment and to sense their physical location relative to environmental elements, as well as to orient themselves during conversation with others. In mobility training, students learn to move around efficiently in their environment. The ability to understand their surroundings and move around with confidence is an important skill for educational as well as social reasons. In addition to basic mobility training, various electronic devices are available to guide the movement of visually impaired persons. These aids range from laser canes to an electronic probe held in the hand that uses vibration signals to indicate how far it is from objects. Daily living skills include self-care, such as eating, bathing, dressing and household chores. These skills are learned by unimpaired children through observation but must be taught to children who are visually impaired.

Visually impaired children need special instruction to develop skills that will enable them to compensate for their lack of vision when learning subject matter. These skills include braille reading and writing, print reading, use of special equipment, listening, and sight utilization. Braille is the primary medium for those who do not have enough sight to read print, although new machines are becoming available that can convert any written material into sound or tactile sensations. Braille writing requires much more space than other writing; thus, books and materials are heavy and require a great deal of storage space. Writing in braille is done with a machine somewhat like a typewriter, or with a slate and stylus. A slate and stylus is a portable device with a metal or plastic frame, with a pointed steel stylus that is used to hand-punch braille dots in paper placed between a top part with holes and a bottom part with indentations corresponding to the holes.

If children have enough vision to read print, they can be provided with books in large type and/or optical aids to enlarge regular type. They are then taught to read in the same way as children with unimpaired vision. However, visually impaired children can be expected to read at a much slower rate and consequently may progress more slowly in certain academic subjects than those with normal vision; often, such children may be able to see only a few letters at a time or may constantly have to adjust the optical aid. The physical environment for reading is as important as the size of print or the visual aid to be used. Printed material or writing on a chalkboard must have sharp contrast between the letters and the background paper or board; the background should be clear and eliminate glare. Teachers should not be concerned if children with low vision hold their reading material closer to their eyes than normal, or at a different angle, if these are techniques that help them see. These children should be seated in an area of the classroom that allows maximum use of their vision and should be provided with special adaptations of materials used as visual aids (e.g., maps, charts). All material presented visually also should be explained verbally to assist in seeing and understanding.

In addition to braille writing equipment, new technology for direct print reading has become available. One machine, the Optacon, converts print into letters that can be felt with a finger. The Optacon allows the blind person to read through sensing the forms of letters transmitted by vibrations to the fingertip by a stylus that in essence converts photographed images to tactile sensations. The newest machine, the Kurzweil Reader, converts printed words into synthetic speech.

Visually impaired students need to be taught how to use residual vision most efficiently and effectively and how to develop fully their capacity for skillful listening to facilitate mobility and learning. Barraga (1964), for example, found that special evaluative and training techniques can greatly improve children's use of residual vision even if the impairment is very severe. Similarly, Bischoff (1979) found that listening comprehension can be effectively taught to children with visual impairments and that these skills are useful in improving academic achievement. Tapes of compressed speech or accelerated speech, which provide information at a faster rate, can be used by students with highly developed listening comprehension skills.

Teachers with visually impaired students in their classes need to be always conscious of teaching behavior and its effect on the learning of those disabled students. For example, all instructions and explanations should be given verbally as well as visually. Tactile materials, such as raised-line drawings or concrete objects, should be available as appropriate complements to verbal instruction. Visually impaired students need as many direct experiences with the environment as possible, as well as frequent opportunities to interact with children who can see. When such interactions with the environment are accompanied by verbal explanations, supplied by either an adult or a child, the meaning of the experience becomes clearer. The important principle to follow is to attempt to provide as much information as possible through senses other than vision to supplement or replace what is obtained visually by other students.

Indicators of Intellectual Giftedness

Since Abe does not remember his elementary school years in great detail, early indicators in his case are difficult to identify. His early and intense interest in mathematics was probably such a sign, which went unnoticed because his teachers attempted to teach computation rather than concepts. However, he apparently did not respond exceptionally well to mathematics instruction, nor did he acquire expected computational skills in the early grades.

The most positive indication of Abe's intellectual ability was the fact that with a good teacher, he learned in three months all the mathematics he should have learned in elementary school. He caught up rapidly! In children with any handicap, as well as in children from minority groups, learning rate is one of the best indicators of intellectual giftedness (Leonard, 1978). As in Abe's case, this exceptional rate of learning occurs only when the individual is developmentally ready and when the conditions, particularly the mode of instruction, are conducive.

Abe was able to function very well in the regular classroom, and his achievement seemed to improve after he learned skills such as the reading and writing of braille. In high school, he generally ranked in the top 10 percent, and by college, his grades were mostly As. This pattern of achievement shows that as his "coping" or adapting skills improved, his performance level rose also. Visually impaired individuals with lesser intellectual ability typically show a decline in achievement as the coursework becomes more difficult. This may be due to interaction of the increasing abstractness of the content (Kirk & Gallagher, 1983) with an inability to grasp abstract relationships (Tillman & Osborne, 1969). The fact that as a blind child he was in the top 40 percent of his elementary school classes was indicative of his high cognitive ability. Most research on blind and partially sighted children shows them to be from one and one half to two years below grade level in achievement (Bateman, 1963; Lowenfeld et al., 1969; Caton & Rankin, 1978). Abe's giftedness was evidenced in his ability to achieve at performance levels higher than those of most sighted children and much higher than those of other children blind from birth.

The high school resource teacher apparently noticed Abe's exceptional ability to understand underlying principles. His way of teaching emphasized grasping an idea or concept, with acquisition of the associated skills later. This method of teaching is particularly appropriate for gifted students (Maker, 1982); it matches their natural learning style.

Finally, Abe's development of a new system of mathematics notation in braille was a further indication of his superior intellectual ability. Developing a system useful for mathematicians as well as youngsters required an in-depth understanding of the underlying principles of mathematics as well as a thorough understanding of braille. Furthermore, making the system easily transcribed by individuals who are not familiar with mathematics required exceptional ability in objective analysis, in order to accommodate a range of abilities and needs in creating a functional device.

Other reliable indicators of giftedness in children with visual impairments can be exceptional memory, advanced problem-solving skills, superior verbal communication, and creative production or thought. However, it is necessary to observe or test auditory or tactile rather than visual input or production. For instance, a child who is blind or has low vision could not be expected to show superior written production or to evidence superior memory of a visual image even if that visual image is described verbally. Exceptional problem solving and creativity are likewise evidenced more often through verbal communication rather than written products or physical activity.

A successful attorney who has been legally blind since the age of 9 years is an illustrative example. He graduated cum laude from Harvard Law School and attributes his success to his exceptional memory and powers of concentration. While in law school, he found that the only way he could do the research and other assignments required in his classes was to have someone reading to him from 9 o'clock in the morning until 10 o'clock in the evening. Since it was difficult and time-consuming to take notes on this volume of material, he relied on his exceptional memory in taking examinations and completing writing assignments. As an attorney, he relies on his verbal ability in litigation and in negotiations with legislators in Congress, where he serves as an advocate of programs and services for the disabled. He and others value his ability to "take regulations which are written in 'legalese' and put them in English."

It was interesting to discuss some of the problem-solving skills, especially in physical areas, evidenced by this attorney. Even though he has little vision other than light reception, as a youngster he was taught by his brother to catch a football. He now gives his wife advice about playing tennis by listening to the way the ball hits the racquet. He also pitches for a softball team; he can judge the distance the ball will travel, as well as its angle, by the way he allows it to leave his hand. Obviously, these physical skills were developed with a great deal of practice and analysis of angles, amount of force needed, and perception of auditory cues. In softball games he does have someone standing next to him with a glove to catch balls that are hit directly toward him.

Exceptional memory may be evidenced in various areas. For example, in an interview for entrance into graduate school, a blind biologist was able to identify with complete accuracy every mollusk shell that was given to him. In fact, his ability to make these identifications was greater than that of most sighted biologists.

Identification of Giftedness

Intelligence tests used with sighted children contain many items that are inappropriate for those who are blind or partially sighted. Not only is it important that test items not require visual information or cues, but it is also important to assure that visual experiences are not necessary to develop the concepts that are being tested. This last criterion is especially important if the child has been blind from birth. Very few tests of intelligence have been developed for use with children who are blind or have low vision. Usually, for research and testing purposes, existing tests are adapted by eliminating items that require the use of sight. Most items on the verbal portion of the Weschsler Intelligence Scales (all levels), for example, are used with the visually impaired; the performance sections are omitted because they require good visual ability. Samuel Hayes (1941) developed an adaptation of the Stanford-Binet based on the 1937 version of the Binet; some work has also been done with later versions of this scale, but these need more refinement. The primary problem with many modifications, however, is that the lack of visual experiences may still adversely affect performance on certain items. No norms are available for blind or partially sighted children for comparison purposes.

One test, the *Blind Learning Aptitude Test* (BLAT), has been developed to test the haptic abilities (e.g., touch perception using items such as formboards or shapes with raised dots) of blind children (Newland, 1976). There is little research available on this instrument, but it offers promise as a means of assessment. Embossed geometric figures are used to pose problems to the person being tested, and responses are verbal. Since the BLAT uses touch perception, it can be used as a supplement to verbal tests to obtain more information about learning abilities.

The most valid and reliable information about the cognitive abilities of visually impaired children may be obtained from teachers, parents, and/or the students themselves. Teachers who have had experience working with visually impaired students can make comparisons of the individual's learning ability and rate of learning with those observed for other similarly disabled students. Resource teachers who work only with visually impaired students may be better identifiers of giftedness in such children than regular classroom teachers, whose basis for comparison is often limited because typically they have had only one or two blind or partially sighted children in their classes. Both resource room teachers and regular classroom teachers need to develop an accurate understanding of the characteristics of giftedness and of the factors that can express—or mask—those traits in children with visual impairments. Skilled observations in both regular and special educational settings are needed for accurate identification. In Abe's case, the resource teacher in high school probably recognized his giftedness in regular teaching situations, as suggested by the fact that he supplied advanced mathematics problems to challenge Abe. Abe's adaptation to the regular classroom and his highly motivated ability to solve difficult, challenging mathematics problems were early indications of his superior intellectual ability.

All teachers of the visually impaired can recognize giftedness through observation of abilities and traits such as the following: ease and speed in learning braille; use of advanced, qualitatively superior vocabulary and syntax; exceptional memory for information presented verbally; exceptional persistence and intense motivation to know, understand, and achieve mastery; and remarkable originality in finding answers or solutions to problems. It is most helpful to make comparisons of an individual with the visually impaired student population. Disabled students rarely display the traits frequently found on identification checklists or rating scales, such as a preference to work independently, assertiveness, little need for teacher direction, self-confidence, ability to organize people, adaptability to new or unfamiliar situations, and ability and desire to direct the activities of others and other leadership skills. Independence and leadership skills may not develop because the child who is blind or has low vision may lack mobility skills or social skills resulting from lack of experience or self-confidence. Children with low vision who need large print cannot usually be expected to read or learn to read as rapidly as children with unimpaired vision, so their acquisition of new information through reading in all subject areas may occur more slowly than is typical in gifted students, especially in situations requiring a great deal of reading to gain needed information. Teachers may not recognize giftedness in this population if they attribute relative slowness in learning to a low level of intellectual ability rather than to the limitations imposed by the need for large print.

Interviews with parents and with the visually impaired individual also can be useful for gathering information about intellectual ability. Parents can provide information about the child's interests, hobbies, memory, ability to find places after being shown how to get there, understanding of language, curiosity, development of skills or creative techniques for coping with or overcoming visual problems, imagination, and sense of humor. Visually impaired individuals are a good source of information about their own intellectual interests; achievements or products of which they are proud; motivating drives and needs; and perceptions of self, others, and school. Abe, for example, talked readily about his lifelong interest in math and his problems with arithmetic computation in elementary school. If Abe had been asked to share his perceptions and feelings in his youth, teachers would have gained insights into his learning problems and giftedness.

Modified tests of creativity (verbal forms) also can be helpful in identifying giftedness in blind and visually impaired students. Most creativity tests require answers to be written, so visually impaired students must be allowed to give oral responses. Items such as "product improvement" in the *Torrance Tests of Creative Thinking* can be modified so that the student can hold the toy and feel it. Of course a methodological problem exists relative to the comparability of the two methods of administering the tests and the lack of norms common to both. Tisdall, Blackhurst, and Marks (1967) reported that the creative abilities of blind children do not differ significantly from those of sighted children. Additional studies in this area may reveal that appropriately modified tests provide reliable indicators of giftedness in blind children. Currently, however, there is very little information available, and much more creative work is needed to establish the validity and comparability of modified and nonadapted measures.

Potential Interaction between Giftedness and Visual Impairment

When asked how his blindness had affected his development both personally and professionally, Abe replied that he had always felt his lack of access to the printed word had limited the ways he could grow and the career options that were available to him. This limitation also could be viewed as positive: because the alternatives were limited, he focused his energies on developing the area of greatest interest to him—an area in which he could excel. A difficulty some gifted individuals have is their inability to make choices among their many options.

Certainly it is unlikely that Abe would have developed the Nemeth Code if he had not been blind. His intense interest in mathematics, coupled with the obstacle of his blindness, created in him the impetus to develop a system to benefit all blind individuals. Had he not been blind, he probably would not have known the braille system well enough to create a mathematics code based on the system.

Other positive effects of Abe's blindness seem to have resulted from a lifetime of dealing with people who have negative and stereotyping attitudes toward blind people, the frustration of not being encouraged to pursue the career of his choice, and his relationship with important people in his life who believed in his ability regardless of his disability. Abe was an absolutely delightful person to interview. His healthy attitudes toward his disability and toward the people who misunderstood his abilities and needs were very refreshing. Rather than becoming upset or angry with obstructive people, he used what he termed "a reasoned, quiet approach." For example, instead of waging a battle for his "right" to take college courses, he simply showed educators that he was capable of taking the courses. Rather than making individuals feel defensive about their obstructive behavior, thereby creating even more negative attitudes, Abe took a calm and rational approach, which clearly demonstrated the need for more appropriate assessments of the capabilities of blind people. Not only was his approach to the situation a positive one for himself, but it contributed to increased opportunities for others similarly disabled. Even without his disability, Abe's positive attitudes and perceptiveness about human relationships might have developed, but he probably would not have made such a contribution to the lives of visually impaired persons.

A negative consequence of Abe's visual disability was the great frustration he experienced initially because of the lack of encouragement and opportunity to pursue his intense interest in math. Even though he knew he had the ability to learn mathematics and to develop his own system for taking notes during lectures, his professors discouraged him from enrolling because of the difficulties they believed he (and they) would face. Unlike Myron, who was highly motivated by obstruction to prove that he could successfully do what he was told he could not do, Abe responded to a lack of encouragement by changing his direction and entering a master's degree program in another field, psychology. Upon receiving his graduate degree, Abe could not get a job in that field and ultimately returned to mathematics in a doctoral program. Thus, his career in mathematics was delayed for a significant period until he completed his doctorate in his middle to late 30s. In the interim, Abe had experienced the acute frustration of not being able to study and work in his chosen field of interest, not being able to support his wife (which at that time was more important socially than it is now), and not being able to find employment commensurate with his intellectual ability and academic training.

SPECIFIC GUIDELINES

The most important guideline for all groups working with the visually impaired is to believe that blindness or low vision and giftedness can exist in the same person. Acceptance of this basic principle will facilitate implementation of the following general recommendations for management of gifted visually impaired individuals: encouraging independence, providing as many resources and varied experiences as possible, holding high but realistic expectations for performance, and providing an intellectually challenging academic program. More specific suggestions for several groups are provided in the following sections.

Family and Friends

It is most important that family members and friends facilitate the growth and achievement of a visually impaired youngster by inhibiting their natural tendency to protect the child with a visual problem and by encouraging the child's independent, active exploration of the environment. Exploration of the environment is important for both physical and cognitive growth. As Piaget has demonstrated, children's active interactions with the environment are important at very early ages in order for them to develop a cognitive foundation for concept formation. Many studies have shown that the cognitive development of both blind and low-vision children lags behind that of sighted children (Gottesman, 1971, 1973, 1976; Simpkins & Stephens, 1974). Most researchers attribute this developmental delay to a restricted opportunity for interaction rather than to the visual impairment itself.

Allowing and encouraging independence and exploration means taking risks and allowing children to do so. If parents and other family members are fearful of injury, this fear will be communicated to the child, who then will become fearful and unwilling to explore the environment. When developed early in life, this fear is difficult to overcome later. Children learning to crawl, for example, should be put in a room in which they can freely explore the environment without danger. All objects that could be dangerous should be removed, but furniture, toys, and other typical items must be available for children to touch and to navigate around. It is helpful first to show and tell the child what is in the room and then to allow free exploration.

Blind or low-vision children encountering a new environment should be encouraged to explore it by touching the furniture or other objects as these are being described. Descriptions of what is going on in the neighborhood and the names of streets or stores, the direction of walking, and any other important information are helpful in orienting a child to the environment. Once children are familiar with the neighborhood and other specific environments, they should be encouraged to play with friends, go to the park, or go to the store independently.

The principle of active interaction should be extended beyond physical environments to people. Visually impaired children should be encouraged to touch the faces of family members to find out what laughing, smiling, frowning, and other expressions may be like. They may need to touch the faces or throats of family members, teachers, or speech therapists to find out how to make speech sounds if they are having difficulty learning some words or sounds.

Another important principle to remember is that children need to get as much information as possible through senses other than vision to supplement or substitute for visual input. Taste, touch, smell, and hearing need to be used when possible. Children should be encouraged to listen to records, to the radio, to television, and to tapes. A sighted person should be available to explain what is happening on television, if necessary, and to read aloud and to describe the pictures in books. As early as possible, materials from various agencies supplying special services for the visually impaired should be provided.

Systematic attention to the physical development of visually impaired children also is important because they are apt not to exercise appropriately. Certain physical activities are difficult to learn because the lack of sight prevents observing and imitating others. Direct instruction, through describing necessary movements or watching the child, explaining when mistakes are made, and assisting in correcting mistakes, may be required.

Several kinds of physical activity do not require sight. Swimming in a pool can be taught rather easily, and aerobics, weight-lifting, and exercise classes are also helpful. In many communities, camps and other nonschool programs provide both children and adults the opportunity to learn and enjoy many sports in which they have previously not been able to participate, such as skiing, running, or canoeing.

Finally, children should be encouraged to develop their own ways of coping with or overcoming their disability, either through interaction with older children or adults with a similar disability or through use of creative problem-solving discussions. Families should not discourage the use of any strategy of adaptation that works—that produces desired results for the child.

Education Professionals and Assistance

Unless a child needs extensive services for an associated disability, there seems to be no reason why a blind or partially sighted child who is gifted should not be placed in a program appropriate for gifted students. Resource room or consulting teacher services can be provided so the child receives instruction in braille, in the use of specialized equipment, and in the development of orientation and mobility. In a gifted program, the student has an opportunity to interact with other children with similar intellectual abilities in discussions, debates, and research projects. Such programs provide a curriculum at an appropriate level of complexity as well as an instruction method that accommodates their accelerated learning rate and distinct learning style. Activities designed to develop abstract reasoning and other "higher levels of thinking" are especially important in order to combat the effects of visual impairment on cognitive development.

When conducting discussions and providing instruction to students with visual impairments, it is important to make certain that sufficient concrete and manipulative experiences have been provided before attempting to present an abstract concept. For example, abstract science concepts of sinking and floating are difficult for a blind child to grasp or conceptualize if "hands-on," direct experiences have not been provided. Such experiences can be gained in the Elementary Science Study (ESS) curriculum (e.g., a unit such as "Clay Boats"), or in the Science Activities for the Visually Impaired (SAVI) curriculum. Blind or visually impaired children can be paired with sighted children to do experiments that facilitate their learning of abstract content.

A technique that is very helpful in teaching blind or visually impaired children is the concept development strategy devised by Hilda Taba (Maker, 1982b). This strategy develops basic thinking skills involved in refining and extending abstract concepts—an area of need in children with visual impairments. The strategy consists of teacher questioning, usually in a group situation, in which children are led through a series of intellectual tasks: they are asked to list items related to a concept; to group these items based on their similarities and to label the groups; to subsume items under different or multiple labels; and then to repeat the grouping, labeling, and subsuming process with completely new groups.

This strategy using concrete objects instead of lists of items provides an effective means of introduction to any subject matter content. Visually impaired children can be encouraged to make groupings based on their perceptions of tactile, auditory, or olfactory attributes, as well as to note the groupings of visual characteristics described by children who can see.

Listening skills and auditory materials are extremely valuable to the learning process for gifted visually impaired students. Since children who are blind or have low vision may read more slowly due to the special materials and equipment used, they may become frustrated. Using tapes with compressed speech or accelerated speech can be helpful. Students also can be encouraged to dictate stories, essays, reports, and other assignments rather than writing them. Obviously, they need to learn to write, in braille or print, or to type as a way of expressing themselves, but their motor skills may lag far behind their verbal skills, causing extreme frustration as they attempt to get ideas on paper. Therefore they should be provided with many opportunities to express these ideas without being dependent on their motor skills.

Community Services and Agencies

Community agencies and organizations can provide valuable services through supplying or procuring materials such as tapes, braille books, and manipulative materials for use in classrooms. Museums or historical societies, for example, can provide replicas or models of objects to classrooms. Interactive displays or models and replicas that can be touched are valuable educational aids.

City parks and recreation areas often are made accessible to the physically handicapped. These areas should also include equipment designed for, or easily used by, children with visual impairments. Camp programs and other recreational opportunities should be made available to this population of children by accommodating their special needs. It is important that visually impaired children not be separated from others in these programs. They can be provided with special instruction or assistance while in a group of nonhandicapped children.

Opportunities to learn the skills of arts and crafts in the community are valuable enrichment experiences for all students. Visually impaired students need much opportunity to develop their creative expression through other than a visual medium. Clay and other tactile media can be a rewarding means of expression.

Other brief suggestions for community service agencies follow:

1. Provide auditory material to supplement all visual displays such as tape recordings that can be activated at the touch of a button or that play continuously.
2. Select counselors, social workers, or case workers who are familiar with bright people who have visual problems.
3. Organize "big brother" or "big sister" or other mentorship programs in which older, successful people of a variety of ages are paired with children who have a similar disability.
4. Organize parent support groups in which those with similar situations can discuss problems and solutions.
5. Provide scholarships or internship opportunities for bright visually impaired students, and encourage them to compete for scholarships with those who have normal vision.
6. Hire capable visually impaired individuals, and make certain that the abilities of these individuals are shown in a positive light to other employees and supervisors.
7. Provide inservice training to staff members unfamiliar with either giftedness or visual impairments.

CONCLUSION

Abe's case provides significant insights into the development of home and educational provisions that can facilitate success in an intellectually gifted individual with a severe visual impairment present from birth. Many of his experiences involved negative stereotypes of and attitudes toward visually impaired persons conveyed by others misinformed about and/or unfamiliar with the capabilities of blind individuals. The possibility that Abe could be intellectually gifted did not occur to them.

The most important ways to facilitate the development of gifted potential in visually impaired persons are first, to believe in their intellectual capabilities, and second, to provide an environment that will attempt to "make up" for the lack of visual stimuli while challenging their intellect. The routine use of simple techniques, such as describing the environment and other people, is important in supplying the interactions and experiences needed by blind individuals. Such descriptions, when combined with discussions about the reasons and implications for what is described, can at the same time challenge and develop superior intellectual abilities.

Chapter Reaction

Anne L. Corn, Ed.D.

During the past several years, I have come to believe that all individuals who are gifted and who have a disability share common threads of experiences. Abe expressed many of these experiences and therefore is representative of the population. As a totally blind individual, however, he may not have had the same experiences as those of most visually impaired individuals who are gifted; only about 15 percent of the legally blind population is totally blind.

Abe has an attitude toward work apparently shared by other successful gifted handicapped people: that with enough hard work, he will be able to attain his goals. He also fought to make sure that others did not expect less of him than he could accomplish. He appreciated realistic expectations of others in regard to not only academic achievements but also to the development of social abilities.

Significant others in Abe's life encouraged Abe to appreciate and develop his capabilities. An internal locus of control and a belief by others in his abilities seem to be the ingredients for his success. In addition, Abe emphasized the need for having a teacher who "understood how to teach blind children." When his teacher could explain concepts and principles, Abe seemed to be able to make "mental leaps."

Abe did not demonstrate "giftedness" during his early schooling. By high school, however, he was in the top 10 percent of his class, and in college he achieved excellent grades. Some of Abe's recommendations regarding educational opportunities for visually handicapped children stem from his own educational experiences. Fortunately, today, materials and equipment are more readily available to children. Technology has advanced to the degree that gifted blind children have, in some school districts, such devices as paperless braillers, which function as word processors, and spoken output for computers. The gifted student who is blind thus now has greater opportunity to compete academically with his peers.

Abe commented that "The educational system did nothing but put obstacles in my way." Still, Abe seemed to have a healthy outlook on others' inadequacies. His actions demonstrated that he did not become angry or discouraged when those he encountered, peers or authority figures, were ignorant of his needs or capabilities. Rather, he used such events in his life as opportunities to educate: with an understanding of how he could function, their apparent prejudice would diminish. Unfortunately, Abe had a difficult time initially finding work, even though he had a degree that would provide sighted peers with easy access to

Exhibit 3–1 Ten Guidelines for Avoiding Stereotypical Messages

Stereotyping Message	Guideline
"You're so smart; I don't know why you want to play with those handicapped children." "If you keep up the good marks you will be in a position where you won't have to ask anyone for help."	1. Encourage the gift without denying the disability.
"Billy is blind, but he's a genius. It's okay that he's a loner; he probably likes it that way."	2. Help the child to develop as a whole; each child is more than the sum of a gift and a disability.
"Why does she always make it more difficult for herself? Kathy has no arms, and she now wants to take the chemistry lab."	3. Expose the gifted handicapped child to as much enrichment and opportunity as you would the able-bodied gifted child (as appropriate and least restrictive).
"George needs so much help just getting around. How could he be a tutor?"	4. Helping is a two-way street. It is as important for the child to help others as it is to learn to ask for and receive assistance.
"You may get high grades, but don't expect to get a summer job as a sales person."	5. Help the child to develop marketable skills (and work experience) in addition to those geared to a specific gift or talent.
"You must be brilliant; you're in college, and you can't even hear."	6. Praise and appraise realistically. Flattery or overpraise do not benefit the child, whereas realism and encouragement will have positive results.
"You're supposed to be so smart; I guess you won't need any accommodations for reading assignments. This honors class reads two books a week."	7. Appreciate the additional efforts which are required by the child to work with his/her disability.
"Jane doesn't have to learn to go to the store until she's at least 15. After all, she can't easily be understood."	8. Encourage risk-taking and problem-solving behaviors within safe and ability-appropriate parameters.
"Jeff is such a handsome and bright child. Of course he'll want to be the poster child to show what the handicapped can do."	9. Avoid reacting to the child as a phenomenon or placing such a child on display (without appropriate permission).
"You're so smart—why do you want to play with those deaf children? You know how people react to groups of the deaf."	10. Help the child to explore self-identity as a handicapped individual and to meet appropriate role models.

employment. Still, he persisted; such persistence is a trait characteristic of the successful individual who has gifts and disabilities.

Abe emphasized that the society fails to appreciate how difficult it is to achieve personal goals—that only the achievement attained is considered. The degree to which society appreciates achievement by those who are disabled may still be either underestimated or overstated. The concept of achievement "in spite of his handicap" seems to persist.

Abe sees his blindness as an inhibitor to intellectual growth. He stated that if he could read more freely, he would be able to " . . . grow quicker or faster or in more directions." The frustrations he encounters in obtaining access to the printed word are understandable. Abe's other weakness is related to his self-proclaimed lack of ability to "create immediately." Both weaknesses to which Abe refers relate to his utilization of his intellectual capacities. Perhaps it is because of his giftedness that he finds his perceived weaknesses in the intellectual domain.

There is little revealed about Abe's social life. The reader learns that he is married and that he had parents who expected him to be with his peers. The cofunctioning of disability and giftedness I have found to affect social development to the greatest extent. In one interview, a 26-year-old with a Ph.D. who was also blind from birth was asked, "Do you ever think of yourself as both gifted and handicapped?" This individual answered, "It's a difficult combination, a volatile mix. I think the intellect develops too quickly while the handicap retards social development. The gaps grows wider. I'm now catching up with myself, but when I'm unsure in a social situation, I revert to being the intellectual computer."

As a former teacher of blind and low-vision children and as an educator who prepares teachers to work with children who are blind or who have low vision, I found this case study to be very poignant. I have taught and used the Nemeth Code. I have the utmost respect for Dr. Nemeth and was pleased to gain insight about the man who provided this valuable tool.

For the benefit of those parenting or serving the gifted handicapped, the accompanying Exhibit 3–1 presents commonly heard stereotyping messages and ten guidelines for avoiding the attitudes expressed in these messages.

*   *   *   *   *

Anne L. Corn is Associate Professor of Special Education at the University of Texas, Austin. As a high-achieving visually impaired educator, Dr. Corn has provided significant leadership to the development of the field of gifted handicapped education. She chaired for several years the CEC/TAG Committee on Gifted Handicapped, which produced the seminal position paper and stimulated early dialogue. Dr. Corn currently is president of the CEC division for education of the visually impaired.

Chapter Reaction

Sandra Ruconich, Ed.D.

Some aspects of Abe Nemeth's case are typical. His public school attendance is typical of today's visually impaired gifted students, though most Depression-Era blind students were educated in schools for the blind. Other typical aspects of the case study include being discouraged from pursuing a career different from those pursued by the majority of visually impaired people of the time, a willingness to work hard, a good attitude toward his handicap, and a mentor or friend providing constructive positive and negative feedback to the gifted visually impaired person and/or to the family. In addition, certainly many of the most useful and practical developments that aid the blind have been created by altruistic visually impaired gifted people who initially just wanted to solve their own problems.

Other aspects of the case are less typical—Abe's "top of the class" academic performance, for instance. Boredom with the subject matter or its presentation is a common problem. Sometimes this boredom is occasioned by teachers who teach "equipment instead of concepts"; sometimes it is encouraged by environments in schools for the blind, where the increasing number of multihandicapped students with intellectual disabilities results in an emphasis on rote learning and a dearth of intellectual challenge and competition. Not all parents curb their overprotectiveness, maintain high expectations, and/or help with homework. Not all visually impaired gifted persons are superior in all areas (e.g., popular notions notwithstanding, all blind people are not extraordinary musicians!).

As this chapter points out, visually impaired gifted people must be encouraged to believe in themselves and in what they can accomplish. Professionals, family, and friends can help gifted persons view themselves positively and realistically—capitalizing on strengths, remediating and/or minimizing weaknesses, and developing effective coping strategies. In addition, mobility training should begin at the earliest opportunity (preschool, if possible) and continue through high school or until the child is as independent as ability permits. The sighted public (e.g., potential colleagues, teachers, employers) tends to perceive the ability to travel efficiently and independently as the most visible measure of competence. Intelligent risk taking also should be taught early in a manner commensurate with concerns about the child's level of understanding, experience, maturity, and safety; and, whenever possible, by experiencing the natural consequences of actions taken (e.g., action: touching hot iron; consequence: burned finger). Physical, mental, emotional, and spiritual risks are a lifelong reality, especially for the visually impaired, and gradual experiences with successful and unsuccessful risk taking can be an excellent preparation for creative, fulfilling adult life.

Wise and caring educators can help visually impaired gifted students so much! Teachers of the gifted and teachers of the visually impaired who share students should compare notes frequently so that each better understands the other's discipline and its interactive effects, what to expect of the child, and how to provide the highest-quality coordinated services. Gifted visually impaired students should be expected to do no more and no less than their gifted seeing peers; the teacher of the gifted should show no partiality toward a visually impaired student and should not tolerate a superior attitude or manipulativeness, whether displayed by blind or sighted students. Even students with additional handicaps should be mainstreamed as quickly as possible; like other gifted visually impaired students, they will live in a sighted world, and the more quickly they enter that world, the more quickly they will become a part of it. It is important to add, however, that mainstreaming any student without the provision of proper services (e.g., visits by a qualified itinerant or resource teacher, books in a medium the student can use appropriately) may result in unnecessary failure. A commitment to mainstreaming, ingenuity, and careful planning can make such services possible.

This chapter lists technological devices that gifted visually impaired students should know how to use. To that list I would add microcomputers, the devices that enable visually impaired people to communicate with computers on site and via telephone, word-processing programs, and printers. Computers can be equipped with braille, voice, large print, and/or Optacon readout. Each kind of readout provides unique advantages and limitations that must be carefully weighed when considering which device or technology will best meet the student's needs. Factors such as how the device is to be used, the medium in which the student works best with information, the device's cost-benefit ratio, portability requirements, and the speed with which information must be accessed also should be considered.

Appropriately equipped computers can enable visually impaired people to do independent research. This is because the number of magazine articles, encyclopedias, and other reference materials made accessible by using small computers linked by phone to large computers continues to increase, and the price of this information, especially during evenings and weekends, is becoming more affordable. Word-processing programs and printers can make writing, particularly for braille readers, far quicker, more efficient, and, as sighted writers have found, higher in quality because of the ease of changing a phrase without the necessity of retyping the entire page on which it appears. Papers can be written using either braille or regular typewriter keyboards, and editing and proofreading can be done via any or all of the readouts just mentioned; a printer can then be used to print the finished product for the teacher, allowing the student total independence throughout the process and producing a result that teacher and student can access with equal ease.

A word to parents: Any parents, you in particular, have one of the most difficult jobs in the world. If you're like my parents, you will sometimes overprotect, sometimes underprotect, sometimes make mistakes; yet above all, you will love. And, like my parents, you will learn that if you provide a loving, nurturing, stimulating environment in which your child can feel secure enough to venture out on his or her own, the child will be likely to do so, secure in the knowledge that loving arms will be there to comfort and encourage. Remember, too, that loving is not always easy, that it can stifle as well as nourish, and that on occasion the highest form of loving is letting go.

As Abe Nemeth's teacher demonstrated, every gifted visually impaired person, like all people everywhere, deserves to be judged as an individual. Some may be gifted in all areas; some may exhibit superior ability in certain areas while needing remedial work in others. Those of us who work with the gifted visually impaired in any capacity have the exciting and difficult challenge of giving them the tools to become independent, competent, confident adults who have the inner strength and maturity to do what they want to do, regardless of the obstacles they face—and then making sure *we* step out of the way!

*   *   *   *   *

Sandra Ruconich is Director of Technical Education for the Hadley School for the Blind in Winnetka, Illinois. A very gifted educator who was one of the first mainstreamed blind students in the state of Washington, Dr. Ruconich earned her doctorate in special education at George Peabody College of Vanderbilt University under the mentorship of Sam Ashcroft.

Chapter 4

Gifted Persons with Severe Physical Impairment

A CASE STUDY: HERB

During the interview for this case study, Herb's personal charm and wit were immediately evident. His quick smile and the twinkle in his eyes, made the experience extremely pleasant. Most memorable however, was his incredible ability to say in two words what ordinary people would take several sentences to explain.

Herb is classified as a quadriplegic. He has no use of his hands or legs and uses an electric wheelchair. Because of his severe physical disability, he must have a full-time attendant. His condition of cerebral palsy has resulted in difficulties in the use of most muscles, including those needed for speech. That is one reason why he packs so much meaning into only a few well-chosen words. Herb has practiced choosing carefully both the words he speaks and those he writes, because both speaking and writing are very laborious tasks for him.

Initially, many of his words are difficult to understand because his speech patterns are unique. However, when the listener gets used to his way of pronouncing sounds and words, understanding him is not difficult. Since Herb cannot hold a pencil or pen, he must type rather than write. However, he does not have enough control over the muscles in his hands to be able to type with his fingers—so he uses the toes of his left foot! He reports that he can type at least eight words per minute using this method.

There is nothing disabled about Herb's mind. In his words, "the mind is the most important part of the body . . . the physical part can be handled by a robot." Herb has a bachelor's degree in Earth Science from Southern Illinois University and a master's degree from Northeastern Illinois University.

Herb is in his early 30s and is employed as a physical scientist for the National Weather Service in Rosemont, Illinois. At the Weather Service, he writes monthly, weekly, and yearly climate summaries as well as monthly storm data summaries for Illinois. According to Herb and those who work with him, he is constantly trying to figure out new and better ways to get his job done. In 1977, his efforts were recognized, and he was named one of the ten Outstanding Handicapped Federal Employees of the Year.

Herb is not married and lives with his mother, who is retired. His mother, who completed eighth grade, was formerly an attendant at a school for the handicapped, and his father, who completed tenth grade, was a waiter.

Although when interviewed he was relatively happy with his job, Herb now believes that he has been denied promotions, and is extremely anxious to make a change to a position with more responsibilities and with a higher salary. As he mentioned many times during his interview, Herb is very aware of his dependence on his family and desires most to support himself without assistance from anyone else. He would like to be able to earn enough money to have his own apartment or home and to hire his own attendant. He then would not feel as burdensome to his family.

It also seems important to Herb that he work toward better employment opportunities for all handicapped individuals. He is currently active in numerous handicapped consumer organizations. For instance, he is employment chairman of the Foundation for the Handicapped in Science, employment chairman for the Congress of Organizations of the Physically Handicapped, and vice-president of the Illinois Developmental Disabilities Advocacy Authority. He is also a board member of the state handicapped housing committee organization in Illinois and serves on the boards of many handicapped consumer organizations.

Personal View of Self

Self-Perceived Strengths

Herb sees himself as intellectually very capable. He ranked in the top half of his class academically in elementary school (with a C+ average), in the top quarter in high school (with a B average), and even higher in college, where he had a B+ average. Herb has never doubted his intellectual ability, but he knows his physical limitations. His physical disabilities greatly limited his achievement in school until he was able to develop coping skills to overcome them.

Interestingly enough, even though he attended a school for the handicapped, in which presumably attitudes are positive and teachers understand the problems caused by a physical disability, Herb was allowed by only one teacher to type his homework in class. At a very early age (approximately 3 or 4 years), he learned that he had more control over his feet than his hands, and he learned to type with his toes. However, the teachers would not allow him to type with his toes in class. To do his homework—indeed, to do the necessary work that others were able to complete at school—he had to stay up very late at night, often without the approval of his parents.

Herb was asked what the most significant events were that helped or hindered him in realizing his potential. He described one of the most important events to have been winning high awards in two state-level science fairs. His science teacher in high school, also a handicapped person, had recognized Herb's potential and had encouraged him to develop projects that could be entered in the science fair. The teacher helped by reviewing drafts of papers and suggesting corrections, but Herb did most of the work himself, including retyping the papers as many as five times each. According to Herb, the principal of the school was not particularly supportive of his entry in the science fairs but at least allowed him to do so. Since his speech was so difficult to understand, it was necessary for him to get interpreters to speak for him. He spent hours training another student in what to say about his experiments. After each success, he was elated about winning, but knew also that there was more work ahead and a next step to complete. According to Herb, he could not "let his happiness get out of hand."

Herb feels that these events were significant for several reasons: they were helpful in showing others that he had the ability to compete with nonhandicapped students; they reaffirmed to himself his intellectual and scientific ability; and they better prepared him for college, especially for editing his many term papers repeatedly, as he says he had to "before they made sense." Science fairs also were important events to his parents, teachers, and others at the school because they demonstrated his capability for academic work and outstanding achievement in science. No one at home or at school seemed to recognize his intellectual ability prior to his work for the science fairs, since it was obscured by his physical disability and difficulties in speaking.

In addition to his scientific aptitude, a second area of strength cited by Herb is his persistence. He sees himself as one who continually seeks ways to do more and to accomplish a higher quality of work on the job. This persistence was most important in two related achievements: completing a college education and obtaining employment in his field. Because of his severe physical handicap, Herb had difficulty securing financial support for his education from the Division of Vocational Rehabilitation (DVR). Since DVR officials make decisions based on their judgment of individual potential for employment after graduation, the rehabilitation counselors were reluctant to recommend financial support for someone with such an extensive and severe physical disability.

Herb described his long fight with DVR for support as one of the events that helped him become aware of his potential, as well as his capacity for persistence. When he first approached DVR about going to college, Herb was told that he should consider a trade school or some other kind of vocational training because his chances of getting a job would be much better and the training would not take nearly so long. Since he was interested in a career in science and knew he had the ability to succeed in that field, Herb was not willing to acquiesce to DVR's recommendation. However, his family was unable to pay for a college education in addition to the full-time attendant he would need while away from home, so he persisted in seeking financial aid.

Finally, after many letters had been written to various counselors and officials, DVR agreed to pay for Herb's education if first he took a college-level course by correspondence and did well. He subsequently enrolled in a correspondence course even though it was very difficult for him. As the reader may know, correspondence courses usually require a great deal of writing, and since Herb only could type about eight words a minute, writing was a painstakingly slow task. It took him a year to finish one course working almost fulltime on it! He did well in the course, but DVR would not honor its previous commitment and suggested that he take all his courses by correspondence. If it took him a year to do one course, imagine how long it would take to get a bachelor's degree!

Herb then secured the names of all individuals in the state who had any authority over the allocation of money and wrote to them. In his letters, he explained the situation and told them all about himself so that no one could say later that he had held back any information. After numerous letters had passed back and forth, DVR agreed to support Herb's education, so he prepared to go to Southern Illinois University (SIU) at Carbondale, a school noted then for its barrier-free campus. His brother agreed to be his attendant. However, at the last minute, officials at DVR changed their minds and told him they did not believe he would ever be able to get a job. Herb was devastated, but he would not give up. Since he already had tried all the official avenues, he felt there was only one more route to take— involvement of the media to publicize his case and put pressure on DVR. He wrote to several radio and television commentators about his situation. One television commentator became very interested and pursued his story publicly. After the publicity, he was given a chance by DVR in the form of financial support on a trial basis for one semester. If he passed all his courses, they would continue to support him.

Herb worked very hard in school and made all As and Bs, except for a C in English. After the first semester, he again had a confrontation with DVR. They decided that his grades were not high enough. Again, he would not give up. He went back to all the individuals who had been supportive of his case, including the television commentator who had helped him before. Owing to his persistence, eventually he was provided the financial assistance he needed.

A second example of Herb's persistence, as well as his foresight, is his story of how he was able to find employment. Knowing that he would have difficulty obtaining a job, he felt that he should plan ahead. Therefore, in his third year of college he started doing volunteer work for the National Weather Service. His rationale was that if he proved to them he could do the work and do it well, they would have no basis for denying him a job later. For two years he worked for the agency for very little pay, working consistently during the academic year and vacations. Three weeks after graduation, his efforts were rewarded: Herb was employed by the National Weather Service in Illinois.

A third area of strength is Herb's writing ability. He enjoys writing and has written several plays and short stories, mostly on the subject of being handicapped.

Self-Perceived Weaknesses

Herb perceives his weaknesses as being mainly in the area of physical skills. He realizes, very painfully at times, the limitations placed on him by his disability. When he was asked if he thought his career or job would be different if he had not been handicapped, his answer was, "I would not have had to be twice as good and wouldn't have to prove myself over, and over, and over, and over. [I] would be climbing the ladder well above where I am now." In the last year of school—indeed, during much of his educational career—Herb was concerned about whether he would be able to get a job. It was, and still is, very important to him that he be "a useful member of society," and that he be able to support himself. He does not want to be dependent on his family or on society for his livelihood.

Herb's physical limitations are severe. Since the cerebral palsy has affected all his limbs, he is confined to a wheelchair and must be pushed by someone or use an electric chair. He can move himself backward by pushing his feet against the floor, but this movement is very difficult for him, and he cannot move himself very far. His cerebral palsy is both spastic and athetoid, meaning that some movements are tense and jerky (spastic) while others are involuntary and purposeless (athetoid). His throat, mouth, and diaphragm muscles are affected, which results in difficulties in speaking clearly. Herb is unable to care for his personal needs or to get from place to place without assistance, so he needs a full-time attendant.

As described earlier, from an educational point of view these disabilities cause him to be unable to write, turn pages in a book, operate in a science laboratory, or even type with his hands. Since he does have more control over his feet and legs, he can turn pages and type with his toes. In school, he also needed an aide or attendant to help him accomplish personal self-care, eating, and doing his schoolwork. Since his speech is difficult to understand, he often must repeat words numerous times, although some of his colleagues or others used to his unique speech patterns often can communicate for him.

Herb believes that he and his family needed a great deal more support and understanding from the professionals in their lives than they actually received. When his parents took him as an infant to be evaluated, many of the doctors seemed to have no idea what to suggest to the family. They apparently were unable or unwilling to make any predictions about his intellectual ability or physical potential. Some even suggested at this early stage that he would need to be institutionalized for life. What the family seemed to need was a physician, therapist, or counselor who could freely, honestly, and accurately discuss cerebral palsy and its possible effects. Even if the doctors could not give an accurate evaluation of his intellectual potential, for example, they could at least have indicated to the family that, although many individuals with cerebral palsy are mentally retarded, there also are many with average intelligence and some who are very bright and intellectually gifted. As Herb became older, and more accurate techniques for assessment became available, more precise estimates of his future physical and mental characteristics could have been provided. Counselors, therapists, or physicians also could have advised the family about how to provide a more nurturing and challenging environment so that his intellectual and physical abilities would develop fully. Family members needed answers to questions like these: What kinds of physical exercises should he do? What kinds of toys could he be given? How often should he be read to? What kinds of educational materials might be helpful?

Herb also feels that he needed more opportunities in school for intellectual recognition and challenge. Very few of his teachers could see beyond the physical disability and recognize or encourage the development of his intellectual abilities. He believes that a major factor in the lack of attention to his intellectual needs was his placement in a school for handicapped children rather than in a school or class where there were nonhandicapped students. There were two aspects of the problem: the expectations of the teachers and the expectations of the other students.

According to Herb, most of his teachers had had very little or no experience with handicapped individuals who were gifted. They did not understand how to encourage disabled students to perform at the highest levels of their intellectual capabilities. Herb recalls that the teachers had very low expectations for the intellectual performance of all the handicapped students, many of whom had multiple handicaps, including mental retardation. In addition, graduates of their school were only very rarely successful in careers or advanced academic pursuits. Similarly, peer expectations for achievement were generally low in that educational setting. In a special school or class for disabled students, students tend to have limited or lowered expectations for their own performance, both physically and mentally. Since their peers, teachers, and parents often do not have high expectations for intellectual and career achievements, each disabled individual tends to develop a very limited view of personal abilities and future possibilities for achievement.

Interestingly enough, Herb feels that even when some graduates of a school for handicapped persons do become successful, their achievements do not have the impact they should have on school personnel. He has stated (Hoffman, 1976, pp. 1–2):

> . . . the handicapped persons who develop drive and won't take ''no''
> for an answer are the only ones that beat the system and go on to make

something out of their lives. However, these persons are often labeled by teachers, parents, and rehabilitation specialists as "special," thus putting them above the other students. Most of the other students do not feel they will ever be "special," and, therefore, they are not encouraged by [the preferential treatment of] those few "special" persons.

Herb feels that he would have gained the most benefit from going to a school where there were both nonhandicapped and handicapped students and teachers. In such a setting, the student with a disability can be given a variety of perspectives and can be helped to find his or her own place, depending on personal motivation and ability. He has expressed these feelings very strongly (Hoffman, 1976, p. 2):

The teachers who are handicapped themselves make the greatest contribution to disabled students. If they are lucky enough to teach in a school that has both "normal" and handicapped students, the contribution is even greater. These teachers can teach the handicapped students from their own experiences and will often make the students work twice as hard as "normal" teachers do, for they know that if a handicapped child is ever going to get ahead in society, he will have to be twice as knowledgeable as a "normal" child. The handicapped teacher will imprint on the minds of the "normal" student that the disabled are the same as anyone else except that they are physically limited. When these students grow up and find employment, they will have more understanding toward the physically handicapped and will perhaps try to change the attitudes toward the disabled. In the long run, I feel it will be the attitudes of our society that will have to be changed if the physically handicapped are going to be able to live a life that is as "normal" and fruitful as possible.

After graduating from high school, Herb felt he still needed more realistic expectations for his potential physical and intellectual performance. Although he recognized his physical limitations and the need to have full-time care, he also recognized his high intellectual abilities. He knew he was capable of getting a college degree (or degrees) and of becoming a productive member of the scientific community. He needed other people to recognize this potential also, so that they would provide opportunities to help him achieve his goals.

Herb has a very strong need to be independent—to be able to support himself and to be a productive contributor. This need for independence has been a driving force throughout most of his life. As a youngster he wanted to prove that he had the ability to succeed in intellectual areas so he could go to college. He wanted to go to college in order to earn the educational degree that would allow him to pursue a career in which he knew he could utilize his abilities and achieve success. Part of his motivation to achieve also has been financial need, as previously discussed; the services of the full-time attendant he needs are a continuous expense, beyond the amount needed by most people to survive and live comfortably. His emotional needs require that he earn a salary that will permit him to be independent of financial assistance from his family.

A recurring theme in Herb's discussions about himself and his career is his need and desperate desire to be a "productive member of society." Herb not only wants to be independent, but he expresses a need to give something back. Society and its institutions need to provide opportunities for such people to fulfill their individual potential and also make valuable contributions.

Personal View of Perceptions and Treatment by Others

Herb feels that, in general, others have perceived him as handicapped or disabled rather than capable and highly intelligent. People tend to view his physical disabilities as more important or salient than his mental abilities. Some individuals even assume that, because he has a severe physical disability, he must also be mentally retarded; they do not even consider the possibility that someone with cerebral palsy may be bright or intellectually gifted. In general, educators, his parents, employers or potential employers, and others have conveyed low expectations for his achievement in every area. Consequently, he has felt a need to be even more successful in school and on the job than a nonhandicapped person in order to "prove himself" a capable individual. There were, however, in Herb's experiences, some people who were able to recognize that his intelligence, innovativeness, and persistence would enable him not only to cope with his disability but to overcome many of its limitations.

Facilitators

As described earlier, Herb feels that his teachers who were handicapped were most helpful and encouraging to him. They were the ones who recognized his intellectual ability in spite of his physical disability. The first facilitator was his third-grade teacher, who allowed him to type with his toes in the classroom. She encouraged him to persist in developing his typing skills and allowed him to do his schoolwork in class whenever possible so that she could assist him if necessary.

The next facilitator Herb identified was his high school science teachers. He was allowed to take a science lab course that allowed him to learn more about a subject of great interest to him. In the course, he observed the other students while they performed experiments. The science teacher encouraged Herb to enter science fairs and assisted him in developing scientific papers for submission by reading and editing them. The result of this teacher's encouragement must have been very rewarding to both of them, since Herb won high awards in two state science fairs. The effect on Herb of winning the awards was tremendous. His self-confidence was remarkably enhanced by the experience, but he was careful not to exaggerate his achievement nor to forget the painful self-discipline required to achieve it.

The third teacher who facilitated Herb's development and achievement was his high school English teacher. After winning awards in the science fairs, Herb remarked that his achievement had proved that his English teacher was right: he would be able to do whatever he set out to do, but it would not be easy. Among other things, he would have to be prepared to stay up late many nights to type painstakingly for hours. This teacher significantly influenced him in another way: she taught him that writing letters could help him get what he wanted out of life. She told her students that they could always write letters, regardless of any disability, including a severe speech impediment. If there was no response, they could write again and again. The overall effect of this teacher's influence was to strengthen Herb's desire to pursue a college degree, get a job, and be successful in his chosen career.

Herb has described these three teachers and their contributions to his career and life in a very special way (Hoffman, 1976, pp. 2–3):

> It might seem ironic that three teachers who had the most impact upon my career, as well as my life, were all handicapped. The first was an elementary school teacher in an all-handicapped school [who] had the understanding that I could contribute more if I were allowed to type with my foot (which I did at home) in class. The other two handicapped teachers were a high school English and a high school science teacher. My English teacher got polio rather late in life, and besides being very good (but hard) as a teacher, she taught us that our physical limitations did not mean that we could not be useful instead of sitting at home and vegetating. She taught us how the power of letter writing could be used to obtain what we wanted out of life. Later this became the way I got the Division of Vocational Rehabilitation to finance my college education and it was also how I became employed. When she was asked to retire because her teaching was not what the school wanted, I received my first look at what society could do if they didn't like someone. This could not happen today—or could it?
>
> Since I was always interested in science; I guess I worked rather hard at it, and even though I could not use my hands for lab experience, I watched my fellow students. Sometimes I was able to tell them how to conduct an experiment. My science teacher, who was handicapped himself, understood this concept the best: it is more important for a scientist to know how and why an experiment is done than to physically

go through the motions, which a robot can do. This teacher also encouraged me to enter science fairs and spent many long hours with me going over the science papers I wrote. I became the first handicapped student to attend a city and statewide science fair—but not with the approval of the school principal. Since my speech defect made it hard for persons to understand me, when it became time for me to explain my science project, I found a fellow student to talk for me. Many hours were spent training him about my project and what to say.

Another teacher who was a facilitator of Herb's development was a college geography instructor, who allowed Herb to find his own ways of doing the same work as that accomplished by other students using a typewriter at home. He was not denied the opportunity to take the course but was told to use his own creativity to figure out alternative ways of learning. He learned to draw graphs, make charts, and "do lab work" at home on his typewriter.

Herb felt that his handicap caused these teachers' expectations for him to be higher than if he had not been handicapped, but he could not explain why. They talked to him about his future expectations and about setting realistic goals. These teachers also talked to other people about his abilities, and their improved attitudes and treatment caused him to raise his own aspirations and to increase his effort to achieve.

The only family member Herb perceived to have been a facilitator was his brother, who served as his attendant while Herb was in college, assisting him in getting to classes or work. When Herb started to work for the Weather Service, his brother helped him overcome many of the problems he encountered because of his co-workers' lack of attention to his special needs. For instance, his brother cut up his sandwiches in his packed lunch so that he could eat without assistance at his desk.

Another facilitator Herb identified was the television commentator who was sympathetic to his plea for the opportunity to pursue a college education. With this man's help, DVR was persuaded to give Herb a chance. This commentator made a significant contribution in two ways: first, he was a key individual in Herb's successful "last chance" effort to obtain a college education, and second, he showed that persons in the general public desired to give handicapped people a chance to succeed educationally.

One other individual, a professor at Southern Illinois University, also facilitated Herb's access to college by supporting openly his right to be given a chance and to show what he was capable of achieving academically. This professor wrote a persuasive letter of support for Herb's college attendance and would not change it, even when pressured to do so by officials at DVR. The professor said that life is like a dice game: "You never know if you'll win or lose, but you have to try."

Although Herb views his parents more as obstructors than facilitators of his development, because they gave him little encouragement or support in relation to his higher educational goals. Herb is grateful to them for keeping him at home and refusing to place him in an institution at birth. When Herb was approximately one year old, a physician told his parents that his "mind was OK"—that he should be allowed to do as many things as he could, and should go to school as soon as possible. Herb cites this physician's insight as one of the most significant factors affecting his life. All other events and opportunities were then made possible. His parents began treating him as if he were capable of learning; they bought him a typewriter at about three years of age so that he could learn to type, and as advised, they sent him to school as early as possible. Typing remains his major means of communication and an important enabler of his independence and determination to achieve success and make a contribution.

Obstructors

Herb identified many obstructors in his life. The most significant probably were his parents, although many teachers seriously impeded his development by their lack of insight. Herb states that his parents did not think he could complete college or high school, and they gave him little encouragement to try or to set higher goals. They even indicated they thought the reason he made good grades in college was that his brother helped him with his homework. When asked if anyone in his family supplemented his educational program, he said they had not provided a tutor, assistance with homework, or any other experiences to enhance or increase his learning. In fact, he often had to wait until they were asleep to do his homework because they disapproved of his late hours spent in typing or reading. He feels that their low expectations had the effect of increasing his motivation and elevating his aspirations.

Many teachers were perceived by Herb as obstructors to his development and achievement. All but one teacher in elementary school would not allow him to type his assignments or do his schoolwork in class by typing with his toes. As previously discussed, Herb consequently was forced to work long, late hours at home on his assignments. In high school, he tried to read at school by putting the book on his desk and turning the pages with his mouth, but that took too long and was rather messy! In addition to difficulty in completing tasks, Herb did not feel a sense of belonging in his elementary and secondary school classes—he felt like an outsider. In retrospect, he feels that the attitudes of teachers and peers prepared him for the barriers he would have to face after school and made him even more determined to "make it."

A major barrier was created in Herb's life by policies and officials of the Division of Vocational Rehabilitation (DVR). The DVR is a state agency that administers funds allocated for assisting handicapped individuals in getting training or educational experiences that will enhance their opportunities for employment. Many of the details of Herb's long fight with DVR are described earlier in this chapter, so only a few points need be highlighted here. One of the first problems he encountered was the counselor's attempt to make him change careers. This case worker tried to convince him that vocational training would be more appropriate than a college education because it would take much less time and would greatly increase his chances of employment. The case worker also tried to discourage him from going into meteorology because, "You can never talk on TV."

Herb also encountered problems with DVR because of his unwillingness to give up when denied support for a college education. He felt that the case workers tried very hard to prevent him from receiving financial aid. He was later told that someone wrote letters to individuals who had submitted letters of support in his behalf and suggested that they had not included complete information about Herb; these supporters felt they were put under pressure to change their recommendations. Luckily no one obliged, and Herb was allowed to pursue his college education. He completed his baccalaureate program in a little over four years and secured his current position with the Weather Service only three weeks after graduation.

Herb also regards his employers as obstructors to his achievement. He feels that he has been denied promotions and recognition because of his disability and that he has had to prove himself much more qualified than nondisabled workers in order to receive equal opportunities, recognition, and rewards for his work. He was the first severely physically handicapped person hired by the Weather Service, so they did not quite know how to deal with him. Their solution was to leave him alone and provide no extra assistance except to install a restroom in his office with a transfer bar on the wall. Thus, Herb had to learn ways to do things on his own, including ways to get around, since no extra space was cleared to allow him to get around the office space in his wheelchair. On the positive side, however, he is pleased that the Weather Service hired him. Being employed and able to support himself financially is crucial to Herb's self-concept and self-esteem because it has helped him feel more independent, even though it is still necessary for him to live with his mother.

It is interesting to note that both the facilitators and obstructors in Herb's life had a similar impact on his motivation to achieve. Both types of behavior caused him to raise his aspirations and to intensify his determination to succeed. Those who facilitated his achievement provided reinforcement or validation of his own belief in his potential for success. They not only helped him sustain belief in his ability but increased his motivation to succeed because he wanted to prove their judgments were accurate and to reward them for having confidence in him. Those who obstructed his progress made him even more determined to prove that he was capable so he could demonstrate their judgment wrong. Thus, Herb was persistently motivated to succeed so that he could prove his worth to himself, to those who believed in his abilities, and to the nonbelieving obstructors.

Statement of Specific Needs

Home and Family

Families need counseling in how a handicapped child can maximize abilities and minimize disabilities. For example, what exercises are important to do? When should they be done? How long should they be continued? Perhaps one of the most important needs of the family is emphasis on allowing and expecting the child to do as many things as possible independently. Being protective usually is not helpful, and it often is resented by a bright or gifted child with or without a handicap. Often a gifted handicapped child is more resentful of being protected than is a nondisabled gifted child due to the continual frustration of not being able to demonstrate their abilities. Finally, parents and families need information about adults with similar handicapping conditions who have been able to "overcome" or manage their disabilities to achieve personal and career success. Parents need to know high achievements are possible so that they can formulate more realistic, positive expectations for their child.

Medical Assessment

Herb indicated that it is most important that medical professionals provide the disabled person and the family with an honest and accurate assessment of all intellectual and physical abilities. His parents visited many doctors before finding one who could provide the information they needed. Herb and his family also needed to know what medication or therapy would help to improve his level of functioning.

Education

Herb supplied numerous recommendations regarding the educational needs of an individual with a similar disabling condition. One of the most important needs is to be educated with nondisabled children as well as with those who are disabled. Children with disabilities need exposure to some teachers who are handicapped and some who are not. For these reasons, he recommends mainstreaming even the most severely physically handicapped children.

In mainstream educational settings, however, appropriate modifications must be made to accommodate the disabilities. For example, science laboratories or the procedures for participating in laboratory courses and taking exams need to be modified. During laboratory work, handicapped students can observe others conducting an experiment rather than actually carry it out themselves; they can assist their fellow students in the work by giving and explaining instructions, or they can write papers describing the procedures for experiments, predicting the results, and explaining reasons for variation in results. Handicapped students can demonstrate mastery of knowledge and skills by designing their own experiments, predicting results, and having someone else conduct the tests.

The most important recommendation, however, is for educators to look beyond a disability and recognize strengths and capabilities as well. Educators must try to eliminate stereotypic assumptions that limit what a disabled person can do; each student should be given opportunities to *demonstrate* what he or she can (and cannot) accomplish, both academically and physically.

Community

When asked for recommendations he would offer to the community, Herb suggested that basic educational courses be provided for the public that develop accurate understandings of the problems and capabilities of handicapped people. These courses should be provided for children as well as adults. The community, especially employers and potential employers of handicapped persons, must be educated about what handicapped individuals can do if given opportunity and support; they need to become more aware of the successes and high achievements of disabled people; and they also need to realize that a little modification can make the difference between successful employment and failure. For example, when Herb applied for a hydrology position within the same office, he was told after a five-minute interview that he could not handle the job.

DISCUSSION

A physical disability may result from a wide variety of conditions, including childhood cancer, heart conditions, epilepsy, and cystic fibrosis to cerebral palsy, muscular dystrophy, and juvenile rheumatoid arthritis. Pless and Douglas (1971) developed a classification system for physical disabilities based on type, duration, and severity. Types of disability include motor (interferes primarily with motor function), sensory (interferes with vision, hearing, or speech), and cosmetic (predominantly affects social interaction). With regard to duration, a disability may be permanent, indefinite (may terminate at a later date), or temporary. Degree of severity ranges from mild (prevents participation in strenuous activities), to moderate (interferes with normal daily activities), to severe (requires prolonged period of immobilization, absence from school, or placement in special schools). For the purpose of this discussion, the authors have chosen to consider only those physical conditions that often result in permanent, moderate to severe motor impairments. The following discussion centers on cerebral palsy, since this disorder often produces severe disability in many functional areas. For further information about physical disorders, the reader is referred to Bleck and Nagel (1975), Cruickshank (1976), and Umbreit (1983).

Cerebral Palsy

Cerebral palsy usually is included as a category of physical disability or impairment because the major problems associated with the disorder are physical in origin. Cerebral palsy is caused by damage to the brain, which can occur before, during, or after birth. A variety of factors (e.g., maternal rubella, Rh incompatibility, lack of oxygen to the brain, prolonged labor, breech delivery, infections such as encephalitis, or injuries to the head) have been associated with damage to the fetal or infant brain. Damage to different parts of the brain results in different disorders or combinations of disabilities.

There are various methods of classifying conditions of cerebral palsy, but the most common seems to be according to physiology—that is, normal body functions. According to this system (Cruickshank, 1976), there are six types of cerebral palsy: spastic, athetoid, ataxic, rigid, tremor, and mixed. The primary characteristic of the *spastic* type is a loss of involuntary motor control. This causes movement to be tense, jerky, and poorly coordinated. As the child grows, spastic muscles become shorter, and limb deformities result. *Athetoid* cerebral palsy is characterized by fluctuating muscle tone during attempts to move. This results in involuntary, purposeless, irregular movements, especially of the extremities. Since throat and diaphragm muscles are affected, drooling is present and speech is labored. *Ataxia* is characterized mainly by balance problems, but ataxics also have slurred speech, staggering gait, and poor fine and gross motor coordination. *Rigidity* can be described as a severe form of spasticity, its primary characteristic being "equal pull" of flexor and extensor muscles. This makes limbs rigid and hard to bend, but once bent, they tend to remain in that position. The major characteristic of *tremor* is shakiness of a limb that develops on the effort to move; alternate contraction of the flexor and extensor muscles produces this effect. Tremor is characterized by small and rhythmic movements; in contrast, athetoid movements are large and changeable. Although the last category, *mixed*, is seldom used, most people with cerebral palsy have more than one type. The disorder usually is labeled according to the predominating type but may be called "mixed" if none is dominant.

Although the predominant problems seen with cerebral palsy are physical, many affected persons have associated disorders of communication, sensory functioning, and intellectual ability. Convulsive disorders may also be present. Communication disorders include those affecting speech or voice and those causing stuttering and aphasia. The most common are speech disorders, usually caused by problems in controlling muscles used to make speech sounds but also resulting from mental retardation or other forms of cerebral dysfunction. Many individuals with cerebral palsy have hearing or vision problems resulting from the brain damage that caused the cerebral palsy. With regard to intellectual ability, approximately half the individuals with cerebral palsy are reported to have IQs below 70. However, accurate measurement of intelligence in people with communication and/or mobility problems is obviously very difficult. For example, Herb did not do well on any tests except those he could work on at home without a time limit. This was one reason DVR did not see him as capable of completing college. Usually physically or otherwise disabled individuals are not included in test norming samples, so there is no accurate basis for judging their performance. Convulsive disorders affect persons with the spastic type of cerebral palsy most frequently but sometimes are found in the athetoid population.

Medical treatment of cerebral palsy is usually in the form of physical therapy, although medical personnel may be involved in prescribing or fitting assistive and adaptive equipment or in prescribing medication for a convulsive disorder. Physical therapy may be prescribed and supervised by a physician, but it usually is provided by a paraprofessional. The major goal of such treatment is to get the child to exercise muscles as much as possible so that atrophy can be minimized, the greatest possible range of motion can be preserved, and alternative ways of doing tasks can be developed.

Other Physical Disabilities

Cerebral palsy as a physically disabling condition creates needs in gifted persons that are shared with many other types of disabilities that severely impair mobility and control of motor or other body functions. The reader should be aware of the other major forms of disability that may impair the motor skills of gifted individuals.

Other conditions associated with moderate to severe motor impairments include muscular dystrophy, spinal muscular atrophy, polio, spinal cord injuries, spina bifida, osteogenesis imperfecta, arthrogryphosis, and juvenile rheumatoid arthritis. Each of these conditions are described very briefly, with a focus on characteristics that affect their treatment rather than causes or medical diagnoses.

Muscular Dystrophy

Muscular dystrophy is a progressive disease that causes progressive weakening and degeneration of voluntary muscles until they no longer function. In the early stages, symptoms include awkwardness, slowness of movement, difficulty in walking, and frequent falling. Later the affected child is observed to have difficulty getting up after falling, may develop a sway back and protruding abdomen, and begins to tire easily. During the third stage, usually beginning at about the age of 10 years in the most common form in children, the child is totally confined to a wheelchair and finally becomes totally dependent and bedridden. Death is usually caused by heart failure or lung infections. There is no cure for the disease, and IQ scores are reported to be below average. The major treatment is physical therapy, and a school program should be designed to keep these children active. Counseling should be provided for the families, teachers, and the child.

Polio

Polio, a common disease in the past, has become rare since the Salk vaccine was developed. However, because of its infrequency, many children are no longer being vaccinated, so it is now possible that neglect may lead to its re-emergence as a feared disease. Polio is a viral infection that affects cells of the spinal cord; when those cells die, the muscles they serve also ''die''—they become paralyzed. Paralysis may affect all or part of the body, but the disease does not affect intelligence.

Spinal Muscular Atrophy

Spinal muscular atrophy is a disease that affects the spinal cord, resulting in degeneration of motor nerve cells. The primary symptom is weakness, which can range in severity from only slight to as severe as that seen in muscular dystrophy. Other problems may be observed, such as delay in acquisition of motor skills, muscle tightening, and contraction of joints. There is no cure, and children with the disease have normal intelligence but little or no muscle strength. Physical therapy programs and provision of tasks requiring little muscle strength or skill are important educational modifications.

Spinal Cord Injuries

Accidents are the major cause of injuries to the spinal cord. The resulting disability varies according to the extent and level of injury. Generally, paralysis and lack of sensation occur below the point of injury to the spinal cord, so the result can be either paraplegia or quadriplegia. Depending on the injury, the person may recover completely or not at all. Intelligence is not affected. The child can be placed in a regular classroom or in a special school, depending on the type and extent of care needed. Chapter 5 describes this category of disability in detail.

Spina Bifida

There are several forms of the congenital disability known as spina bifida. It results from failure of the bones in a part of the spine to grow together. In the least severe form the only evidence is a growth of hair covering the area. In the most severe form, however, part of the spinal cord protrudes through the opening in the bones, and the exposed cord is constantly subject to trauma, with resulting neurological problems. This form is the most common (Bleck, 1975). In a more moderate form, the spinal cord does not protrude, and there is no neurological impairment.

Spina bifida is often accompanied by other disorders such as hydrocephalus (drainage of cerebrospinal fluid is blocked) and kidney infections; there is also a high incidence of spontaneous (not due to external trauma) dislocation of hips. Most people with the severe form of spina bifida use crutches or wheelchairs and have no bowel or bladder control. Physical, occupational, or speech therapy may be needed, but there is no damage to intelligence unless the pressure of cerebrospinal fluid caused brain damage.

Osteogenesis Imperfecta

In osteogenesis imperfecta, commonly called "brittle bone disease," bones do not grow normally in length and thickness, and they break easily. Associated problems may be dwarfism due to multiple fractures and hearing impairment resulting from deficits in the bones of the ear. There is no cure; intelligence and educational progress are unaffected by the condition. Children may need braces or wheelchairs, and surgery may be necessary to straighten bones. Affected children and their classmates and teachers must be very careful because even simple activities such as using a stapler or shifting body positions can result in a broken bone.

Arthrogryphosis

Stiff joints and weak muscles characterize the disorder known as arthrogryphosis. It is not progressive, intelligence is normal, and the condition ranges from mild to severe. Muscles of the limbs may be small or may fail to develop altogether, causing stiff joints and restricted movement.

Adaptive Equipment for Physically Disabled Persons

Adaptive equipment and aids include three basic types (Melichar, 1977, 1978): *adaptive,* supportive equipment that helps people adapt to their environment; *assistive,* equipment that partially or fully replaces the lost capability in order to assist people in increasing their functional capability; and *rehabilitative,* equipment used in therapy or rehabilitation to help people regain physical functioning they have lost. Devices are classified into six categories according to their purposes:

- existence (used for feeding, grooming, sleeping, fastening clothing)
- communication (special typewriters, hearing aids, machines for dialing telephones)
- in situ motion (braces, splints)
- travel (wheelchairs, canes, walkers, crutches)
- adaptation (cooking utensils for people with one hand, driving aids)
- rehabilitation (used to exercise body parts and to measure physical functioning)

Decisions about the use of adaptive aids should be made carefully because of their potential effect on later functioning. The use of adaptive or assistive equipment leads to dependence on the aid to do a task. Without the aid, an individual may become more independent, which may prevent or retard physical deterioration. Some aids actually restrict movement or body functions. The expense and difficulties associated with the use of certain devices make their overall usefulness questionable, so decisions must be made carefully on an individual basis.

Educational Programs

In the past, the educational needs of physically handicapped individuals took second place to medical needs. Health problems received maximum attention, and the development of appropriate educational programs was of little concern. Physically disabled individuals received treatment in hospitals or state institutions. However, gradually, because of the recent commitment to educating handicapped children in the least restrictive environment (mainstreaming), even the most severely disabled children are being educated in the public schools. Decisions about placement in a regular classroom setting with support services, a special classroom for the disabled, or a special school are usually based on the severity of the disability (including the extent of physical functioning as well as the number and severity of associated problems) and on the availability of personnel to provide for the physical and educational needs of the child. For example, a child with cerebral palsy affecting all four limbs who also is severely retarded, has a hearing loss and occasional convulsions, and needs constant physical care cannot be placed in a regular classroom unless a full-time aide can be assigned. Usually such resources are not available, but one aide can serve several children in a special classroom or in a special school. On the other hand, a child with cerebral palsy affecting all four limbs but with normal intelligence and hearing, poor speech, and limited self-care skills can be placed in a regular classroom if given minimal assistance by a classroom aide, the teacher, or other students.

Often adaptive aids such as automatic page-turners, special typewriters, or other electronic devices can provide the help a teacher needs in the classroom if assistance from support personnel, such as physical therapists, speech therapists, or consulting teachers, is available. Usually, the physically disabled receive services from a team of professionals in a variety of disciplines (e.g., physical and occupational therapy, social work, nursing, psychology, speech therapy, rehabilitation, counseling, and recreation), who attempt to judge how to best meet the needs of the "whole child."

The major task in educational programming for the physically disabled is to adapt learning experiences to allow maximum independence in communication, movement, and academic learning. Adapting tasks requires flexibility and creativity on the part of both the teacher and the student and may also involve the use of mechanical or electronic devices. In a classroom setting, for example, a physically disabled child who cannot write should be allowed to complete assignments in whatever way is possible, such as dictating on tape, typing, or using a work or picture board.

One of the most significant problems often faced by disabled children and their families is the need for hospitalization. Children may require surgery, physical therapy, or other extensive care in the hospital. Hospitalization can be a frightening experience for a young child. In addition, the separation of the child from the family may cause a disruption in the development of infant-mother bonding as well as of emotional ties with the family. Later, extensive and frequent hospitalization disrupts the development of peer relationships. Certainly, hospitalization can cause lowered achievement because of absence from school.

Affective needs of children with severe motor impairments must be addressed either through the educational program itself or by counseling and therapy programs. Very few studies have compared psychological and social adjustment of children with physical disorders to that in children without disabilities. However, Pless and Roghmann (1971) concluded, after a review of research and their own study, that chronically ill children are at risk for psychological and social maladjustment. These researchers found that such children are more often socially isolated and troublesome in school than are healthy children; that the risk is greater if the disorder is more severe or if it is permanent; and that psychiatric disorders are more frequent in those who are chronically ill than in the general population. Children and their families may need counseling or therapy addressing their concept of the disability, the need for and ways to cope with the hospital experience, ways to deal with the reactions and attitudes of others, implications for sexual functioning and interactions, and ways to cope with stress and negative effects on self-esteem and self-image.

Cognitive development needs to be addressed by both parents and educators. Children with severe motor impairments have difficulty *actively* interacting with the environment. Even though they can see, often their visual field is limited because of their restricted movement. More important, however, they may be unable to touch and manipulate toys or other objects to learn how things work. Many are dependent on others for all visual, kinesthetic, and even auditory experiences. Parents and teachers must provide as many varied interactive experiences as possible.

Because of the tendency of educators to focus mainly on the disability, and the fact that many severely physically disabled individuals achieve low scores on intelligence tests, academic expectations for their performance are usually neither high nor realistic. Often the goal of an educational program is "basic survival," with an emphasis on daily living skills and vocational training so that the individual can become self-supporting. Emphasis is placed on the development of physical skills or medical treatment in early childhood programs, sometimes to the exclusion of academic and pre-academic skills. However, more and more educators are beginning to realize that many physically handicapped individuals are very intelligent and should have every opportunity to develop their intellectual and academic skills. They must often be given extra instruction to minimize the effects of extensive hospitalization. Severely disabled individuals may have a better chance of becoming financially self-supporting with an academic degree than with vocational training.

The most important advice for parents is to allow and encourage the child to be as independent as possible. Parents often somehow blame themselves for the child's condition. They need counseling to resolve the feelings of guilt and to learn effective ways of helping their child to develop fully. Guilt, along with a desire to make things easier for the child, may lead to overprotectiveness. Even though the tendency to be protective stems from concern, it can foster dependence. A child will benefit later by learning adaptive methods at an early age, rather than becoming dependent on parents for assistance in all tasks.

Indicators of Intellectual Giftedness

There were very few early indicators of Herb's intellectual ability—at least, few that were noticed. A major one was the fact that at the age of 3 years, Herb had discovered he had more control over his feet than his hands and began to be interested in using them. When his parents bought him a typewriter and enrolled him in school, he started learning how to type.

In elementary school, his achievement was not outstanding. He was in the top half of his classes, with a C + average. In high school, he was in the top quarter of his classes, with approximately a B average, and in college, he maintained better than a B average in both undergraduate and graduate school. One indicator of Herb's exceptional intellectual ability, illustrated by this pattern of academic achievement, is that as he learned or developed skills to compensate for his physical disability, his academic achievement improved.

Another characteristic that could also be perceived as an indicator of intellectual giftedness is Herb's creativity, or ability to develop alternative ways to accomplish everyday tasks. In other words, he has shown an unusual ability to compensate for or cope with his disability.

Perhaps the most important indicator of his intellectual ability was his achievements in science fairs, in which he competed with nonhandicapped students, many of whom had a much more extensive and rigorous background in science than was offered at Herb's special school. Other indicators were his early concern with his future, his ability to set long-range goals for himself, and his ability to develop plans for achieving these goals. Herb became concerned at a very early age about being a "productive member of society." This concern included not only a desire to produce in order to achieve personal independence but also a need to make an impact on, or a contribution to, society. From a very early age, he was interested in science and saw it as an area in which he could turn his interest into a productive career.

Perhaps the most salient trait in Herb that suggests his giftedness is his persistence and motivation to succeed. Even though he does not characterize this motivation as "perverse," as does Myron, their degrees of determination were very similar. Neither was willing to take "no" for an answer when their potential futures and careers were jeopardized. They were persistent in getting the education necessary to actualize their career goals.

Identification of Giftedness

Formal identification of giftedness in a youngster as severely disabled as Herb is difficult if only traditional means are used and may be impossible if standardized tests are not adapted. Three major problems can be identified. First, most intelligence tests require verbal responses, and in some cases lengthy explanations are required for full credit for an answer. Since Herb's speech is labored and difficult to understand even now as an adult, and no doubt has improved considerably since he was a child, high performance on a verbal test would be difficult to achieve. Second, tests that are nonverbal or primarily nonverbal are even less appropriate for severely disabled persons because they require adequate hand use for manipulative tasks. Such tasks are impossible for Herb and are difficult for even those with mildly limited control of their hands. Most intelligence tests are timed, with higher scores awarded if the task is completed early; a failing mark for a specific task may result from slowness. Third, severe disability commonly leads to lack of life experiences, and it is difficult to evaluate the potential effect of this deprivation on test performance. Many physically handicapped individuals are at a cultural or an experiential disadvantage because their disability has limited their ability to explore the world in a normal manner. Thus, such children may lack information about the environment that other children obtain at a relatively early age.

It is possible, however, to adapt tasks on intelligence tests for use by the physically disabled or those with speech and communication problems. Some tests are more easily modified than others. For example, the Peabody Picture Vocabulary Test (PPVT) consists of a word and four pictures. The examiner pronounces the word, and the examinee is required to point to the picture that illustrates the word. If a child does not have the ability to point, the examiner can develop a way for the child to give a signal when the correct picture is indicated. Even the ability to blink, for example, may be adequate. Similarly, the *Ravens Progressive Matrices* and the *Advanced Progressive Matrices* can be easily adapted. On these tests, there are several possibilities for completing a design, and the examinee crosses out or circles the correct one. Again, the examiner can help the child select a usable system for signaling when the appropriate design is noted. Certain subtests or tasks on other tests, such as the WISC–R or Stanford-Binet, may be more easily modifiable than others. Time limits, for example, can be waived. It must be understood, however, that the test norms are not accurate if testing procedures used for norming are not followed. This consideration is pursued further in Chapter 8.

With regard to standardized tests of other abilities such as creativity, critical thinking, and academic achievement, many of the problems are the same as in assessment of intelligence. The figural form of the *Torrance Tests of Creative Thinking* (TTCT), for instance, requires that the examinee be able to use a pencil and paper. The verbal form requires writing or dictating of answers. Even though dictation may be appropriate for some physically handicapped children, the time limits still penalize those with speech deficits. Tests of academic achievement and critical thinking are more easily adapted than tests of creativity since they usually require simply choosing the correct alternative from a list. Typing, pointing, and blinking when a correct answer is identified are all examples of ways the tasks can be accomplished.

The most useful procedures for identifying giftedness in a neurologically impaired or severely physically disabled individual are observational methods in which the *intellectual* performance of the person is compared with that of other similarly disabled individuals rather than norms for a test that was standardized on a nonhandicapped population. Numerous checklists are available for the behaviors that indicate giftedness in students. These can be useful if the observer recognizes that certain behaviors may be masked or may be impossible because of the disability. Other characteristics can be readily observed, and if several children with a similar disability are studied, the observer will gain a better understanding of what to expect.

The most frequently used checklists to identify gifted students are the *Scales for Rating the Behavioral Characteristics of Superior Students* (SRBCSS) (Renzulli, Smith, White, Callahan, & Hartman, 1976). Several examples of characteristics that are observable to differing degrees follow. (a) "Quick mastery and recall of factual information," "keen and alert" observation, and the ability to reason things out are traits that can be observed in a variety of settings with relatively little influence from the disability so long as the affected individual has some means of effective communication. (b) "Unusually advanced vocabulary for age or grade level," the possession of "a large storehouse of information about a variety of topics," and "rapid insight into cause-effect relationships" are traits that can be observed, if effective communication exists, but may be influenced by a lack of experience due to the limitations of mobility. (c) The possession of "good verbal facility" and speech that "is usually understood," an ability to direct the activity in which the individual is involved, and highly developed athletic skills are characteristics that are generally masked by the disability in an individual with cerebral palsy.

One checklist that has been adapted for use with severely and multiply handicapped children is Torrance's (1974) *Checklist of Creative Positives.* White (undated), in a project to identify creative children among a severely physically handicapped population, enlisted the help of teams of practicing artists to develop multiarts experiences in which handicapped children could participate to allow them opportunities to develop and demonstrate their creativity. While children were engaged in these activities, they were observed by artists using characteristics taken from Torrance's checklist. These activities, designed for children with limited physical capabilities, have been successful in eliciting creative behaviors.

Other methods for identification include interviews with parents and teachers, assessment of products, trial placement or diagnostic teaching, and observation of performance in a single event such as a science fair. With product assessment, there must be a realistic evaluation based on the physical and verbal capabilities of the student. In fact, comparison with the work of other similarly handicapped students, if possible, is important. When using diagnostic teaching or trial placement in a program as an identification tool, it is important that the teacher work with the student long enough to become familiar with the specific handicap and to assess accurately the student's characteristic ways of responding. A day or two is often enough time for assessment in a nonhandicapped child, but in one with a severe disability, a week or two is more appropriate. The fact that he performed so well in the science fair competition was very significant in identifying Herb's giftedness. Even if his academic performance had not been outstanding in any other area or at any other time, his performance in this one event was outstanding enough to suggest that he was intellectually gifted.

In summary, identification of a child with extensive cerebral palsy requires adaptation of tasks on standardized tests, recognition of the possible effects of experience on performance, use of tests that can be easily adapted, and extensive use of observational methods or informal procedures. The evaluation team also must collect information about the child's performance from a variety of sources and should observe the child in a variety of settings in order to become familiar with the child as a person as well as a test subject. All this information should be compared with data on performance of other children with similar handicaps.

Potential Interaction between Giftedness and Handicapping Condition

There is an obvious interaction between Herb's giftedness and his handicap. Some of the outcomes are positive, and others have potentially negative effects, especially frustration stemming from the gap between what he would like to do and what he and/or others perceive him as being intellectually capable of doing.

Positive Effects

One of the most obvious positive effects of Herb's giftedness and disability is his ability to say so much in a few words. Herb uses his advanced vocabulary and understanding of abstract terms to speak and write very efficiently and effectively. He practices these skills every day so that his writing as well as his speaking is as clear and precise as possible. These skills are highly desirable in many areas of professional life. A constant need to use language wisely may cause an individual to think about and use abstract concepts to a greater extent. The resulting emphasis on higher-level thought may help to develop more efficient thinking by forcing the development of highly abstract categories for ideas.

Another positive effect of the interaction between Herb's giftedness and his disability is his development of a higher level of creativity. Most theorists believe that creativity needs to be exercised in order to develop. Thus, as Herb coped with the need to accommodate his disability and developed alternative ways to accomplish various tasks, his cognitive characteristics of flexibility, creative problem solving, and innovativeness were rapidly developed to new heights. The continual need to come up with unusual answers to dilemmas or improved solutions to problems further accelerated and enhanced the development of his creative abilities. It is interesting to note that in the project designed to identify creativity in a severely and multiply handicapped population (White, undated), there was a much higher percentage of creative students in this handicapped group than usually found in a nonhandicapped group. This greater percentage may be due to the constant need of handicapped people to be creative problem solvers (A. White, personal communication, August 1981).

As a gifted individual with high aspirations for himself and a personal need to develop goals and plans at an early age, and as a handicapped person who realized his limitations in activities of daily living and particularly in career choices, Herb developed a high degree of persistence, determination, and motivation to succeed. His determination to be successful and his early planning for a career were probably two of the most positive outcomes of the interaction between his giftedness and his handicapping condition.

Another positive product of the interaction between Herb's disability and giftedness has been his diligent effort to make societal changes to benefit other handicapped people. He views these efforts as a logical response to his personal experience with severe disability and as a consequence of his natural desire to "adapt, improve, and modify institutions, objects, and systems." Herb has been an influential leader in the movement to make educational programs more accessible to disabled persons and to sensitize the general public to the specific needs of physically handicapped individuals.

Negative Effects

In addition to the positive effects of the interplay between Herb's giftedness and the disabling condition, there are some negative ones. As a young child with curiosity about "what makes things and people 'tick'," Herb endured many frustrating moments because of his difficulty in communicating. Frustration also resulted from an early, strong need for independence coupled with severe limitations on his physical ability to explore, to take care of himself, or to work on projects and assignments.

Like many other gifted individuals, Herb has set high standards for his achievement. As is typical of many intellectually gifted persons, he tends to be overly self-critical and not easily satisfied with his speed of task completion or quality of products; these tendencies are exacerbated by the limitations imposed by his disability. Acute frustration caused by the interactive effect of a keen desire to achieve perfection and the need to accept what may be perceived as imperfect abilities and accomplishments is a vulnerability of all young gifted children without disabilities; the resulting emotional stress is significantly greater in gifted children with severe and/or multiple handicaps.

Most intellectually gifted people are keen and alert observers, perceptive of relationships and consequences, and prone to be exceptionally sensitive to details, including the reactions of others. Like it or not, physical appearance has a major impact on social interactions and relationships. When children or adults encounter a disabled person with physical traits similar to those created by cerebral palsy, their natural reactions often are not positive. They may avoid interacting with the disabled person, stare uncontrollably, make humorous comments to relieve embarrassment, or try to hide their true reactions behind expressionless, tense faces. A less observant or sensitive individual is not as adversely affected by these reactions as is a gifted person. This vulnerability to acute social discomfort is exacerbated for persons like Herb, who highly value social interaction and relationships. Sensing the discomfort or rejection of others is particularly painful for a disabled person who enjoys using wit and humor to make others happy and who values relationships that are relaxed, accepting, and mutually rewarding.

SPECIFIC GUIDELINES

The following specific guidelines for working more effectively with gifted individuals who have a severe motor impairment are based on the reported effects of being both intellectually gifted and severely disabled. These recommendations must take into account variations in the degree and nature of the disability, specific strengths or exceptional abilities, and significant personality traits. Thus, information gained from the research literature as well as from interviews with other bright, successful adults with cerebral palsy and other physical disabilities provides the foundation and framework for the discussion.

Parents, Siblings, Neighbors, and Friends

The most important underlying recommendations for parents, close relatives, neighbors, and friends are to encourage and allow independence, and to develop and communicate realistically high expectations. Both of these recommendations stem from the authors' belief that a person with a handicap is *different,* not *inferior.* Behavior congruent with this belief will encourage independence in the person with the handicapping condition and will reveal realistically high expectations in that person.

Some examples of specific ways parents and others can encourage independence are the following: (a) purchase books or toys that the child can use independently; (b) teach the child to use communication aids or devices as early as possible; and (c) rather than restricting the child from certain activities because of the risk of injury posed by the disability, discuss the possible dangers and urge caution, but allow the child to participate.

With regard to expectations, the child's various specific abilities should be carefully observed during stimulating learning opportunities of increasing difficulty; expectations should be gradually raised in response to improved performance. Uneven achievement is to be expected, and as higher levels of ability are observed, parents' expectations should be tentatively adjusted until a pattern is established; these revised expectations should be communicated in appropriately small steps so that the child's feelings of success are sustained. Expectations for one child must never be based on the performance of another disabled person, because each possesses a unique set of attributes.

It is critically important that expectations or goals be realistic and attainable. Parents should talk with successful adults who have handicapping conditions similar to their child's to obtain a helpful perspective; such persons can provide useful suggestions regarding appropriate, facilitative guidance and assistance. It also can be very beneficial to provide opportunities for a handicapped youngster to interact and develop a personal relationship with a successful adult who has a similar disabling condition.

Families must seek information regarding available adaptive aids. The decision to purchase and use a specific aid should take into consideration the risk of dependence. For example, an adaptive aid provided to a child early in life may inhibit the child's development by fostering dependence on the aid rather than encouraging the use of existing motor skills. Parents and families also should seek professional counsel regarding ways to encourage the development of intellectual ability or giftedness in a physically disabled child. Some suggestions follow:

- reading books to the child
- selecting educational toys that can be used by a child with limited muscle control
- providing opportunities to watch television and films and to listen to tapes and records
- allowing as much freedom to explore as possible

Providing early education and speech therapy and encouraging cognitive abilities and academic interests are ways to stimulate the development of gifts and talents as well as to demonstrate high expectations for the child's intellectual achievement.

Parents, neighbors, and siblings can facilitate the identification of talents and exceptional abilities by observing the child's development and then conferring with other adults familiar with the expected developmental abilities of similarly disabled children of the same age. Some possible early indicators of giftedness are unusual skills in coping with or adapting to a disability, early interest in speaking or communicating, an unusually intense desire to be independent, and an early interest or ability in reading.

Some other general suggestions for those who are in contact with a physically disabled individual seem obvious but nevertheless deserve mention. Persons should speak directly to the disabled individual rather than to others nearby, even if the disability involves difficulty in verbal communication. Offers of assistance in daily tasks are appropriate, but the disabled person should be asked for suggestions of how help can be given (e.g., "I will be happy to help you if you would like my assistance; just let me know if and how I can help."). Concerned persons can also volunteer to assist in other ways such as taking notes in class, helping with pronunciation of words, and listening during rehearsal of a presentation.

Educational Professionals

As with parents, siblings, neighbors, and friends, two of the most important recommendations for educational professionals and aides involve formation of realistically high expectations and encouragement of independence. Educators must look beyond the handicapping condition to the possibility of high intellectual ability. A disability in one area is not necessarily associated with a disability in another area; nor does a specific disability preclude the possibility of giftedness in another area. For example, a speech deficit does not always result from intellectual or hearing problems. Educators should not "talk down" to children with cerebral palsy and a speech deficit as though they were mentally impaired. In such children, the receptive vocabulary is probably much larger than the expressive vocabulary. Furthermore, the use of simplified language to communicate with the child does not stimulate the development of more advanced expressive language.

Handicapped students must be allowed to "test their limits." This requires the provision of intellectually challenging activities, both those that can result in failure and those in which the student can achieve success. Self-testing of limits also demonstrates abilities and limits to the teacher, who can then design more appropriate experiences. Most often, for this population of gifted students who are physically disabled, the expectations for physical performance are too high, whereas the expectations for intellectual achievement are too low.

As Herb recommended, physically handicapped students need to be main-streamed as much as possible. They need to be educated with other students who have high expectations for their own performance. Teachers who work with both the disabled and nondisabled tend to have higher expectations for students than those who work only with the disabled. If teachers are to work more effectively with disabled students, they need information about adults who have the same type of disability and who have been successful. Whenever possible, these disabled adults should work closely with teachers and should be invited to interact with students or to serve as mentors for them. Getting to know a disabled adult who has "made it" can be an effective way to raise the expectations of both teachers and students. Disabled adults can provide assistance in identifying coping strategies or skills that can be useful in overcoming a disability.

With regard to the teaching of coping skills, educators can be most helpful by developing in students an attitude of "self-advocacy." Rather than depending on others to assist them or blaming others for their lack of success, many successful handicapped adults feel they must control their own destiny. Researchers (Maker et al., 1978) have catalogued and described strategies used by handicapped scientists who are successful in their careers. Similar techniques and attitudes can be developed in handicapped students.

A related recommendation is to encourage the development of strengths and to provide many opportunities for challenges in these areas. Often educators are so concerned with the areas of difficulty and the provision of remedial activities that they neglect the development of areas of strength, which may compensate effectively for the weaknesses and may become avenues for career development. Disabled children should be encouraged to compete with nondisabled children, especially in their areas of strength.

When necessary, academic tasks designed for nondisabled students should be adapted to allow disabled children to participate. It is important to emphasize, however, that the objective of adaptation is not to make the task *easier* but to make it *possible*. For example, the general idea behind Herb's recommendations for modification of laboratory courses and assignments is that teachers need to be flexible about the exact form or method of an assignment or learning experience while addressing specific objectives. Concepts can be acquired in many ways, and handicapped students should be allowed to use ingenuity in developing alternative assignments or methods for achieving the objectives of a course. Students also should be encouraged to use whatever abilities and skills they possess to accomplish a task; they should never be discouraged from using unusual adaptive skills, such as typing with the toes or turning pages with the teeth.

Educators need to become highly skilled observers. They need to be familiar with a child's unique speech patterns so they can understand the child and/or teach the child's classmates how to understand. They need to notice what specific tasks individual students do well and what they do not do well. They need to compare the performance of one handicapped child with that of another but must not assume that the same disability will lead to identical behavior. Teachers must use their observations to identify exceptional creativity and intellectual abilities as well as to note areas needing remedial instruction.

In advising gifted students with disabilities, it is more effective to identify alternatives than to suggest a specific course of action. An educator offering alternatives is perceived as an accepting advocate who respects the students' abilities. If a handicapped student perceives a teacher as an obstructive influence because of negative attitudes and low expectations conveyed, the student is apt to reject any advice from the teacher, to behave in a way to prove that the educator is wrong, or to avoid even listening to the advice. If the advice is presented in the context of identifying and selecting alternatives, the gifted handicapped person usually will be more willing to listen and consider alternatives. For example, if a physically handicapped student is having trouble completing writing assignments in high school or college, a teacher or counselor should first assist the student in identifying the problem and its possible causes, through asking questions and listening rather than offering answers. When the problem and possible causes have been identified (e.g., not enough time to complete the work because the student types too slowly), together the teacher and the student can "brainstorm" alternative solutions. Possibilities include reducing the number of academic classes taken, balancing writing courses with nonwriting courses, taking some grades of incomplete, and allowing some assignments to be taped rather than written. Some of the alternatives, such as taking a reduced load or taking an incomplete grade, might be viewed by the student as a "put-down" if presented as advice rather than as alternatives to be considered.

A similar approach of identifying alternatives must be taken by counselors, especially those involved in assisting with career choices. The choice of a lifetime career is a personal decision that involves consideration of interests and skills along with the demands and opportunities presented by a particular career. Counselors often ignore the specific interests and cognitive skills of the severely disabled individual and consider only the limitations imposed by the handicap. If both counselor and client take a problem-solving approach to identifying career alternatives that relate to personal interests, utilize intellectual strengths, and require minimal skill in areas affected by the disability, a more satisfying process will result in an optimal outcome.

Institutions of higher education preparing teachers and other educational personnel must ensure that their graduates have accurate knowledge about the needs and characteristics of handicapped students. Most important, all educators must understand that intellectual giftedness can be expected to occur with the same frequency in the disabled population as that in the nondisabled population. Accurate information about giftedness, disabilities, and appropriate accommodation of individual differences should be integrated into coursework and the clinical training of *all* educators.

Medical Personnel

Medical personnel need to be knowledgeable about severe motor impairments and their implications for education as well as for health, since they are the professionals to whom a family first turns for guidance and information. Medical professionals should be able to refer a family to specific agencies or organizations for special assistance. If unable to provide such information, physicians, nurses, and therapists should at least provide informational brochures or pamphlets that give accurate answers to questions, and they should refer the family to general community resources for securing additional assistance.

Medical personnel can provide a valuable service to parents and to educators by presenting information in workshops or classes on such topics as causes and effects of specific disabilities, appropriate physical exercises, uses of adaptive aids or devices, and ways to provide a more challenging and nurturing environment for disabled children. Together child development specialists and medical personnel can assist parents in understanding what to expect during their child's early years of growth and how to provide the best environment for optimum development.

Community Services and Agencies

The most important recommendation for community services and agencies is to foster *awareness* of the needs and characteristics of gifted people with physical disabilities. Implementing this recommendation requires making certain that all employees possess an understanding of the characteristics and needs of gifted individuals with disabilities, and also disseminating printed information and providing educational programs for the general public that will develop awareness and motivate needed changes. All employees should participate in workshops designed to inform them about handicapping conditions and to develop accurate understanding of the needs and abilities of gifted disabled people in relation to employment in the agency or to services rendered. For example, in Herb's situation, information could have been provided to DVR counselors about physically handicapped individuals successful in specific careers, the types of careers in which success is based on intellectual ability rather than physical ability, and the high achievements of some physically disabled individuals. In turn, these counselors would have become more effective in working with handicapped persons because they would have more accurate information and could disseminate this information to other agencies or the families of individuals they counseled. Had Herb's DVR counselor known more about the field of meteorology for example, he would not have believed all meteorologists must talk on television or radio.

DVR and other agencies that provide scholarships or other financial support to individuals with disabilities need to develop methods for making decisions that take into account the intellectual abilities of a client in order to estimate more accurately overall ''employability'' and the capability for successful performance of the job in spite of a handicapping condition. Severely disabled individuals sometimes need a chance to prove they can cope and achieve in a specific role. Moreover, when agency officials evaluate the individual's academic progress, it is important to consider the influence of the disability on specific performance areas, along with the need for those skills in the chosen career. For instance, in Herb's case, high grades in English composition were not as important as those in geology; his job at the National Weather Service requires skills in technical writing rather than in literary writing.

Awareness workshops need to be provided for employers and potential employers of handicapped individuals. Employers need to be aware of the potential abilities and limitations of individuals and need to know what they can do to facilitate the development of their employees' skills. Some specific suggestions follow:

- recognition of exceptional abilities as well as disabilities
- development of understanding of the need for on-the-job support and counseling
- awareness of the need to send disabled as well as nondisabled individuals to conferences and meetings
- development of understanding of the need to help those with disabilities feel accepted and respected as equal members of the staff

Community agencies can be instrumental in providing support services such as group living facilities, in which handicapped adults can share attendants and facilities that they cannot afford individually. The availability of such alternative residences can reduce tension in homes, provide relief to parents, and develop feelings of independence in the disabled adult.

Community and religious groups that sponsor programs for youth should integrate disabled children into their regular programs rather than forming separate groups for them. Special Boy Scout and Girl Scout troops for handicapped children, for example, defeat the purpose of the activity and do not provide a setting in which stereotyped notions about handicapped persons can be overcome.

CONCLUSION

Obviously, not all gifted individuals with neurological impairments or physical disabilities will be like Herb. They will have different abilities and disabilities. However, many characteristics will be similar. Recommendations Herb made were remarkably similar to those voiced by other bright and gifted individuals with cerebral palsy.

According to Herb and others like him, their most important needs result from the tendency of every segment of society to assume that an individual with a physical handicap is not capable of achieving at as high a level as a nondisabled person. The general public seems unaware that a disabled individual's willingness to work, determination to succeed, and intellectual ability may well compensate for any lack of physical skills.

Chapter Reaction

S.J. Obringer, Ed.D.

"A child's speech is his window of the mind," wrote a prominent speech and language clinician. With regard to the highly intelligent cerebral palsied student, this is a very prejudicial statement.

The cerebral palsy population is a very heterogeneous group of persons in whom degree of involvement ranges from slight to extreme in both physical and intellectual characteristics. Generally, those individuals with the subclassification of athetosis and ataxia display higher intellectual abilities than those with the subclassification of spasticity or rigidity. However, wide variance is observed in all subgroups.

In the infant or toddler, professionals tend to assess intelligence almost exclusively through the motoric channel—that is, through the observation of smiling, hand grasping, and other early signs of normal gross motor coordination. Because these early signs certainly are delayed or even absent in the cerebral palsy infant, a number of professionals either label intellectual potential incorrectly or make no comment at all. To compound this problem, there is little correlation between the degree of physical involvement and that of intellectual retardation. Therefore, it is not uncommon to find individuals such as Herb with a severe muscular incoordination but with no intellectual impairment—in fact, with superior intellectual ability.

Because few school psychologists or psychometrists have an in-depth knowledge of cerebral palsy, intellectual assessment often involves only crude estimates. For this reason, a number of very intellectually endowed individuals go unnoticed or are mislabeled because of low scores on intelligence tests.

As with Herb, it is not uncommon that individuals with neuromuscular disorders show more ability in the later stages of school. Apparently, neat work, quick verbal responses, and physical prowess are highly rewarded in the elementary and junior high grades. As problem solving and abstract thinking replace the former, the intellectual ability of cerebral palsied students becomes better understood. This becomes even more apparent during the post-secondary or higher education years.

Parents need immediate information when the child is born, not only for self-understanding but for helpful procedures to foster both physical and intellectual growth in their cerebral-palsied child. Informative books such as Finnie's (1968) *Handling the Young Cerebral Palsy Child at Home,* or short chapters on cerebral palsy from current textbooks on developmental disabilities (Cruickshank, 1976; Umbreit, 1983; Bleck and Nagel, 1975), answer many questions and remove some of the myths or stereotypes faced by the parents. Information gained directly by reading is often much more valuable than that presented in office sessions between parent and physician or parent and school psychologist.

Our society tends to put great trust in its physicians. A recent study by Obringer (1984) found that a great many physicians, especially general practitioners and family practitioners, felt inadequate to deal with the developmentally disabled child. The areas of least expertise were reported to be in family counseling and career counseling. It appears that Herb was confronted by this lack of expertise at several points in his life. The services of an informed physician, or, better yet, of a developmental disability clinic with a multidisciplinary team are essential to parents of the motor-handicapped child. Such services should provide an honest and realistic view of the child's future with applicable recommendations.

Giftedness can be present in any motor-impaired individual. Professionals, especially medical and psychoeducational, need to be aware of this possibility because giftedness is often masked by factors normally associated with delayed intellectual development and performance. Like other gifted persons, motor-impaired individuals such as Herb can make significant contributions to both self and society. Unfortunately, there are many "Herbs" who go unnoticed and whose potential contributions to self and society remain dormant.

REFERENCES

Bleck, E.E., & Nagel, D.A. (Eds). (1975). *Physically handicapped children: A medical atlas for teachers*. New York: Grune & Stratton.

Cruickshank, W.M. (1976). *Cerebral palsy: A developmental disability* (3rd ed.). Syracuse: Syracuse University Press.

Finnie, N.R. (1968). *Handling the young cerebral palsy child at home*. London: W. Heinemann Medical Books.

Obringer, S.J. (1984). Survey of physician expertise with developmentally disabled children and attitudes toward mainstreaming. *Educational and Psychological Research, 4*(2), 91–95.

Umbreit, J. (Ed.). (1983). *Physical disabilities and health impairments: An introduction*. Columbus, OH: Merrill.

*   *   *   *   *

S.J. Obringer is a Professor of Curriculum and Instruction at Mississippi State University. The areas of his research activities include mental retardation and related developmental disabilities. Dr. Obringer, who also has a mild form of cerebral palsy, is an impartial hearing officer for the Mississippi State Department of Education and past president and governor of the Mississippi Council for Exceptional Children.

Chapter Reaction

Patrick M. Ghezzi, Ph.D.

One reaction to Herb's story would be to ask, "Why aren't there more people like him?" A satisfactory answer to this question would, of course, point to an environment that with few exceptions militates against optimum development. If the question were asked, "What can be done to optimize the development of the gifted handicapped person?" the answer again would be found in the environment.

Just as it is clear that it is the environment to which one turns for an explanation of behavior, so too is it clear that in order to optimize development one must focus attention on educational environments. From this point of view one could ask, "What would such an environment look like?" The answer to this question would require a lengthy response, focusing upon at least five essential ingredients for creating an effective learning environment. These would be: (1) establishing individualized goals in behavioral terms, (2) assessing current functioning relative to these goals, (3) applying the principles of learning, (4) monitoring the effectiveness of instruction, and (5) arranging conditions to promote maintenance and generalization of the gains achieved.

Of the five ingredients indicated above, one in particular stands out as being especially relevant to gifted handicapped students. Assessing current functioning by administering standardized, norm-referenced tests usually provides no *instructionally* relevant information about the student's level of functioning. Further, this type of assessment often generates a label that can be detrimental to the development and well-being of the child. The use of criterion-referenced tests and direct observational recording techniques avoids the potential damage of labeling, while simultaneously providing instructionally relevant information.

A final point relates to the home environment. *Active* parent participation is imperative. Ideally, training in the home would begin at an early age, and later, would be coordinated with school training by the teacher. The aim here, as always, would be to optimize development, or as Herb puts it, to create the circumstances under which he, and his peers, can eventually become "a useful member of society."

*　　*　　*　　*　　*

Dr. Ghezzi is currently Visiting Assistant Professor in the Department of Special Education at The University of Arizona. In collaboration with Drs. Sidney W. Bijou and John Umbreit, he is presently conducting research on language development in normal and handicapped children.

Chapter 5

Gifted Adults Incurring Severe Disabilities

This chapter is unique in that the authors invited the subject of the case study, John Robertson, to write his own story and to discuss the issues relative to rehabilitation and higher education. John, an education professional who as an undergraduate incurred a severe disability, has distinguished himself among his university colleagues as an exceptional scholar, both in the expression of personal insights and in the ability to formulate objective analyses. The authors believe that this chapter, a unique blend of a personal story and an objective analysis, will stimulate the reader's thinking and understanding of the issues involved to a degree not possible with a discussion by an outside observer.

* * * * *

Writing my own case study created some difficulties that do not occur when one's experience is described by a more objective observer. The first difficulty I had to overcome was a tendency toward self-critical analysis that could be a barrier to self-expression. Another difficulty has been my desire for self-disclosure while maintaining the objectivity necessary for any scholarly analysis and insights that I might contribute to the field of knowledge about giftedness in individuals with handicapping conditions. I have struggled with these difficulties continuously in writing this chapter.

John Robertson

* * * * *

A CASE STUDY: JOHN

A disabling condition that occurs in adulthood creates a powerful psychological need to develop unimpaired abilities, perhaps exceptional potential or giftedness not before recognized or developed. The growth of my intellectual abilities occurred in my early adult years *because* of my physical disability, *not in spite of it!*

I have been a quadriplegic since I was 25 years of age, owing to a spinal cord injury that resulted from an automobile accident in 1972. I have no motor function and only partial sensory ability in my lower extremities, and I use a motorized wheelchair for mobility. My upper body is impaired with loss of muscle response to about the mid-chest. My arms and hands have functional loss with no tricep muscle response and minimal grasp and no voluntary finger movement. Besides a wheelchair, I use some simple adaptive devices to aid me in holding writing and eating utensils. I employ an aide to assist me in my daily personal care consisting of bathing, dressing, and grooming. Once I am prepared for the day I am, for the most part, self-sufficient. I am married; it is important for the reader to know that my wife is also a quadriplegic owing to a spinal cord injury, although her functional ability is markedly higher than my own. We live in our own more than slightly mortgaged home in suburbia.

Though my wife is a quadriplegic, we are independent and self-sufficient, largely because of her efforts. By independent and self-sufficient, I mean that we maintain our own care or, at least in my case, instruct that care. The majority of our efforts are done collectively and, owing to my wife's strength of will and determination, we are relatively free from the restraints of dependency on others in our daily activities.

At present I am a doctoral student in Higher Education Administration at a major state university. I am employed as a counselor in the Office of Teacher Education with primary responsibility for working with undergraduates who are experiencing academic difficulty or need career counseling. My career goal is to become an administrator in higher education with responsibility for student affairs. My personal objective is to be in a position to enhance the educational experiences of individual students through responsive, sensitive administrative leadership.

My accomplishments in the development of my intellectual or academic abilities I attribute to the following: (a) the recognition of my potential abilities brought about by the sudden incurrence of severe disabilities, (b) the opportunity through rehabilitation services and higher education to develop those neglected abilities, and (c) the support and encouragement of individuals who assisted me in my efforts. In order to understand my story, it is important to know something about my childhood and my early pattern of academic underachievement.

I am the oldest of five children from an urban, Catholic background. My parents' educational profile is typical of those who lived through the Depression of the 1930s: my mother is a graduate from high school; my father finished school through the eighth grade. Now divorced and remarried, my mother is a supervisor at a women's alcoholic treatment facility. My father has worked in construction as a heavy equipment operator for over 30 years.

In the time and place of my growing up, education was seen as an assurance of social mobility, a key to a better life. The expected social rewards for education were assumed to provide incentives for students to strive to achieve in school. However, many students in my community, including me, tended to perceive an education as a desired but unattainable goal. My peers and I gave great "lip service" to the goals of achieving entrance to higher education while avoiding anything that would put us in close proximity to schoolwork. This was the result of our perception of the unspoken "knowledge" that college was only for the selected elite. Consequently, I completed high school with a mediocre academic record; was advised by my school counselor to go to work, not college, as I was considering; and enlisted in the Navy, in which I was trained to be an aviation electronics technician.

My development up to the point that I acquired my disability could be categorized as academic underachievement based on the discrepancy between (a) my intellectual ability and potential for academic achievement and (b) the level of my performance in school. Accompanying a pattern of academic underachievement was my inability to focus on one particular area of interest because of my impulse to strive to learn as much as I could about everything in life. For me, exploration of each new area of knowledge always has been an exciting adventure, creating new interests and directions to further diffuse my overabundant intellectual energies.

At the time I incurred my disability, I was just beginning to develop a general area of academic concentration in political science and history as an undergraduate student. After the accident and five years of rehabilitation training, another three years of study was required before I finished my undergraduate general studies (liberal arts) program and received a bachelor's degree. Within two years after that, I also obtained a master's degree in Educational Administration; my work for this program included an internship in a university Career Planning and Placement Center.

Personal View of Self

In discussing what I perceive to be my strengths and weaknesses, I have responded in terms of three classifications: (a) those characteristics evident in me from birth, (b) those specifically created by the disabling condition, and (c) those that are the product of interaction between inherent characteristics and those created by the disabling condition. It has been difficult for me to describe accurately my self-perceived characteristics because it is difficult to recall life before the accident. As a consequence of my rehabilitation experience, I believe an individual who suddenly becomes severely disabled must, in a real sense, become a *new* person by completely restructuring his or her self-image. A new "personhood" must be developed by building on an innate sense of Self to develop all salvageable and dormant resources (i.e., potentialities, abilities, traits). For me, this required help from others in order to identify and strengthen those abilities that I had not previously recognized and developed. Therefore, much of what I describe as my characteristics was learned from others who observed and assessed my abilities and traits.

Unlike other case study subjects described in this book, I have spent almost three-fourths of my existence free from severe disability. My disability was created in an instant of time—on one side of which I had a normally functioning body and on the other side, a profound disability. As in most young adults, my self-image prior to the automobile accident was influenced significantly by my physical attributes and abilities and by a sense of relative freedom from medical concerns. My accident changed all that and the way I looked at myself, others, and my environment.

The impact of suddenly becoming permanently and severely disabled is such a traumatic life experience, so profound in its effect, that all my attempts at adequate description have felt unsatisfactory. It must be enough to say that the events of my accident had the subsequent effect of so altering my perception of self and others and of my reality that it became difficult to perceive in memory the person before the trauma as being in any way the same person that I am today. Of course, I am essentially the same "person" with the same fundamental strengths and weaknesses of personality, the same intellectual skills and potential cognitive abilities; what changed were my perceptions, my *physical* abilities, and my desire to develop intellectual skills and abilities.

Coping with a severe disability requires the combined, concerted efforts of many people. The most important efforts, of course, are those of the individual who has become disabled. One way in which others may help the newly disabled person is in objectively assessing strengths which can be developed. Ideally, gifted potential will be identified and developed early in life so that, in the event of severe trauma, individuals are aware of those gifts that can help them not only to cope but to adjust and compensate in the process of rehabilitation. However, all too often individuals are unaware of those abilities; they need assistance in identifying their strengths. The identification and development of my exceptional intellectual abilities late in life nevertheless have enabled me to adapt more effectively than others, to contribute much more to the world in which I live than I would have, and to enrich my life and the lives of those with whom I come in contact. It is unquestionably the responsibility of all persons involved in the rehabilitation process to seek to identify and guide the development of all potential intellectual abilities that may enrich the life experiences of the person who must live with permanent and severe disabling conditions.

Self-Perceived Strengths

In addressing specific self-perceptions that I feel have been dominant influences in bringing me to my present stage of personal and professional development, I have several attributes and abilities that could be considered as both strengths and weaknesses. From the perspective of having contributed significantly to the growth of my intellectual abilities, these self-perceptions definitely are strengths. From the perspective of emotional vulnerability, they could be regarded also as weaknesses. I identify my strengths as those characteristics that have motivated and enabled my growth: persistence, drive to be creative, problem-solving skills, adaptability, and a strong desire to make a positive impact that will advance and enhance individual human life experiences. Additional important influencing characteristics are my diversity of interests and my tendency toward perfectionism.

Others perceive me as exceptionally persistent, and I know that I have a tenacious drive to achieve goals that I have set. Combined with considerable patience, these two attributes add up to a persistence that often enables me to succeed in attaining my goal. This is a positive attribute, but it does produce some negative effects on social relations when other members of the activity group do not have the same drive.

My drive to express myself creatively has always been a source of positive feelings about myself. My artistic potential was the first area of creativity to be developed and provided me an opportunity to enjoy expressing feelings and ideas in constructive, effective ways. My artistic ability brought personal satisfaction until my need to communicate ideas and feelings outran my ability to express those feelings through painting. I then turned to other forms of creative expression, such as writing prose and poetry, to fill the gap left by my sense of inability to express myself satisfactorily through art.

Another important strength I have is the ability to solve problems; that is, I have developed the ability to identify problems or causes of problems, and to select or create an alternative strategy to provide an effective solution. This skill has been particularly evident and useful in addressing problems created by my disability. A very simple example of this problem-solving skill can be provided by my experience in college after I became disabled, when I needed to develop an effective way to take notes during class. My first method of note-taking was tape-recording lectures and replaying them. I found this method to be an inadequate one because it required listening to large amounts of superfluous information, and it was too time-consuming. Also, not the least of my problems with audiotape was the unbearable idea of again having to listen to an all-too-often uninspired, boring lecture! My next method was to photocopy lecture notes from someone in the class. This method was ineffective for two reasons: first, others often omitted much of what I considered important; and, second, photocopying notes removed me further from active participation in the note-taking process, which decreased my learning. The eventual solution to the problem was to develop an elaborate system of abbreviated note-taking as well as to improve my physical writing speed and legibility. This method of making judicious notations eliminated many of the problems I encountered initially in taking or obtaining lecture notes.

I have always had considerable adaptability—that is, the ability to cope with and compensate for changes in my environment. Obviously the ability to adapt, to change, and to compensate is an essential agent for adjustment to an incurred severely handicapping condition. My ability to cope with and adjust to instability and change in my environment began to be developed in my childhood because of a lack of stability in my home. Since I became disabled, that ability to adjust and to cope with change has of necessity developed further. It seems to me that my ability to adapt to the changes I have experienced has been a product of the combined abilities to perceive the necessity for specific adaptations, to analyze and evaluate alternatives, and to develop strategies for implementing those alternatives. I do know my ability to adapt to change has been essential for my survival as well as my achievement.

I consider my most significant strength to be my intense desire and total commitment to contribute to the enhancement of the life experiences of others. That is to say, I am highly motivated—actually *driven*—to contribute to the enhancement of individual and collective life experiences through education. I see education as the ideal medium and method by which to accomplish my goals. My sensitivity and desire to enhance life experiences of others has been heightened by the experience of being exposed to so much human devastation in hospitals and rehabilitation centers. This experience has increased my passion for developing educational programs and creating educational activities to better life circumstances. Perhaps the desire to contribute to the improvement of the human condition gives a perfect transition to what I see as weaknesses because they are related to my ambitious, though somewhat idealistic and unrealistic, goals.

Self-Perceived Weaknesses

I identify as an inherent weakness my tendency to strive for perfection. When driven by unrealistic expectations, perfectionism can lead to counterproductive activities and can pose a real deterrent to healthy growth and self-satisfaction. For me, the striving for perfection is a weakness because of the intense frustration that it fosters. As described later in the chapter, frustration can be the most powerfully debilitating effect of the interaction that occurs between exceptional intellectual abilities or potentialities and a severely handicapping condition. Intense frustration caused by my inability to achieve personal goals at the desired level of perfection or mastery is probably the most pervasive and interfering outcome of my disabling condition.

Another personal weakness I have identified is a tendency toward procrastination, although this tendency has diminished since my disability. Simply, in reflection it seems to me that I began to use procrastination in childhood as a mechanism to avoid the uncomfortable feelings created by the incongruence or gap between the levels of my intellectual abilities and my developed skills. For example, as a child I understood much more than I was able to communicate in any way. The imbalance between my sensitive perceptions and developed communication skills resulted in my denial of a need to communicate and in avoidance of situations requiring effort to communicate feelings and understandings. My tendency to procrastinate has diminished as my drive to succeed or to communicate effectively has become greater than the urge to avoid negative feelings and discomfort.

Another personal characteristic that I see now as a weakness has been the diversity of my interests. In my undergraduate years, each semester was an ordeal of feverish activity to gain as much knowledge as I could from each new course. The result of this diffusion of interests was my neglecting to declare an undergraduate major while pursuing three different areas of concentration; in the end, the only bachelor's degree I qualified for was a liberal arts degree in General Studies. My disabling conditions served in two ways to focus my career goals and educational objectives. First, my disability effectively eliminated many alternatives, a fact that made me value highly those areas remaining. Second, and even more important, my disability created the *need for focus*, to have specific career goals and objectives following a precise or clear path while cutting down on extraneous and unproductive efforts.

Personal Needs

In considering my personal needs relative to both strengths and weaknesses that continue to influence my achievement and level of self-fulfillment, I have identified three very broad areas. The first area is the need for some control over what I regard as my external and internal environments. Another broad area of need is to accommodate the deficiencies created by my disabling condition. The third area of need can be labeled "support" needs. These three areas of need are neither unique to disabled persons nor all-inclusive of special needs, but my disability has particularly increased their importance to me and my sense of urgency to satisfy them.

The need to have some reasonable sense of control over environmental conditions is a significant need for me and for others who have severely handicapping conditions. My condition represents an almost total loss of control over both what occurs in the external environment and internally, within my body. My external physical and social environment is determined by accessibility; that is, physical barriers continuously limit where I am able to go. Overcoming these barriers to accessibility is a continuous, tedious process requiring not only the efforts of disabled people individually and in groups but the assistance of federal, state, and local government through legislation and enforcement.

Another aspect of limited access and the loss of control over the external environment caused by a physically disabling condition is the restricted number of alternatives available to changing residential locations or to travel. Nondisabled people tend to take for granted their ability to control generally the external environment, so it may be difficult for them to understand the effects of missed opportunities, severe inconveniences, and pervasive loss of control that are inevitable consequences of a severely handicapping physical condition.

Persons with severe physical disability might reasonably be expected to have more control over their internal environment, that is, the internal physical and psychological aspects of self. However, suddenly becoming severely disabled has devastating impact on the ability to control not only body functions but psychological conditions. Instantly becoming profoundly and permanently physically disabled creates unrelenting fear, anxiety, insecurity, and a sense of hopelessness and helplessness that can be devastating in its psychological effects. I have been able, with the help of skilled professionals, to develop understandings of the interaction that occurs between my emotions and my disabling condition. I have needed professional guidance to gain the understanding of my emotional reactions to aspects of the disability and to develop my ability to cope. The loss of self-worth experienced and the need to restructure completely both self-image and the criteria used for self-evaluation make it very difficult to regain any sense of internal control over the psyche without guidance. I find that I still must continuously cope with negative feelings and the psychological implications of being severely physically disabled. For me the intense need to gain *some* feeling of control over life situations is a source of motivation to develop my strengths, especially my unimpaired intellectual abilities. It is only with the continuous refinement of my skills in problem solving, leadership, communication and interpersonal relations that I ensure some control over my environment and life situations.

Accommodating or compensating for deficiencies that develop because of a severely disabling condition is the second significant personal need. To develop all remaining abilities to their fullest potential is an essential way to counteract the effects of limitations and deficiencies. For example, I have focused on developing and refining my verbal skills because I must be able to instruct and illustrate verbally what I can no longer do physically. Equally important to me has been the development of my ability to quickly and correctly identify and solve problems.

Physical disability generally limits energies and, as a consequence, reduces the amount of activity that can be performed to complete a task or solve a problem, which makes it imperative to develop efficiency in problem solving. Accommodation for deficiencies also includes the development of abilities to direct and coordinate the efforts of those rendering personal care. This involves developing leadership and management abilities to assert control over methods, procedures, and activities that can no longer be achieved personally because of the disability. Refined verbal and written skills, leadership abilities, problem-solving skills, and sensitive understanding of interpersonal interaction are all needed skills to compensate for such handicapping conditions.

The third and probably the *most* significant need for me, and for other individuals acquiring severely physically handicapping conditions, is the need for psychological and physical support. Without the acceptance and assistance of my wife and extended family, I would not have been able to survive either the initial impact or the long-term effects of my disabling condition. My family provided aid and comfort in the early stages of my disability. My wife has provided the love, positive caring, and understanding necessary for me to accomplish my goals and develop my academic potential to my present level of achievement. In the early stages of my acquired disability, my family's willingness to learn new ways of doing things, to accommodate my dependency, and to support psychologically my physical rehabilitation were essential to my initial survival.

My wife appeared in my life and began to supply psychological support at a time when my family's support had started to become a deterrent to my development. My family had begun to react as is typical of families confronted with a member becoming severely disabled. As a consequence of sharing the disabled person's pain and frustration, family members begin to perform tasks that their disabled relative is still capable of achieving without help, or to provide excessive assistance because they cannot bear to observe the struggle. The unfortunate result of such responses is that the disabled person does not develop necessary simple skills for more independent physical accomplishments, or for achieving emotional stability, and consequently becomes increasingly dependent on the family and others providing unconstructive aid. It is difficult for members of a family, or anyone interacting with a disabled individual, to know when help is appropriate or not constructive. Such was the case in my family situation; my family was providing aid to the point that I was not developing essential skills for more independent living, and as a matter of fact, the skills I had were beginning to atrophy.

It was only through the efforts of my wife that my skills were enhanced and developed. My wife's ability to assess objectively my potential abilities and to identify my developmental progress stems from her personal experience with her own similar disability plus her exceptional sensitivity, good intuition and judgment, and extraordinary drive. At the time of our marriage, I had been a quadriplegic for two years, but her disability had been incurred almost ten years before. She had gone through stages of adjustment I had not reached as yet, and she had developed skills I had not even identified, let alone developed. She was able, as a consequence, to assess my specific needs and guide me through the painful process of rehabilitation.

It is not an overstatement to say that the psychological support my wife has provided me has been the most significant external factor contributing to the development of my academic abilities. By the powerful influence of her strong will, drive, and determined effort to see me overcome many effects of my disabling condition, she forced and nurtured the development of my skills. For example, shortly after we were married I had to undergo several extensive corrective orthopedic surgical procedures, which meant long hospital stays exceeding six to eight months at a time. My wife found out that there was a community college near the hospital and encouraged me to enroll in a course in history, a subject I love. After I finally agreed, my wife made audiotapes of the lectures, which she played for me while I lay in the hospital bed. Hour after hour, she read textbook material aloud and made notes for me at my direction—a particularly unrewarding task for her because she has no great passion for history. I passed the course and received credit for it. That incident kept alive my belief in my ability to overcome the circumstances and achieve something at a point in time when that belief was at its lowest ebb and nearly extinguished. I have observed time and time again, while in rehabilitation facilities and hospitals, that human beings who do not have "encouragers" or "support systems" lose faith in themselves, hope in the process, and vital potentialities. Often the will to live is lost because of the lack of encouraging reinforcement and validation from loved ones and those who care. My blessing has been to have not only support but exceptional encouragement in all my efforts.

Through all efforts to attain my career and life goals as an individual with a severely handicapping condition, my needs have centered on finding effective ways to accommodate the disabling condition, gaining control over my self and life, and receiving psychological support from others. These needs are not unique to me, or to any other disabled person; they are common to all human beings. The unique aspect of these needs relative to a disabled person is the critical importance of their fulfillment to overcoming the difficult life situations created by the disabling condition.

Today, I see myself as an individual who is highly competent academically, having a strong desire not only to achieve but to excel. I want to contribute to the enhancement of life experiences through a role in the shaping of policies and programs that affect important aspects of the human condition.

Personal View of Perceptions and Treatment by Others

I believe I have been fortunate to have had many persons I can describe as facilitators, who believed in and encouraged the development of my potential. For purposes of discussion, I have separated facilitators of my growth into those significant in my early development—that is, before I acquired my disability—and those who have been influential since my disability. I have further separated these facilitators according to the environmental setting in which they most influenced me: home, school, or community. This section of the chapter also addresses those I have come to regard as obstructors, who erected barriers to my development. These obstructors, real and/or perceived, also are discussed in terms of time (before and after incurring my disability) and environmental setting.

Early Facilitators and Obstructors

I regard as facilitators those persons contributing in significant, positive ways to the development of my potential intellectual and academic abilities. The earliest impact of significance on my growth, of course, was provided by my parents. Though far from being ideal parents or creating a stable home environment, they each supplied part of the foundation for my later growth. My father instilled in me a belief in unlimited possibilities, emphasizing that each individual has potentials that can be developed only through persistent, consistent personal effort. My mother recognized my academic potential early and encouraged its development. She not only gave praise for early writing and artistic efforts but supplied the necessary materials. She encouraged the family to visit museums and used passes to take us to symphony concerts, although she never showed much personal interest. It was her belief that my brothers and I should be exposed to the arts, to "culture." It is important to understand that these were unusual activities in the context of our neighborhood and our peers. My parents, each in a different way, recognized and affirmed my intellectual potential.

Those in my elementary and secondary school experiences who facilitated the development of my potential were those who recognized my special abilities and nurtured their growth. Although there were many facilitators in the educational setting, my memory focuses on two as most significant. The first was my eighth-grade history teacher, who, through her perception of my interest and potential and her teaching methods, developed my exceptional ability in history and gave me my first sense of potential for scholastic success. That specific experience represents a turning point in my beliefs about my academic abilities. The other facilitator in my early academic background was my art teacher in junior and senior high school. Through his recognition of my creative abilities and his effort to develop my artistic giftedness, he enabled me to develop a form of creative expression that has been an invaluable outlet for my deep emotions at different times in my life. These two early facilitators in the educational environment both identified, believed in, and gave special attention to the development of my special abilities. Their impact has stayed with me and has helped me believe in my abilities.

Facilitators in the community environment are much more difficult to identify. In a sense, the community was facilitative of my growth in terms of the collective values placed on education and the fact that the community presented no great obstacles to my early development. In my particular community, the church and religious education were significant facilitators of individual growth. Without elaboration it is necessary only to say that religious education provided a foundation of beliefs in the sanctity of human life, of awareness of the potential gifts within human beings, and of how to cope with adversity—especially necessary to my later development.

A lack of knowledge of giftedness in general can be identified as a major obstructor in my early educational and community environments. As a result of their lack of understanding regarding intellectual giftedness, some individuals became obstructors in that they reinforced through their inappropriately low expectations my tendency to underachieve academically. For example, in my senior year I was advised by my high school guidance counselor not to pursue a college education but rather to seek a job in one of the steel mills and perhaps get some vocational training. Of course the general lack of knowledge about giftedness, and especially gifted underachievers, at that time was more responsible for that poor advice than was a lack of sensitivity.

Facilitators and Facilitating Factors after Becoming Disabled

As I reflect on my experience after becoming disabled, I can identify some general factors that were facilitative of the development of my gifted potential. First, a major facilitator was the fact that I am highly verbal and have a disability that neither inhibits my communication verbally nor is grossly disfiguring. Disabilities that are grossly disfiguring and/or impede communication skills severely limit an individual's rehabilitation because the ability to communicate ideas, feelings, and needs is critical to the rehabilitation process and to recognition of potential abilities. Also, individuals with profoundly disfiguring disabling conditions, such as certain types of cerebral palsy and individuals with severe burns or birth defects that result in disfigurement, unfortunately make others around them uncomfortable, and consequently they do not benefit fully from the rehabilitation process. It is psychologically painful for sensitive people to undergo gross disfigurement or catastrophic body distortions. I have been fortunate in that the disfigurement of my body gradually acquired with my disability is not of a degree that causes people to shy away. In addition, being highly verbal makes communication a facilitator of my development.

Facilitators in my home environment after my disability were my parents and brothers, who supplied nurturing love and concern. Through the initial stages of my disability my family gave the emotional support, physical aid, and caring that enabled me to survive the initial stages of my disabling condition. Then, as described earlier, my wife facilitated most significantly my growth through her ability to understand the process of adjusting to a severe disability and to see beyond present situations to envision my future potential.

Unfortunately, a newly disabled person cannot expect much support from old friends. Generally, when individuals suddenly become severely disabled they tend to lose contact with friends they had before the accident or illness occurred. The reason for this tendency is the fact that friendships are based on mutual values, interests, and concerns. Those commonalities are eliminated, at least temporarily, by the disability. My case illustrates the point: the disabling condition gave me a totally different focus on life; my priorities and values changed radically from those of my friends. Life-threatening implications took precedence over all relationships in the beginning of my rehabilitation, and the continuing need to cope with the disability has created distance from prior friends. For me, there was a shying away from old friends because relationships formed before I became disabled represented the past, and coping effectively with a traumatic disability requires letting go of the past and beginning a new life. What needs to happen ideally is for disabled individuals to develop new friendships.

"The past" represents a potentially destructive force to the disabled person because it tends to divert energy away from dealing with the important issues and needs related to the current condition of life. Living life through past relationships, when times were "better" and conditions were more "normal," is not constructive. It takes great effort to resist the natural tendency to live in the past after becoming disabled. One of the ways that I have resisted that tendency is to sacrifice many friendships.

Individual educators who have facilitated the development of my potential since I became disabled are again difficult to identify. Generally, however, in higher education I have encountered many sensitive and perceptive persons who have encouraged the development of my academic potential. In university study, particularly graduate school, the investment of time and energy required of me and individual professors to develop further my academic potential has been much greater than for other students. That is, because of my limitations I have to invest great amounts of effort to develop my abilities, and the deeper my commitment to my career goals in education, the greater the investment. My drive to achieve has forced me to seek out those professors in higher education who would be helpful to me in developing my abilities and attaining my educational and career goals.

As in education, in the community setting it is difficult to identify specific individuals who have been facilitators of my development. It is in the community context that I identify facilitators in the rehabilitation process. In general, those individuals who have enhanced the growth of my potential have been those persons who have identified my specific academic abilities and have helped me focus my energies on the definition and strengthening of those potentials. The goal of all persons involved in rehabilitation activities is to develop the individual's potential, so it is difficult to single out any one person who was especially significant. It is important to say that there have been many people who have been significant contributors to my rehabilitation: medical professionals, vocational trainers, and counselors.

Obstructors after Acquiring the Disability

Although I can recall several individuals whose interaction with me created a serious impediment to my development after becoming disabled, I believe the great obstructors have been characteristics of insensitivity, ignorance, and rigid, uncreative thought generally manifested in individuals and institutions I encountered while dealing with the conditions of my disability. In reflecting on these obstructors in my experiences, I tend to perceive the principal obstructor to be an attitude of conservatism. This conservatism is an obstructor to the rehabilitation of disabled persons because of the value it places on productivity and earned rights in a society. The elements I perceive necessary for effective rehabilitation include creative, innovative thinking and experimentation with different approaches to solving problems. These elements are lost or significantly impeded when unduly conservative thought prevails.

If they are to address effectively the problems of severely disabled individuals, government agencies and social institutions must be proactive rather than simply reactive; innovative and creative rather than tradition-bound; and flexible and willing to redirect or modify efforts rather than rigid and reluctant to change. However, agencies and institutions serving individuals with profound disabilities tend to be large bureaucracies, which are by nature conservative. Such conservatism is unfortunate, because these bureaucracies providing services for disabled individuals have great impact on the lives of disabled people. For me, a significant obstructor to development in the rehabilitation process has been government agencies with an entrenched conservatism and inflexibility.

I must add that I am talking about the *structure* of agencies, rather than the individuals who work within them. The vast majority of individuals who work in rehabilitation agencies and government agencies providing services for disabled people are very sensitive to the needs of the disabled population. It is the system in which they work that inhibits the expression of that sensitivity and creates barriers to sensitive and creative action.

Statement of Specific Needs

The specific needs of gifted adults with severely disabling conditions have been discussed throughout this chapter but are summarized here. In terms of the family and home environment of individuals becoming severely disabled, I have identified several important needs. First, as has been stated earlier, the impact of suddenly being severely, permanently disabled affects not only the disabled individual but the family. The implications of having a severely disabled family member can test family unity, strength, and stability. For the disabled individual there is a greater need for family stability and support, especially through the early stages of disability.

The importance of psychological and physical support cannot be emphasized enough. This support is essential for survival. In the home environment, as in other environments, there needs to be a basic understanding and knowledge of giftedness and of how that affects or interacts with the individual's disabling condition. If a person who has become disabled has been identified as having gifted potential before acquiring the disability, family awareness of the possible consequences of interaction between the individual's giftedness and the handicapping condition can help them understand the behaviors that may result from that interaction. This knowledge can contribute to more realistic expectations for the disabled individual that affirm the giftedness and the potential ability to accommodate the impairment so that achievement can occur.

In the first stages of a disability the needs of the gifted disabled individual in the medical setting are similar to those of a nongifted person. That is, all medical efforts are directed toward stabilizing the disabling condition and providing treatment necessary to maintain and to strengthen physiological functioning. It is only after the initial impact of the disabling condition that the needs of the gifted disabled individual in services from medical professionals become unique. At this point, the patient needs the services of medical professionals who understand the nature of giftedness and are committed to cooperating with other professionals in evaluating and directing activities designed to utilize fully and develop gifted potential. Medical professionals all too often leave the responsibility for assessment of reasonable goals for rehabilitation to other professionals and limit their involvement to specific aspects of medical treatment. There is a need for medical professionals to be involved in and to provide input through all stages of a gifted disabled individual's development, especially in the assessment of educational programs and the physical requirements of activities they entail, and in formulating the overall prognosis.

The needs of individuals with gifted potential and severely handicapping conditions in the school setting include professionals with accurate knowledge about the educational implications of the disability and the giftedness. This need requires educational professionals to be sensitive to and knowledgeable of the potential interactions between the attributes of the individual's giftedness and the disabling conditions. It is a responsibility of educators in school settings to be sensitive to needs not only for physical barrier removal but for identifying and fulfilling the intellectual and social needs necessary to maximize the individual's gifted potential.

In the community there is a need for awareness of the barriers to access that exist, architectural barriers preventing physical access to buildings and barriers preventing access to the opportunities for participation in community activities.

The latter category includes failure to encourage the participation of disabled persons. In some communities it is assumed that the community responsibility ends with eliminating physical barriers; too often there is a total lack of encouragement of or opportunity for participation by disabled individuals in community events.

DISCUSSION

I believe there are some accurate ways to describe how society has viewed *all* severely disabled people, not just those with spinal cord injuries. In general, it seems individuals with severely handicapping conditions have been viewed to varying degrees in the following ways: (a) as burdens to the society that is responsible for their comfort and care; (b) as naive children who need to be protected from the world rather than given opportunity for active participation; (c) as objects of pity and charity, a view that regards severely disabled persons in terms of abnormality and differences instead of similarities to others; (d) as manifestations of the work of a wrathful and vengeful deity and, occasionally, as retribution for evil doings. Granted, these perspectives and views are historical and generalized, but in my experience it has been evident that society has been slow to eliminate them.

With the growth of social activism and social awareness in the 1960s and 1970s came a sensitivity to and awareness of the rights of disabled persons to physical access to facilities and also rights to full development of their potential for active participation in society. With this awareness has come the elimination of many architectural and attitudinal barriers. Society needs to be in the continuous process of becoming aware of the needs of disabled persons and selecting the most appropriate plans of action. Currently it seems society is in danger of again being guilty of "benign neglect" because of the assumption that all social or environmental barriers to severely disabled persons have been eliminated. In reality these barriers, both physical and attitudinal, exist, continue to be erected, and constantly need to be recognized and eliminated.

Description of the Disabling Condition

It is estimated that in the United States there are 500,000 individuals with spinal cord injuries, with approximately 15,000 new cases each year. The major causes of injury to spinal cords have been automobile accidents, war-related activities, and sports accidents, most often in diving.

Although there has been some dramatic medical research, spinal cord injuries or nerve damage to the spinal cord have been considered permanent. The nerves in the spinal cord do not have the regenerative capacity of the peripheral nerves located outside the spinal cord. Researchers have not been able to identify why spinal cord nerve tissue does not regenerate. As a consequence, individuals who have spinal cord injuries, in the majority of cases, are considered to be permanently impaired in motor and sensory function. There are a variety of complex physical, psychological, and emotional implications of spinal cord injury. The following discussion provides a general overview of the complexities of these implications.

The physical consequences of spinal cord injuries are motor and sensory impairment. The degree of impairment is determined by the location and extent of damage to the spinal cord. In very general terms, the closer to the head an injury occurs, the more extensively the body is affected. Individuals who have spinal cord damage at the level of the upper back, called the upper thoracic region, generally are quadriplegic—that is, they have impairment involving all four limbs. Persons with spinal cord injuries below the upper thoracic region generally are paraplegic—that is, they have impairment in the lower half of their bodies. The implications derived from the level of injury to the spinal cord are important in determining the amount of self-sufficiency an individual can expect to attain. For many quadriplegics it is difficult to gain a significant degree of self-sufficiency.

Besides the motor impairment involved, there are other medical consequences of spinal cord injuries, which fall into three major categories:

- diminished respiratory capacity
- susceptibility to kidney infection and/or dysfunction, including kidney stone formation
- complications arising from lack of active use of muscles and tendons

Diminished respiratory capacity is a serious medical problem for those with higher-level spinal cord injury because the involvement of chest muscles results in an inability to expand the lungs or expel inhaled material. At higher levels of injury, special provisions, such as periodic use of a respirator, may be necessary.

The next potentially major medical consequence of spinal cord injury is kidney dysfunction, produced by infection or calcium deposit formation. Typically, an individual with a spinal cord injury has frequent incidents of kidney infection, which can result in high blood pressure and/or fluid retention. Spinal cord–injured people must take long-term treatments of antibiotics to help counteract kidney and urinary tract infections.

The last major medical problem for the spinal cord–injured person is a consequence of muscle inactivity, which causes muscles and tendons to atrophy. The effects of muscle inactivity can to some extent be minimized by exercise requiring passive muscle movement to maintain flexibility. Muscles and tendons start to shorten because of a lack of use, and contractions, which are very painful if sensation has not been affected by the spinal cord injury, occur. These contractions occur mainly in the extremities—arms, legs, fingers, and hands—and can cause functional problems, such as an inability to open and close the hand, leaving the person with permanently clasped fingers.

It is important to understand that there are wide variations and differences among individuals in the functional disabilities and other medical problems associated with spinal cord injury. However, spinal cord injury always has a devastating impact on both body functions and life conditions.

Although the medical problems caused by spinal cord injury are immediately life-threatening, it is the psychological and social consequences that ultimately determine the individual's survival. Adequate discussion of the complex processes of adjustment, both psychological and social, to an instantaneously profoundly handicapping condition cannot be provided in the space of a chapter. It is, however, necessary to provide the reader with some insights into the psychological impact of suddenly becoming disabled.

Generally, individuals who suffer severe trauma that results in a profound and permanent disability have stages of readjustment in which they must rebuild their self-perceptions; they suddenly have a different self-image that they unequivocally reject. Individuals acquiring a physically disabling condition must develop new sets of values by which to define themselves, others, and their environment. Every aspect of self-perception is changed totally. The psychological impact can be described as traumatic, so without helpful direction and guidance there is high probability that the individual will not be able to become psychologically healthy in terms of self-concept, self-esteem, and perception of others and of reality.

After my accident I found myself on an emotional "island" with no visible reference points, with nothing in my experience to draw upon to give me a more secure or confident perspective. My feelings were typical of the isolation, insecurity, and total bewilderment experienced by individuals who suddenly become disabled. Depression, periods of unrealistic expectations of self and others, denial, and self-delusion regarding the future become very serious problems. Finding emotional balance, even self-assessment of overall psychological state, requires a continuous groping through the murky waters of emotional and psychological disorientation. Without the help of sensitive professionals, individuals easily become suicidal, lethargic, or manic-depressive, or develop any number of psychological maladjustments. It is painful for me to recall the feelings of total confusion and disorientation that came with my disability.

The environment and social implications, as distinct from psychological and emotional consequences, of becoming severely disabled are more specific and straightforward. These environmental and social implications can be summarized by the phrase "opportunity to access." When an individual becomes severely disabled, especially when the use of a wheelchair becomes necessary for mobility, there are environmental limitations on opportunities to access programs, places, and people. Barriers to physical access severely limit the affected individual's ability to function within the environment. Of course, the limited access to facilities also has the obvious social consequence of barring participation or restricting opportunity to engage in social activities and functions.

Efforts to eliminate the recognizable environmental limitations have misled society's institutions and individuals into believing most barriers to access have been eliminated. Unfortunately, what in reality has happened is that only the most identifiable, significant, and obvious barriers are eliminated. Many barriers to the use of services and facilities, such as those of public buildings, educational institutions, and large businesses, have been eliminated. In spite of these improvements, it still is not unusual for a disabled person who uses a wheelchair to confront daily physical barriers that deny access to public facilities.

Social implications of the disabling condition, not directly related to physical environmental limitations and barriers to access, involve a general lack of knowledge and understanding of disabling conditions derived from personal interaction with disabled people. A consequence of the general lack of social interaction between disabled and nondisabled individuals is the creation in disabled persons of feelings of isolation and rejection by society. These feelings become psychological barriers in both groups. Every day, as with the physical environmental barriers, I face the social implications of my disability; it is a constant struggle against the feelings of loneliness, isolation, and disengagement from much of the normal social interactions.

Rehabilitation Following Spinal Cord Injury

The treatment of a patient with spinal cord injury, or any severely disabling condition, involves an extensive rehabilitation process. Rehabilitation usually involves hospitalization, medical treatment, physical therapy, psychological therapy, and vocational/educational therapy. Rehabilitation efforts focus on different aspects at different times and in different settings, as determined by various professionals involved in the process. Although there is no one definition of rehabilitation, a working definition I find functionally valuable is the process that encompasses a variety of components designed to bring physical, psychological, social, and environmental adjustment and improvement to profoundly disabling life conditions. The process and progress of rehabilitation varies according to the extent of the disability and the efforts of the disabled person, and according to differing philosophies and technical approaches espoused by the professionals providing services.

It is the general aim of rehabilitation to make an individual as independent as possible. In the past, the emphasis in rehabilitation has been on helping disabled individuals become productive members of society by developing their employ-ability. Programs were designed and directed toward the goal of producing individuals with marketable skills, often at the expense of neglected intellectual abilities. My initial rehabilitation program emphasized the immediate identifica-tion of an employable skill, such as using a calculator or becoming proficient at using a typewriter or computer keyboard. In recent years, program emphases have seemed to shift toward more use of vocational guidance or career counseling, which employs test instruments to provide a profile of the individual's interests and abilities to guide the development of appropriate educational/vocational programs. This shift in emphasis is placing much more importance on higher education as a possible vehicle for rehabilitation.

The emphasis in rehabilitation through higher education has not shifted away from employability as an outcome, however. Unfortunately, rehabilitation pro-grams often fail to assist individuals in accurately establishing realistic life goals, so they often formulate unrealistic expectations regarding employment oppor-tunities that may result from having a college degree. The popularity of the shift in emphasis from occupational training in rehabilitation centers to educational train-ing programs in higher education seems to be related to the ease of administration created by well-defined, structured curriculum; explicit time requirements with precise outcomes; and standardized methods of evaluating individual progress in the program. It is only recently that college-based vocational/educational training has become popular for severely disabled persons, with more tailoring of educa-tional and training goals to individual interests, needs, and abilities.

Educational Expectations and Programming

As I stated earlier in the chapter, becoming severely disabled focused my energy on identifying and developing special potential within me. That is, becoming severely disabled created the imperative that I develop all potential and unaffected abilities in order to survive. It sparked in me the first significant amount of motivation to actively pursue educational goals.

Educational opportunities for disabled persons are critically influenced by the policies and values of the agencies and professionals delivering rehabilitative services. Government agencies tend to be most influential since they are the major funding source for rehabilitation programs and services. These agencies are empowered to dictate the direction and focus of individual educational programs. For example, a government agency's policy and values may result in an emphasis on training programs centered on experiential, "hands-on" training for vocational trades through internships and apprenticeships. On the other hand, a government agency may value higher education as a suitable path to vocational rehabilitation and, in fact, may prefer highly structured professional programs that lead to certification or licensure.

Too often educational programs are approved for an individual by an agency primarily to accommodate bureaucratic needs or desires for a program that is clearly defined and narrow in scope—one that provides defensible and measurable objectives, has consistent curriculum structure, and delineates the time requirements for program completion. The type of program approved may be incompatible with the educational activities necessary for the disabled person to maximize intellectual abilities and potential for academic achievement and professional contributions. Both the disabled person and the rehabilitation professional may be unaware of academic potential and consequently the inappropriateness of the selected program.

To serve adequately gifted individuals who are severely disabled, the personnel implementing rehabilitation programs must engage in open-minded problem solving using creative, innovative, and nontraditional ideas. Without variety and flexibility in approaches, it is unlikely that programs will be created or selected that will optimally develop the special abilities and the intellectual giftedness of the disabled person. Flexibility often is diminished in governmental agencies and bureaucratic institutions by their need for accountability, consistency, administrative control, measurable results, and complete documentation to justify all services rendered. These needs result in such practices as unnecessarily slow responses to requests, inflexible procedures, and rigid application of eligibility criteria.

Disabled individuals may fail to pursue programs that nourish their intellectual abilities because they may feel that there is no alternative other than to acquiesce to the desires of educational program developers. As a result, they may enter into training programs that have vocational goals incompatible with personal interests, values, and abilities. The need for a specific rationale for an educational or rehabilitation program, justified by documentation of ability through standardized testing, may discriminate against many persons for whom the measurement may not be either predictive of future success or accurately reflective of ability. Although the limited value of standardized tests in making educational decisions about an individual is recognized, tests continue to be used inappropriately as the sole justification for program funding. This tendency results in the placement of gifted individuals with disabling conditions in programs that are inappropriate, understimulating, and unchallenging relative to their personal desires and giftedness. For these reasons, it is important that appropriately trained educators in higher education be responsible for more accurate assessment of individual abilities and selection of appropriate educational goals and programs.

Indicators of Intellectual Giftedness

Early recognition of giftedness is critical to the full development of gifted potential. There are reliable indicators of cognitive ability that can guide a search for intellectual giftedness in youngsters. My own case illustrates some possibilities.

The first indicator of my special abilities was my drive to express myself creatively, both in artistic and literary (poetic) forms. As I reflect on my childhood, it was the drive, the inner direction and compulsion to be creative, that were natural indicators of my potential intellectual abilities. Artistic creativity alone may not have been an indicator, but in conjunction with other creative behavior, it apparently was a reliable indicator of gifted potential. Other primary indicators of my potential cognitive abilities were my natural skills in communication, oral and written, and my intense desire or drive to communicate effectively with others. Another indication of my giftedness were my advanced problem-solving skills, which included exceptional capacities for analytical and creative thinking. My problem-solving abilities or competencies were evidenced not only in the academic realm but in interpersonal relationships and the ability to analyze social interaction.

Intellectual giftedness, or the potential for intellectual achievement, was manifested in some other personal characteristics, I believe. Two attributes that have been associated with intellectual giftedness (Whitmore, 1980) are my tendency toward unhealthy levels of perfectionism, accompanying acute self-criticism, and oversensitivity to the feelings and needs of others. Another characteristic, common to many gifted youngsters, was my diffused wide range of interests and a difficulty in focusing my energies on one particular area with a goal of mastery or developing expertise. The last characteristic I can identify as a possible indicator of giftedness is my compelling drive to use all my abilities to impact positively on the human condition. I have always found myself gravitating toward social activism to eliminate inequities, intolerance, and suffering I perceive existing in our society.

Major obstacles to the identification of intellectual giftedness in severely disabled adults fall into three major categories. The first category of obstacles are related to an inability to recognize giftedness because of ignorance about its characteristics and nature. The second category of obstacles pertains to failure to consider or look for possible cognitive strengths or superior intellectual attributes in severely disabled persons. The third category contains obstacles to identification that result from rigidity and uncreative thought—that is, rigid and inaccurate expectations for both gifted and disabled persons, inflexibly bonded to traditional methods of identifying and serving both groups.

The assessment methods and procedures used to identify intellectual giftedness and to evaluate the potential for achievement in rehabilitation by disabled individuals must be continually questioned and improved. New, more effective methods of assessment must include reports, by trained observers, derived from opportunities to observe the individual's intellectual abilities manifested in an educational setting.

Potential Interaction between Giftedness and the Incurred Disability

It is difficult to categorize the interactions between characteristics of giftedness and a severe disability as having totally positive or negative impact on the affected person. The complex interactions that occur can have equally constructive and destructive effects. For example, my tendency toward perfectionism has had positive impact in that it has made me continually strive to better all my efforts, to refine my activities, and to reject merely adequate goals or achievement. Negative effects of my perfectionism have been the frustration induced and my tendency to expend undesirably large amounts of limited energies refining small details and insignificant activities. The latter has been a destructive consequence for me in that it often has depleted my limited energy needed for more important tasks.

The complexity of the interactions between a disability and giftedness is increased by the range of individual variations relative to the specific profile of gifted attributes as well as the degree and nature of the limitations imposed by the disabling condition. Therefore, all possible interactions and effects cannot be identified precisely. The interaction between gifted characteristics and conditions of disability in my own case serves to illustrate some potential effects of this interaction on life experiences of the severely disabled adult. The following discussion presents some specific categories of effect on life conditions; both positive and negative aspects of each category are considered simultaneously as appropriate.

Frustration

The most significant and pervasive product of interaction between my giftedness and my disability has been intense frustration. Frustration for me is a product of the great gap between my cognitive perception of a desired outcome or goal and my severe limitations in actual physical ability and energy to realize that goal. In general, frustration increases commensurate with the distance between my desired actions or goals and the actual level of my ability to perform, as affected by the interfering physical limitations. I perceive intellectual giftedness as a mixed blessing because the increased perception of possibilities and motivation to achieve intensifies extreme levels of frustration created by the disabling conditions and heightened awareness of the significance of the goals.

Psychologists have explained frustration as a consequence of blocked or unrealized needs and goals; it is irrational in most of its manifestations, can be severely debilitating in its psychological and physical effects, and is difficult to accommodate and control by traditional methods of compensating and coping. Many adults becoming disabled have abandoned their goals because of seemingly insurmountable barriers and unbearably intense frustration required to pursue them.

In my personal life there are countless examples of frustration and its effects. Daily I am faced with restrictions interfering with attaining goals or satisfying needs. I must cope continually with my tendency to avoid difficult goal-directed activities, to eliminate the goal altogether, or to alter my goal(s) and deny my needs. If I succumb to those emotional tendencies, the consequences can be more debilitating than any relief obtained. Therefore, I have developed a variety of strategies to overcome frustration or to modify its debilitating effects.

First of all, the extent to which I have been successful in compensating for the personal effects of continuous, acute frustration seems to have been directly related to my problem-solving ability. I continuously engage in a process of identifying specific barriers to goal achievement and evaluating alternative courses of action I can take to circumvent frustration and increase the possibility of success. An everyday example of coping with frustration is trying to guide a nondisabled person to do a ''simple'' mechanical operation or physical task that I am unable to do, such as tying a necktie. To reduce frustration in the process I develop very precise steps to explain the task, even to the extent of writing them out in clear, understandable order, going through each step one by one until the task is learned. The effect for me is to reduce frustration by making the activity a manageable training task instead of an impossible physical task. By making a problem or an activity one that draws upon my intellectual resources, I have de-emphasized my inability and emphasized my abilities. The psychological consequence is to strengthen my motivation to persevere.

Other methods I have used to reduce the effects of frustration involve altering my objectives or goals in terms of the levels of aspiration and importance, or accepting an alternative goal as a substitute. These methods are illustrated by how I coped with blocked educational and professional goals that I had set before my accident. Before acquiring my disability, I had intended to study in Europe for a career in international relations. My disability made that goal unattainable because of the related physical, emotional, and economic limitations. Although it might have been possible to gain sufficient financial resources to accomplish my goal after becoming disabled, the difficulties involved in travel, including securing personal care, and gaining physical access to many buildings and sites, were too great for me to confront. So I altered my plans and set goals in an alternative field of study with different educational, career, and life objectives. My new goal fortunately has resulted in a plan for my career and life aspirations that is completely compatible with my abilities, values, and personality. I have found it important to evaluate carefully the decision to change a goal because there is a danger of restricting myself unnecessarily, or in ways that would be counterproductive—a danger of using the frustration involved as a excuse not to pursue a particular goal.

My cognitive ability to perceive and understand the circumstances and the necessity for accomplishing particular goals contributes both to heightened frustration and to my ability to limit the negative effects of that frustration. That is, through having a clear understanding of the rationale for specific activities and desired outcomes, I may be able to reduce feelings of frustration through rationalization and reflection. The following anecdote illustrates a rehabilitation activity that created in me an abundance of intense frustration and how I used rational understanding of the necessity and long-term advantages of that activity to reduce the crippling levels of frustration and to persevere until I achieved the goal.

One of the first areas of rehabilitation activity is to develop what is called "aids to daily living," commonly referred to as ADL. The objective of ADL activities is to develop in the disabled person as much independence as possible. The first of ADL activities was learning to feed myself. Because of severely limited muscle function and weakness, the "simple" task of bringing a spoon from a plate to my mouth was a seemingly insurmountable task. The activity was made into an ordeal by the use of a swivel spoon (a spoon that is hinged so that the bowl of the spoon remains level at any angle). The apparatus works well but has one major flaw: the spoon bowl has a tendency to become highly unstable, swinging back and forth with the slightest uneven movement. Since my hand and arm muscles were weak, they had a tendency to tremble with exertion and fatigue; as a consequence, any contents of the spoon would spill out because of the frantic swinging action of the swiveling bowl. After several weeks of continuously trying to put food onto the spoon, after locating the plate from my horizontal position in bed, I was ready to try to put food into my mouth.

As the time came closer for my attempt to feed myself, my determination was piqued. I knew this was an important step to becoming more independent and an obstacle that I had to overcome. It was my misfortune that my first attempt to put food into my mouth was on a day when spaghetti was on the cafeteria menu! The idea of attempting to put spaghetti noodles on an extremely unstable swivel spoon, and then trying carefully to bring the contents to my mouth, was enough to cloud from my mind any positive value of the activity. The first several passes at the lukewarm noodles gave no promise for success; the frustration and tension mounted. The harder I concentrated, the more my arms trembled and the more frantically the swivel spoon swung, dumping its contents. Noodles slipped from the spoon, leaving traces of greasy tomato sauce on the floor, tray, my lap, and shirt. But I tried again. Success was a short, cold spaghetti noodle on the end of a shaky spoon that reached my mouth just as both my strength and my faith were waning away. The accomplishment was insignificant to others, but I knew it was a great step toward independence.

Though there were many frustrating hours before I was able to manage a complete meal independently, my ability to perceive the significance of this initial success, and to focus on the implications for my future, helped me temper feelings of frustration and despair to persist in my efforts. This small incident in the rehabilitation process does illustrate how knowledge and understanding of the significance of an activity has helped me manage, control, and reduce frustration and its consequences.

To summarize, for me the most effective means of managing frustration caused by the interaction of intellectual giftedness and my disabling condition have been the following:

- being able to analyze and evaluate in a creative problem-solving process
- changing the levels of aspiration or priority, or choosing an alternative acceptable goal
- analyzing and understanding the necessity of the activities to temper the feelings of frustration and to sustain motivation to persist

These tactics have enabled me to reduce and manage unavoidable feelings of intense frustration.

Social Isolation

Conditions of severe disability inevitably create feelings of social isolation, separateness, and aloneness because of diminished opportunities for interpersonal interaction. When intellectual giftedness is an attribute of the disabled person, the consequence may be greater feelings of isolation and loneliness that result from high motivation to communicate, to relate, and to be socially influential. Severe limitations on social interaction also has significant consequences for the development of superior communication skills and for the growth of possible leadership abilities in persons with gifted intellectual potential.

Like most gifted youngsters (American Association for Gifted Children, 1978), it seems I have always felt different from most of my family, friends, and associates because my perceptions, understandings, and conclusions so often were different. My perceptions have not necessarily been better or clearer than those of others, just different. For me, feeling different has been at times difficult and uncomfortable throughout my life. The visible, verifiable physical difference my disability created in early adulthood, combined with my already existing feelings of difference, creates at times almost unbearable feelings of separation and loneliness.

In my case, limited social participation was the result of a protective home environment in my childhood and the reduction of opportunities in adulthood to interact socially, created by long hospital stays and severely limited mobility. The effect of my insufficient social participation was the development of unrealistic expectations for social relationships after the rehabilitation and difficulty in perceiving accurately the various roles of individuals in different social environments. One example that comes to my mind was my first experience as a graduate intern in a college office setting. I expected individuals to be open about their feelings and attitudes toward me and my actions. I had come from hospital settings and a home environment in which people were used to my difference, and in which

I had become accustomed to open, frank interactions without many constraints. I expected my new fellow employees to understand, with little explanation, my needs and feelings in the office setting. I focused my attention on the tasks and the responsibilities I had in the office and failed to develop any interpersonal relationships. The result was disastrous. Because I failed to communicate with them and to develop personal relationships, the unexpressed discomfort—related to my difference—of my co-workers and supervisors eventually became manifested in ill feelings and misunderstandings. I was perceived as being aloof, cold, rigid, and not very cooperative.

Though the office experience taught me a lot, it was unnecessarily painful and did intensify my feelings of isolation and desire to withdraw socially. It took over a year for me to venture again into an employment setting, partially because of not wanting to re-create those feelings of isolation and difference. I believe that as a result of that experience, in subsequent years I have developed more realistic and responsive interpersonal skills, with greater sensitivity to and understanding of the behavior and feelings of others. A completely different set of work experiences has resulted from my later efforts to communicate my needs, to build personal relationships, and to help co-workers become comfortable with me.

Dependence, Lack of Control

I was used to being independent when my accident occurred. Being self-sufficient had become a vital part of my self-image. After being injured, I rigorously fought losing that independence. A fierce desire to be independent has been described as a characteristic of intellectually gifted children, and it certainly has been characteristic of my personality.

After becoming disabled, I became part of an environment that required me to be almost totally dependent on others for every aspect of my survival. The result was a pervasive sense of helplessness and a total loss of feeling of being able to control any aspect of my being. These feelings of extreme dependence and loss of control in turn fostered feelings of despair and futility that had to be controlled in order for any progress to be made through rehabilitation. My disability had totally incapacitated me; that is, I had lost control over all body functions and voluntary muscle movements. Therefore, I was totally dependent on others for all physical activities. This complete dependence was particularly frustrating as my condition stabilized and I started to comprehend with agony the permanence and totality of my condition.

The hospital environment initially required for the severely disabled unintentionally fosters dependency and destroys any sense of personal efficacy. Hospitals are institutions that of necessity demand control. From the moment a patient enters a hospital, procedures are taken to exert control over that patient. These controls range from insisting on the wearing of identification tags to the regulation and control of all aspects of life, such as when and what can be eaten, when medications are given and prescribed, times for sleep, and times for activity. Beneficial interaction between hospital personnel and patients who understand the medical aspects of their condition is rare, because the medical profession generally operates on the assumption that its members alone know what is best for patients—that only medical professionals understand what is appropriate and that only they can provide treatment. When confronted with a patient questioning orders for medication or therapeutic treatment, hospital personnel tend to tighten controls further.

Hospitals have ways of enforcing their wishes upon individual patients that would be considered inappropriate in other settings. These enforcement behaviors are seen as not only appropriate in the hospital context but as the responsibility of competent hospital personnel. For example, when I refused to take a particular test or treatment because I did not understand the rationale for it or believed that the test was being duplicated, all services to me were stopped until there was resolution of the conflict to the satisfaction of the staff. That is, all personal care services were suspended: bathing, dressing, and sometimes meals were delayed, and medications were cancelled. The patient learns that, although a particular treatment or test may indeed be inappropriate or unnecessary, it is important to weigh the possible consequences of questioning or refusing to follow the directions given. Usually the patient's conclusion is that it is better to comply than to face the consequences.

These characteristics of a hospital environment rapidly develop in the patient feelings of helplessness and powerlessness. Ironically, even in rehabilitation hospitals, where there is an emphasis on developing individual independence, personnel still carry out treatment with the same institutional needs for control and conformity. It is only through continuous effort of the disabled person to become an increasingly active participant in all aspects of daily activities that the effects of being in such controlling environments, which foster dependence, can be overcome. The intellectually gifted person seems more naturally to resist such treatment and to persevere until some sense of efficacy is regained.

Although my physical abilities have increased with therapy and I have consequently gained some control over internal and external environments, I still am dependent and always will be dependent on others to aid me in physically managing my life. The difference today is that I understand what I can control in my life and how I can use my abilities to maintain some degree of control. I am able to direct all of the personal care activities that I am unable to perform physically myself; I am able to train individuals and to explain step-by-step procedures for helping maintain my physical condition. This is a result of continuous effort to gain independence combined with the knowledge and acceptance of my actual limitations. It is a process that continues and is a result of understanding gained through analysis of my abilities and continuous learning experiences.

Limited Energy

The limited amount of physical and psychological energy associated with an acquired severe disability produces a negative effect on the gifted individual's tendency to pursue intellectual interests. No longer can I maintain and pursue the wide range of interests I once had, because I no longer have the energy required. My limited energy creates for me the need to prioritize my interests to determine which ones I will pursue. Consequently, I focus my energies now on more specific objectives, courses of study, and educational activities that will most effectively help me achieve my academic and career goals. This requires very clear and precise thinking about my direction and long-term plans.

Another product of the interaction between my diversity of interests and limited energies is the need to become increasingly efficient in my activities and procedures. No longer do I have the luxury of expending energies frivolously or unnecessarily. My energy has become a precious commodity that I preserve and reserve for what I consider are the most important activities. There is a danger in this, obviously, if priorities are misdirected or if too much emphasis in one area sacrifices other important areas. For example, if I invest too much energy in educational or career activities, it is likely that I will not have enough energy to pursue important interpersonal relationships and social activities. I see the need to evaluate continuously how I expend my energies and how I can use my resources most effectively to accomplish my life goals.

Coping, Adapting

My creative abilities have significantly influenced my rehabilitation and the impact of my disability. Artistic creativity has enabled me to express deep feelings that, because of my disability, I had limited ways of expressing. Artistic creativity, especially through painting, has provided both a useful diversion from daily physical rehabilitation activities and an outlet for pent-up feelings.

Besides artistic creativity discussed earlier as an outlet for expressing feelings, my imagination and ability to be innovative have enabled me to survive some of the most difficult times during the rehabilitation process. For example, during the first several years of my disability I spent much of my time lying on a Foster frame (a type of bed that is used to change the position of a person without disturbing the body alignment; the only possible positions on most of these devices are face up and face down, alternating every two hours). Many months passed during which I was either flat on my back or on my stomach, with only the floor or ceiling within my visual field. I began to think of ways to design and shape devices to improve the conditions of patients like me. I invented in my mind wheelchairs with casters designed to reduce the turning radius, utensils shaped for more effective use, an arrangement of mirrors to enable me to watch television and to observe faces when turned toward the floor, and devices to allow me to hold books and turn pages. All of these "inventions," implemented or not, came from mental activities that helped me pass many tedious hours and gave me a sense of active participation in my treatment. My creative imagination distracted me from feelings of fear and disrupted the boredom of that period of hospitalization.

Creativity has helped me to continue expressing emotions and feelings through painting. I have de-emphasized painting recently because the energy required has effectively eliminated it as my major creative communication tool, but I have begun to engage more in creative communication through writing and public speaking in a variety of settings. I have found I am able to use my creativity to communicate more effectively, and it brings to me a unique sense of satisfaction and worth.

Analytical problem-solving skills also have significantly influenced my ability to adapt and cope with my disability. I define one such skill as the ability to identify the problem and to assess the significance and implications of the problem situation. A second skill for problem solving is the ability to develop alternatives, to create a variety of courses of action. The third aspect of problem solving is implementing those courses of action. This activity involves being the catalyst for activity—providing leadership, definition, and direction for the efforts—and supervising the process. A fourth problem-solving skill is evaluating the action. This activity requires judging whether the problem has been solved and evaluating the necessity for further action to achieve desired goals. This ability to analyze and solve problems permeates the content of this chapter. Superior problem-solving skills are significant facilitators of rehabilitation because they enable the affected individual to develop strategies for adapting and coping with the disability and for designing ways to foster the growth of gifted abilities.

Another characteristic of gifted potential that has facilitated adaptation and coping is my tenacity and drive. I have an ability to stick to a project to see it through its end, sometimes to a fault. When this stubborn characteristic interacts with my physical limitations, it results in an ability to be persistent in striving to achieve a desired goal or objective. Although I am tenacious, I have not always been so consistently. That is, my disability has made it imperative that I control not only the direction but the intensity of my drive to achieve a particular objective. What can happen, and has happened to me, is that I have been driven toward achieving a specific goal at the expense of physical health and interpersonal relationships, with a singular vision that can certainly be a destructive element. This drive is by far more constructive than destructive in its effect; it has been invaluable throughout my disability and has enabled me to accomplish goals and activities that, without being stubbornly driven, I would not have accomplished.

These interactions of gifted characteristics and my disabling condition have both positive and negative implications, depending on varying circumstances. Generally, the consequences of possessing gifted potential have been enhanced feelings of self-worth; an ability to clearly analyze myself and my situation, to adapt and to cope; and motivation to nurture my abilities and to pursue my goals. On the negative side, attributes of giftedness have intensified my frustration, my discontent with being so dependent, and my sense of social discomfort and isolation.

SPECIFIC GUIDELINES

Family and Friends

The first, and to me the most striking, need of a newly disabled individual to be met by family and friends is for assistance in minimizing feelings of social isolation and in developing new relationships and interpersonal skills. I have seen very assertive, gregarious, and extroverted adult personalities almost totally withdraw after suffering a severe and traumatic disability. Feelings of isolation or wanting to withdraw from social interaction may be difficult to recognize in the disabled adult in the highly protective environments of hospitals, rehabilitation settings, or homes, in which individuals feel protected and comfortable. A lack of manifestation is the primary reason those feelings of social isolation have tended to be overlooked in the rehabilitation process. It also may be assumed erroneously that an individual who has been identified as intellectually gifted will have no difficulty developing the ability to interact socially or to re-establish interpersonal relationships. Thus, a primary area of need is ignored by family and friends.

As I mentioned earlier, I have always struggled with uncomfortable feelings of being different, and the obvious physical difference after injury created an overwhelming impulse to withdraw and avoid the unbearable pain of social interaction. Family members and friends frequently do not perceive the social discomfort and the impulse to withdraw and therefore do not address adequately the individual's need for supportive assistance. They also can be helpful by sensitizing professionals to the disabled adult's social needs.

Family members and friends may have an important role in guiding the newly disabled adult in a search for effective ways to adapt to the handicapping conditions and to nurture the growth of gifted potential. One way to help is by guiding the individual to focus mental energies on exploring a limited number of alternatives from which to choose ultimately a specific path for long-range development of gifted abilities. Any person, but especially the severely disabled, needs a helpful companion in the search for ways to experience life to its fullest potential, to develop fully special abilities, and to enhance contributions and life satisfactions.

Certainly the psychological support of family members and friends can provide some comfort and strength as the individual experiences the emotional shock, the intense frustration, and the impulse to totally withdraw evoked by the newly acquired condition. The support of loving persons can prevent severe mental illness from developing. In my hospital visits I have seen intense frustration and denial—an inability to accept, to accommodate, and to cope with a severe disability—result in suicide, catatonic withdrawal, and chemical dependency. It is extremely difficult for me to communicate an accurate sense of the psychological consequences of a permanently, profoundly disabling condition. Although the pain of altered roles and expectations for the future significantly affects all persons close to the injured adult, strength must come from a support system of loved ones so that the patient can direct energies toward physical survival.

To provide the needed psychological support and appropriate assistance, family members and significant others must recognize the exceptional potential of the gifted disabled individual. They must be as much aware of the person's intellectual potential as the medical/physical problems of the disabling condition, and also must understand the potential interaction between the individual's giftedness and the disabling condition. Parents and providers of support are the major facilitators of treatment programs, so their active direction is essential to the identification and development of gifted abilities.

The specific roles of parents and supporters of gifted disabled individuals vary according to how well each gifted disabled person is able to assume responsibility for personal care. However, all support persons assume the following roles: (a) rigorous observers of the individual's behavior, (b) primary facilitators of the individual's gifted potential, and (c) coordinators of services (medical, physical, and educational) for the gifted disabled person. To fulfill those roles effectively, parents and other supporters must be equipped with information and understanding, gained from medical, psychological, educational, and social service professionals, regarding the person's potential and limitations, reasonable expectations, alternative methods of facilitating rehabilitation, and resources available to stimulate or guide the development of the gifted disabled individual's abilities. The more accurate and extensive the information, the better prepared parents or supporters are to fulfill the roles effectively. A critical factor to the rehabilitation process consequently is the ability of parents or supporters to judge the extent to which information provided by professionals is accurate and sufficient, and whether or not services being rendered are appropriate.

Medical and Rehabilitation Professionals

Professionals trained to help individuals recover from severe injury and to adapt to specific handicaps resulting from the injury also must have adequate and accurate information in order to evaluate individual potential much more accurately than has been the case in the past. The need for complete information has always been recognized in the medical community and in the rehabilitation process, but this need has been addressed in ways that have not been adequate. The need for complete information about disabled individuals has led to the use of a multidisciplinary team approach to assessment.

Although the concept of team assessment as the basis of the design of effective rehabilitation and educational programs is sound, there are some drawbacks that tend to develop in implementation. I have participated in many team assessments, in which my roles ranged from objective evaluator of program development to the object of the evaluation process. The major flaw I have observed in the team approach is that the primary objectives—that is, the welfare of the individual and the assessment and development of strategies for the development of individual abilities—tend to be obscured in the process.

The fragmented evaluative reports of a variety of professionals on the team tend to provide bits and pieces of information. For example, medical representatives on evaluative teams usually consist of several physicians in different specialties, nurses, and physical therapists. Their respective emphases tend to be on the physical aspects of their specialty, and although they are concerned with the emotional stability of the individual, they are much more concerned with the effect of emotions on the physical condition than with the patient's overall emotional well-being. The other representatives on these evaluative teams are typically occupational therapists, social workers, at least one psychological evaluator, and most often an educational or vocational specialist. What happens is that these team members evaluate individuals from their own limited perspectives through a collection of reports and charts. There is little chance of interaction among professionals to integrate perspectives on this information, little consideration of how one aspect of the condition affects another, and little attention to how a specific physical condition may alter the emotional stability and motivation of an individual.

A fragmentation of information and focus is one negative aspect of the team approach. Another is that these professionals typically have strict time demands, so team meetings are arranged to maximize the use of time. Consequently, whatever might be gained by the team approach is lost to generalizations based on brief reports and made for the sake of expedience. Time is a destructive force in the team approach; even with modifications, many of the advantages of the team approach are lost. Another unintended consequence of team evaluation is the tendency to depersonalize or to dehumanize the individual being evaluated—an almost inevitable dynamic, especially when any more than a few individuals are being evaluated by the same team of professionals. Furthermore, the observations are made by rehabilitation team members for whom educational program development is but one aspect of the total purpose of the team's evaluation.

My view is that the most effective assessment is achieved by a relatively small evaluation team in which each member has a very focused responsibility, and in which a more integrated view of the total person is emphasized. That is, each individual evaluator should be responsible for accumulating *all* information on a limited number of assessment areas, and the team should integrate all reports into a more accurate picture of the individual's total set of needs and characteristics. Many variations of this approach have been used and evaluated. The only impediment to the practice seems to be the tension created by a need for administrative efficiency at one end and the demand for an individualized approach to the process of holistic rehabilitation on the other end.

Perhaps because of my own career goals, I see treatment in the educational setting as the most significant innovation in rehabilitation. Educational professionals are as important to the process of informing parents and other supporters about the educational implications of the disabling condition for gifted individuals as are medical and social service professionals. Training, informing, and educating parents and significant others may produce significant benefits: (a) helping them understand the disabled individual's potential abilities; (b) having them stimulate the development of the individual's gifted potential; (c) increasing their understanding of the individual's disabling condition and intellectual giftedness, and consequently decreasing their anxiety; and (d) expanding the information base about the individual by their use as skilled observers to record observations of the gifted disabled individual's behavior.

Besides providing information to parents, educational professionals must direct their efforts to providing medical and human service professionals with information about educational programs for gifted disabled individuals. College-based teacher education programs clearly have a responsibility to prepare teachers and administrators for such roles. All professional programs in colleges of education should include accurate understanding of the needs of gifted persons with severely disabling conditions. Programs that increase teacher ability to provide for the needs of gifted students with specific disabilities must develop systematically an accurate understanding of severely handicapping conditions and the nature of giftedness. This understanding is based on more than casual knowledge of physical characteristics and physiological needs that result from a severely disabling condition. It is derived from increased interaction in educational settings with individuals having severely handicapping conditions—at a variety of ages, from different backgrounds, with a diverse range of potential intellectual abilities. The emphasis in professional preparation must be on direct experience with individuals possessing various degrees and types of disabling conditions rather than a simplistic, theoretical understanding of the conditions and their consequences.

CONCLUSION

Despite the heightened sensitivity that has developed in the United States during the last 20 years, a new danger has emerged in the form of a tendency to consider all needs of disabled persons to have been met by the legislation and policies of the

1970s that addressed civil rights. We see the observable signs of accommodation, of opportunity to access experiences and facilities, of sensitivity to the needs of disabled persons. We do not readily see evidence of the underlying attitudes of indifference and resistance toward the mandated removal of physical and attitudinal barriers to the full participation of disabled individuals. Furthermore, most persons are totally unaware of the special needs of disabled individuals with gifted potential. Throughout the spectrum of people that influence the rehabilitation of severely disabled adults—parents, siblings, friends, neighbors, educators, medical and rehabilitation professionals—there must be a sincere desire and diligent effort to identify and meet the special needs created by the disability and to provide creative alternatives by which to enhance the individual's gifted potential.

The education profession clearly must assume responsibility for not only the development but also the implementation of most guidelines for responding to the needs of intellectually gifted persons with specific disabilities. Educators must assume leadership responsibility for accurately informing parents, siblings, neighbors, friends, medical professionals, and all human services professionals in the community about the nature of giftedness and how it interacts with severely disabling conditions. Educators also have responsibility for the process of designing individual educational/vocational programs for disabled gifted individuals, and for developing research and training programs pertinent to the professional field of education for disabled gifted students. If all of us do not continuously reaffirm, in all of our efforts, our commitment to the advancement and enhancement of the human condition, we run the risk of the development of human potential being dropped as a high priority in the minds of educators, human services professionals, and taxpayers. It is my hope that we shall always prize the human condition and the enhancement of all potential in human experience.

Chapter Reaction

Martha Lentz Walker, Ed.D., C.R.C.

Rehabilitation has been largely dependent upon the observations of clinicians for understanding psychosocial adjustment of persons with disabilities. John Robertson's analysis of the interaction of giftedness and severe physical disability is an excellent example of a new path in research, the "laboratory within."

As I am not an expert in giftedness, I cannot say how representative John's experience for this subpopulation might be. I am struck by how harmonious his perceptions are with the clinical folklore of adjustment to disability, particularly his description of the shock of physical loss. The importance of hope has been central in rehabilitation philosophy but has never been so eloquently detailed as in John's description. Family support has long been preached as essential in the adjustment process. John's elaboration of his experience brings the concept of family support to life. These and several other comments are very similar to perceptions reported in autobiographies of persons with disabilities.

My assumption is that those persons who undertake writing an autobiography are intellectually gifted. If this notion is correct, then John Robertson's experience is quite representative. What is valuable in the approach taken in this case study is the research focus. Autobiographies are written for diverse purposes: commercial, inspirational, argumentative. As such, they may be a collection of socially desirable responses, leaving much unexplored. A case study of the quality and nature provided by John Robertson can advance what we know about psychosocial and educational needs of severely disabled persons. The guidelines provide needed structure; his ideas supply a validation of clinical views and insight into what really made a difference in his life.

This case study prompts the hypothesis that a major interaction of giftedness and severe disability is problem solving on a societal level. Persons with severe disabilities still encounter social rejection, despite increased accessibility to "regular" education, community living, and employment. It may be that gifted persons who are severely disabled direct their superior problem-solving abilities toward the attainment of goals that will benefit all severely disabled persons and improve society. For example, I believe the growth of the "independent living movement" in the United States is the story of gifted persons, who are also severely disabled, learning the legislative process and changing the rules for all disabled persons. Persons so severely disabled that they do not have the potential for remunerative employment can now receive services such as housing and transportation, social and recreational activities, and skills training and counseling, provided through public funds. The ideology of independent living requires the leadership of and decision making by consumers. Gifted persons with severe disabilities have seen what had to be done to counteract social isolation on the societal level. I propose that this activism is a positive outcome of the interaction of giftedness and severe disability.

Several points should be added so that readers in the educational community will understand the rehabilitation system. Although John at times experienced the rehabilitation bureaucracy as rigid, users of that system should know that the state–federal program of rehabilitation has been in place since 1920. Had it not been for its ''inflexibility'' and capacity to justify the use of federal dollars on an economic basis, it would not have survived the changes in presidential administrations from Wilson to Reagan.

Fifty years before the Education for All Handicapped Children Act, rehabilitation workers were identifying the developmental possibilities in persons for whom others said nothing could be done. The technology of medical treatment for spinal cord injury came from research and training dollars produced by bureaucrats who made yearly pilgrimages to Congress with the assertion that ''taxpayers were being made out of taxeaters.'' That bureaucracy deserves credit and understanding. Educational leaders should know the history and development of rehabilitation so that all can work together.

That said, I have a final recommendation for those serving gifted persons who have severe disabilities. Only three states in the United States require a master's degree of rehabilitation counselors working in the state agency. These are the persons who make decisions about medical, vocational, and educational programs and invest public money in a course of action. In most states, a client has one chance in nine of receiving services from a qualified rehabilitation counselor. Check the qualifications of the persons with whom your students are working.

I agree with John Robertson that our response to the challenge of gifted persons with severe disabilities is surely a measure of our humanity and ingenuity. Rehabilitation and education are natural partners in this work.

* * * * *

Martha Walker is an Associate Professor at Kent State University in the field of Rehabilitation Counselor Education. She is past president of the National Council on Rehabilitation Education and has served on several national advisory committees, including the Rehabilitation Institute of Chicago's Rehabilitation Research and Training Center.

Chapter Reaction

Joanna Gartner, C.R.C.

In 1973, the year after John Robertson's disability was incurred, a very important piece of legislation came into being that has had an important effect on services for people with disabilities, especially severe disabilities. Had that law been in effect several years earlier, John would probably not have had to confront as many barriers as he has described.

This important legislation was the Rehabilitation Act of 1973 (Public Law 93–112), of which Section 504 mandates:

> . . . all recipients of federal funds must ensure that programs are accessible to qualified handicapped persons. No institution may discriminate against handicapped persons because these programs are inaccessible to, or unusable by, such persons. An institution is not required to make structural changes in existing facilities where other methods are effective in achieving program accessibility.

It is important to realize, however, that the effects of any law may not be felt until long after it has been passed.

As the coordinator of Disabled Student Services at Kent State University, I am pleased to say that this institution was a leader in the nation in establishing services for students with disabilities, beginning in 1964, long before such services were mandated. Since that time, services have been added and available programs have been improved allowing disabled students easier access to activities of the academic setting.

Services in 1964 started under the auspices of the Rehabilitation Counseling Department. In 1970, the program was funded as an official university office as part of the Student Affairs Division, where it remains today.

Over the years, more than 3000 students with various types and degrees of disabilities have attended Kent State. The role of Disabled Student Services is to provide support services ensuring equal educational opportunities. Students are encouraged to participate in all aspects of university life. The kinds of services available to eligible students include the following: attendant, reader, writer, and interpreter referral; class relocation; preferred registration; coordination of admissions, housing, parking, and transportation for new students; equipment repair and loan; liaison with other state agencies; resource library on disability-related materials; pre-enrollment interviews; academic assistance, such as test proctoring

172

and assistance in ordering taped materials; wheelchair repair and loan; and personal and academic counseling.

Numerous institutions throughout the United States provide similar services. This has become apparent through the establishment of a professional organization, the Association on Handicapped Student Service Programs in Post-Secondary Education (AHSSPPE), which promotes equal access for disabled students in higher education. This organization, which started in 1978, now has over 600 members throughout the United States, Canada, and other countries and has been a trend-setter in making society aware of the needs of students with disabilities at the post-secondary level.* The rapid growth of AHSSPPE since 1978 shows that services to students in post-secondary settings have expanded greatly and continue to grow.

Along with the services provided through specific programs and the existing professional organization, there is also a greater awareness of the role state governments must fill in providing financial support to post-secondary institutions to enable them to provide accessible facilities. In the state of Ohio, the Board of Regents has been instrumental in setting aside funds that post-secondary institutions can apply for to make buildings accessible. Repeatedly, Kent State has been granted funds to make more and more buildings barrier-free.

John Robertson's experiences and his concerns about available services and prevailing attitudes in a university setting emphasize an important consideration: the effects of legislation are not felt until a certain amount of time has elapsed after the legislation has been instituted. This is what happened with Section 504 of the Rehabilitation Act. Even though the law was passed the year after John's injury, he did not—nor did others—see the effects of it until the late 1970s and into the 1980s. I think that at last, students are beginning to realize the benefits of that legislation.

I am in agreement with John that one of the major problems to be faced is that of attitudinal barriers. There will always be a continual need to address the attitudes of faculty, staff members, and fellow students; this is true not only in a post-secondary setting but throughout society. Continual awareness of the effects of specific disabilities is always needed. We must continue to work on making others aware of the services that must be provided at the post-secondary level.

*   *   *   *   *

Joanna Gartner is Coordinator of Disabled Student Services at Kent State University. She currently is secretary of the national Association on Handicapped Student Service Programs in Post-Secondary Education and president of the Ohio Valley chapter of AHSSPPE.

---

*The address of AHSSPPE is P.O. Box 21192, Columbus, OH 43221.

Chapter 6

Intellectually Gifted Persons with Specific Learning Disabilities*

A CASE STUDY: MARCIA

> I have never seen myself as an exceptional person. Much of my life I
> have struggled with feelings of failure; I couldn't cope with the idea of
> being a failure. And, somehow I knew I was not really a failure—I knew
> I was smart, not dumb, because I could understand; I just couldn't
> express it.

Marcia's comments illustrate the emotional conflict and struggle many intellectually gifted persons with specific learning disabilities experience in schoolwork
and other tasks, such as grocery shopping. Knowing one comprehends at more advanced levels than many others yet encountering relative failure in seemingly
simple tasks seriously threatens one's self-concept. Marcia is an example of a
gifted person who responded positively to that conflict and threat to self-worth; she
demonstrates fierce determination to succeed and overcome those feelings of
failure. Marcia emphasizes that the disabilities do not go away with age: there is a
continual need to cope with learning difficulties, to adopt new ways of doing
things, and to struggle to maintain belief in self-worth and ability to succeed.

At 37 years of age, Marcia is an anatomical pathologist who has developed and
directed clinical laboratories for two small community hospitals in Missouri. She
also has developed a health club (spa) and is considering developing a center for
holistic, preventive medicine. Marcia lives in a house on four acres of farmland
with her husband, who is a patent lawyer, and two sons—plus many animals she
enjoys raising.

Except for the fact that Marcia's father was in the Air Force, so that the family
moved often during her elementary and secondary school years, her childhood was
quite normal. She was the second child of six, following an older sister she per-

---

*The authors gratefully acknowledge the contributions of Gladys Knott as co-author of this chapter.

175

ceived as a "super achiever"—very popular, talented in voice, and an avid reader. Marcia's younger sister "always got straight As" in school, but her two brothers, who were much younger, were not academic achievers.

Marcia, like most learning-disabled individuals her age, was neither identified as needing special educational services nor given any information to help her understand her extreme difficulties with reading and writing. She regards it, in retrospect, as probably fortunate that she attended parochial schools for 8 of the 12 years of schooling. Most classes, she recalls, were small, with "a lot of individual attention" from the teacher.

After managing a B grade average in high school, Marcia attended a state university and successfully completed a Bachelor of Science degree program in education, majoring in physical education with a minor in biology. After graduating, she attended the university one more year to complete requirements for medical school, which had become her goal. Once admitted to an accredited College of Osteopathic Medicine, Marcia completed successfully the four-year curriculum and was awarded the Doctor of Osteopathy (D.O.) degree, which she describes as "equivalent to the M.D." degree. It is significant that it was during a lecture on dyslexia in medical school that Marcia finally diagnosed and understood the nature of her learning disability.

Having received her D.O. degree, Marcia married and moved to Washington, D.C., where she was employed by the D.C. City Board of Public Health as a school physician to give physicals for athletes, etc. She also worked part time teaching in two city colleges. After a year her first son was born. Subsequently, she completed two years of residency in pathology at George Washington University and had a second son before the family moved to Missouri. During Marcia's residency, in addition to mothering two infant sons, she worked part time in the emergency room of a D.C. general hospital.

In Missouri, Marcia's husband established his law practice. Marcia began a general medical practice, which she found to be exceedingly costly in time, energy, and financial investment, partly because of having two small children. She decided to complete her pathology residency—requiring a total of four years—with emphasis on anatomical pathology and clinical laboratory medicine. Four years later Marcia was under contract with two small community hospitals to establish and direct their clinical laboratories. Integrating her background in physical education and medicine, she developed and managed the health club, in addition to the hospital clinical laboratories.

Personal View of Self

During Marcia's early years of schooling, when her self-concept and motivation for school achievement were forming, she was often confused by an inner sense of being "smart." She felt that she comprehended but also felt failure on assigned academic tasks involving reading and writing. Marcia recalls that elementary teachers made her aware that she was not functioning "up to par," awarded her C grades generally, and admonished her that she was capable of much higher achievement in school. By second grade she skipped school for weeks at a time because she wanted to avoid the painful conflict and negative feelings engendered by schoolwork.

In school, Marcia felt frustrated and angry when she could not read and became confused in doing her work. She puzzled over her difficulty intensely in second grade, when she was in a classroom that contained students in grades one to four. She observed that she could understand easily what the teacher was teaching the third- and fourth-grade students; yet she became confused and failed to do successfully her own easier work. For example, she remembers vividly feeling extremely upset when she converted a column of figures into division and all her answers were marked wrong. She notes that she "never recovered from that in math!"—she still dislikes it and has low self-expectations for success doing it.

Marcia's self-perceptions as a child were adversely influenced by the acute sense of discouragement and frustration she experienced in trying to read. She recalls reading as "an exceeding chore." Although the teacher did not notice, so far as Marcia knows, she herself started noticing in the middle elementary years that she was reversing symbols, numbers, and letters, and also sequences of information. This problem apparently was not recognized by teachers; at least no effort was made to help Marcia understand or correct it. Consequently, Marcia struggled to find some way to cope. One example she remembers is from the fourth grade, when the teacher required four book reports to be given orally to the class. Since Marcia could not read a book, she listened carefully to others and then used her exceptional auditory memory to repeat summaries given the week before. Fortunately, the teacher never recognized the duplication!

Marcia remembers often wondering as a child, "Am I lazy? Why am I not able to read?" She describes the feelings she had about her academic difficulties as "*torture!*" Her academic failure and emotional struggle created in her a feeling of being "out of step, not with the rest of the crowd." Marcia also struggled with feelings of guilt that she was deceptive and to some extent cheating through strategies she had developed in order to cope with expectations and required tasks. She felt trapped between guilt over the use of such strategies (e.g., the "fake book reports") and the equally unacceptable alternative of "flunking," which her forming self-image would not tolerate. In recalling those childhood days, Marcia vividly describes her inability to cope with the idea of failure and her struggle created by sensing exceptional abilities. She remembers her internal conflict and her threatened self-esteem; she would mentally enumerate reasons she was not "really a failure." Marcia was aware she was physically strong and well coordinated, could "trick" her sisters and teachers, and was smart when it came to understanding things and remembering.

Marcia's elementary school record indicates she was an average ("C") student. All through those years, she could not read, except for words or phrases that she connected with context clues to discern meaning. She remembers distinctly that the first book she "really read," cover to cover, was in the ninth grade. It was an exhausting struggle to get through all of it, but she was "driven to read it because it was so engaging." There is a bit of irony in the fact that the book was about a seeing-eye dog! She read several books that year, mostly related to her emerging interest in science and her love of animals. Aside from these books read for personal interest and pleasure, Marcia continued to read in "snatches" as necessary, reading bits of information in order to pass tests and courses. The psychological stress and mental exhaustion induced by the struggle to "really read" was so great that she reserved the effort for personally motivated purposes—she recognized she could not expend such energies regularly in school. Furthermore, if she were to read all assignments, multiples of the total time allocated for all school subjects would be required.

Marcia reports that every year after the ninth grade became easier academically because she had somehow learned to read. She completed high school and college courses by attending classes faithfully, listening carefully, and employing exceptional auditory memory skills in order to remember "*all* content without any notes." Marcia did not read the textbooks, except for a few in biology, but picked out critical bits of information to memorize for tests. She avoided taking subjects that required an extensive amount of reading. With a B average and a score of about 710 on the College Board Examination, Marcia was admitted to a state university as a physical education major. She wanted to go to medical school but refused to take the required mathematics courses. She completed a minor in biology with difficulty only in one course, zoology, in which she "had to read the text." Marcia earned a C + average as a freshman and sophomore and did slightly better in her last two years of college. Her high score on the Medical College Admissions Test (MCAT) gained her admission to medical school so that she could pursue the career of her choice.

Marcia "never considered [herself] much of a student; anyway, if you could make Cs and have some fun, it did not seem worth it to work day and night to get Bs and As." School always was a struggle because of her disabilities. She was motivated to persist with her education, regardless, because "if not, I would be stuck as a housewife or at the bottom of the man's world of careers. Besides, I couldn't file, make change, or spell, so I knew I couldn't make it as a secretary, salesgirl, cashier, or whatever. I had no choice but to become a doctor!"

As an adult Marcia still has to cope daily with her disabilities in her professional and personal life. She regards her disability as severe but has very positive feelings about the fact that it did not prevent her from achieving academic success. Her self-image centers on her ability to understand and make professional contributions while accepting, in proper perspective, her specific difficulties: (a) expressing herself, even socially; (b) perceiving and remembering accurately symbol sequences (e.g., she still tends to dial phone numbers backward); and (c) organizing her work. She describes herself as having the information and knowing how to use it, but often being confused and disorganized and then unable to express herself effectively. She still tends to have right-left mirror image, which produces error in memory for spatial relationships and sequencing; she has to concentrate hard to retain mental images.

Marcia's repertoire of coping skills to compensate for the disabilities seems to be a source of comfort, if not pride, to her. She is aware that her disabilities are much more severe when she is fatigued, so she paces herself. Marcia improved her ability to communicate to others by taking a speech class in college and by seeking instruction on how to outline lectures before she taught. She recognizes that she has "an incredible memory for some things, like tissue slides." For example, she did 100 autopsies, taking only brief notes; she did not write up reports yet remembered accurately for years the specific details. Numbers, especially memory of the sequence, remains her biggest problem in her work, so she has other staff members record those data.

Self-Perceived Strengths

Marcia views her *ability to improvise and adapt* to situations as her primary strength. She feels she can size up a situation well and determine how to interact with it in order to achieve her goal. That special ability she extends to include exceptional perception or intuitive sense of the integrity, the rightness or wrongness, of a situation or a person.

The creative strategies Marcia devised to adapt to the school situation are clear evidence that she was engaging in *creative problem solving*, including some manipulation of persons and events, not typical of the average child of her age. She identifies *perceptual and analytical abilities* as critical elements of her ability to improvise and adapt, which is consistent with identified traits of intellectually gifted children.

The second strength Marcia identifies is *memory*. From early childhood she knew she was exceptionally good at remembering what she heard. She capitalized on her exceptional auditory memory to compensate for her inability to write detailed notes or records, to read thoroughly or skim to review for examinations, or to organize well and search for needed information. This attribute of exceptional memory is typical of intellectually gifted individuals.

Music is the third area of strength Marcia notes. She first taught herself to play the trumpet early one year in secondary school. Then, she literally took home *every* instrument in the school bandroom on loan and taught herself scales and simple melodies. Within a year she was playing in the marching band! Marcia exhibited through her music a highly developed auditory memory as well as musical talent.

The fourth area of strength recognized by Marcia is what she calls "mechanical skills." She notes excellent skills in such tasks as wiring lamps, putting points and plugs in cars, and fixing mechanical objects.

The interview with Marcia revealed several areas of strength that she did not include in her response to the question of what she recognized to be her strengths or areas of special ability. These additional strengths include her drive to succeed, her intense motivation to achieve self-set goals, and her persistence or task commitment. Her determination to succeed despite her disabilities seems exceptionally strong compared to most individuals. Similarly, her motivating curiosity, her intense drive to know and understand, appears to be quite exceptional. In her reflections on school experiences she commented that she had always sensed she had sufficient ability to achieve her goals "if she could get it to work for her." She recalls that she has always been "quite exploratory," especially fascinated with biological things and sought knowledge about biological functions. As an adolescent she wanted to know the inner workings of animals. She remembers an incident that began her interest in medicine as a career. A dog had been hit by a car. A local pharmacist was summoned and said apologetically that he could do nothing for it. It was at that moment that Marcia thought that if she became a physician, she could help in such situations.

Another unquestionably strong personal attribute not identified by Marcia is her creativity. Her exceptional creative abilities were revealed through her situational problem solving as well as music.

In summary, Marcia's perceived cognitive strengths include auditory memory, symbolization, and conceptualization. Her successes in academic achievement, development of musical talent, and mechanical skills performance indicate these strengths, in addition to creative problem solving. The authors also recognize strengths of character, such as motivation, curiosity, perseverance, and personal commitment.

Self-Perceived Weaknesses

Poor organizational skills are pinpointed by Marcia as her major weakness, which causes her considerable annoyance and frustration. She explains that the weakness is related to having moved so many times as a child that the base of information or points of reference for organization were constantly changing. However, Marcia feels her mother made moving a creative, positive experience that actually developed her skills for adaptation to situations!

Marcia also notes as a weakness her *reading difficulty*. She still cannot read with distractions in the environment, such as children playing. Given a quiet, still place to read she can enjoy reading almost any book now, except novels, but she still reads in short periods and relies heavily on context clues for comprehension. She does not read newspapers, except the front page and the commodities/stock market listing to check the price of animals for the farm.

A related difficulty pertains to *writing*. It is particularly difficult for Marcia to prepare lecture notes for teaching, or to outline a plan or chapter. By way of illustration, she reports that it takes her four hours to outline book material for use in one hour of lecture. Furthermore, in order to accomplish the task she must leave the house to eliminate all distractions. Under ideal conditions of quiet and low fatigue level, she may be able to produce about eight pages of outlined lecture notes during a three to four hour period.

In her professional work, Marcia must cope with some *technical difficulties*. She has no problem recognizing patterns but cannot remember figures or details of a sequence necessary in her work as a clinical pathologist. Marcia feels that her interpretive skills offset her technical weaknesses, and she relies on staff assistance to prevent errors. In response to the question of how she would rate or grade her professional self-image, she indicated between a C and B. Then she added that she felt much more successful professionally than domestically; she rates her domestic self-concept as D − because of feelings of failure created by an inability to organize and manage smoothly. That low self-perception may be a reflection also of a perfectionistic trait, or a bent toward high levels of self-criticism. The multiple roles and responsibilities Marcia manages in her daily life, however, indicate that she must be reasonably well organized to be as successful as she has been—especially in the laboratories she directs.

In summary, Marcia perceives her weaknesses to be in the areas of organizational skills, reading, writing, and some technical difficulties in her work related to memory for figures or sequencing. Overall she feels more positive about her professional competence than her domestic abilities because of a pervasive sense of disorganization and failure to manage "smoothly."

Personal Needs

Marcia perceives her foremost need as help with improving her organization or management skills. As a young person she had difficulty even organizing her clothes to figure out what to wear together. She seems to feel totally inept in keeping personal possessions organized in her home, saying, "I don't like distractions, noise, and clutter, but I *can't* control it in my home!" Consequently, because she does not consider herself to be a good housekeeper, she readily admits she feels she is not "such a good mother." Similar comments were not made in reference to her work directing the laboratories, but such feelings of inadequacy may have been a factor in her decision to leave general medicine practice.

Related to the first need is a desire to improve her ability to concentrate and think productively in an environment with some noise and distractions. It is impractical to have to withdraw into isolation in order to complete a "simple" task of writing a note, making out checks to pay bills, or reading a newspaper!

The third need pertains to a negative aspect of Marcia's self-concept, social competence. This negative self-perception was shaped early by feelings that she was not "with it," that she was not socially adequate or acceptable. As a consequence, she prefers not to be in the public eye and does not like to receive attention. She says, with a tinge of regret, and some defensiveness, that she does not have many friends and that she wants it that way. To develop fully her leadership potential in the community, laboratory, or field of science, Marcia needs help in becoming more self-confident socially and more socially effective.

After commenting on her desired lack of friends, Marcia stated that one reason she left the medical practice was to avoid having people emotionally dependent on her. She did not identify a related need, but the comment suggested the possibility that she needs help in dealing with her fear of failing to meet others' needs and/or expectations. Perhaps in her private general practice, the demands for total organization and self-management of all tasks, without a large staff to help, engendered the fear of forgetting a detail or erring in some detail that could have negative consequences for the patient. She may need assistance in coping with the fear of failure that often plagues gifted persons.

The last need expressed by Marcia was related to becoming "more self-sufficient." She wants to be more independent but finds a problem in that people already perceive her as being relatively successful and independent, which she claims she really is not. Apparently, Marcia has rejected positive feedback from others regarding her perceived success and competence and has been inclined to believe that they simply do not see her dependency and incompetence.

Perhaps as an outgrowth of these perceived needs, Marcia dreams of one day being a farmer with a self-sufficient farm. She loves animals and professionally would like to transplant human embryos into animals. She firmly believes that this will be done some day and noted that it was predicted during her sophomore year of college that embryo transplants would occur! She says her recreation is "weird daydreams" in which she manipulates scientific facts to come up with scientific answers to problems and needs. Marcia believes that living in the quiet, isolated environment of a self-sufficient farm would allow her to let her imagination go, experiment in her private laboratory, and fulfill her potential as an innovative scientist.

Personal View of Perceptions and Treatment by Others

Facilitators

The fact that Marcia felt her parents always treated her as capable and encouraged her to try whatever she desired was a significant factor in the development of her self-concept and motivation to succeed. Her mother read to her regularly, which developed in her an appreciation for books and for the ability to read.

In Marcia's adult years, her husband has been her greatest help. He is very proud of her and is a constant source of encouragement, lifting her low self-image. Marcia feels her husband gives "tremendous support domestically and professionally" through being well-organized, an emotional stabilizer, and reassuring. His skills and elements of professional life style complement Marcia's. In addition to being very self-assured and organized, he writes and speaks very well (a natural accompaniment to his work in the law profession).

The only aspect of school experience that was facilitative of Marcia's development as a gifted individual was the experience of being in classrooms with multiple grades. In that context she made comparisons and realized her special comprehension and memory abilities while also developing greater interest in school. She feels blessed in having had a few patient teachers who read lessons aloud to her so that she could learn the material. Her sixth-grade teacher read the entire history book to the class, and a high school English teacher read literature aloud to them. She felt fortunate when such events occurred because it made learning so much easier for her.

One person who was a facilitator by helping her find a way to go to medical school without taking all the mathematics requirements was her college advisor. Without that assistance, she might not have found a way to achieve her goal.

Obstructors

Overall, the entire school experience was a major obstruction to the full development of Marcia's intellectual potential. She received no special help from anyone in the schools. Teachers seemed unaware of her problem, perhaps in part because she moved so often. In the interview, Marcia exclaimed, "I did it in spite of them!" in reference to her ultimate academic and professional success. Marcia gave some illustrative examples of the obstructive behavior of teachers. In second grade she asked the teacher to show her how to write the numbers 1 to 100. The teacher told her she had to do it herself. When Marcia did not do the assigned task, the teacher put her in a closet as punishment for not trying. Finally a classmate taught her how to do it by writing the numbers in columns of ten. Teachers through the years kept saying, "You can do it if you just try!" But, when Marcia asked a teacher, "How?" she was given no help.

Teachers, lacking an understanding of the nature of learning disabilities, failed to help Marcia develop the self-understanding that would allow self-acceptance without guilt for shortcomings. Marcia was given no assistance in devising ways to learn, to complete her schoolwork successfully, or to cope with the conflicting pressures and frustration.

The only other form of obstruction that Marcia recalls occurring was her father's order that she drop out of college and return home after a freshman semester of D grades. That obstruction may have been converted into a positive, facilitating effect because she defied her father and became even more determined to succeed.

Statement of Specific Needs

Having grown up without realizing the nature of her specific disabilities and, consequently, not recognizing her needs, Marcia found it very difficult to respond to questions regarding her specific needs related to other people, agencies, or the community. Aside from the need for emotional support and encouragement from family members, and the understanding that led to realistic expectations, the only needs she recognized were pertaining to teachers. She unquestionably needed teachers who understood the nature of both her giftedness and her specific learning disability—teachers who could skillfully modify her curriculum in relation to how she learned.

In reflecting on the needs question, Marcia commented that it was hard to pinpoint why she became so driven and so intensely motivated to achieve. However, Marcia completed four years of college, four years of medical school, and four years of residency despite the exhausting struggles inherent with learning disabilities. She concludes that the motive probably was the financial security that would permit independence.

DISCUSSION

Traditional and Contemporary Perspectives on Learning Disabilities

Parents and professionals influenced the birth and development of the field of education of the learning disabled. Historically, a plethora of educational research, theories, and programs dates back to the 1800s, but it was during the 1950s and 1960s that awareness of this special population of children was heightened. Generally, this population was described as fitting none of the existing special education categories but requiring special education in one or more academic areas. Formal legislative recognition of learning disabilities began with the 1966 formation of a National Advisory Committee on Handicapped Children, which encouraged the Congress to deal with the special population. The Committee recommended the following definition of learning disabilities:

> Children with special learning disabilities exhibit a disorder in one or more of the basic psychological processes involved in understanding or in using spoken or written language. These may be manifested in disorders of listening, thinking, talking, reading, writing, spelling or arithmetic. They include conditions which have been referred to as

perceptual handicaps, brain injury, minimal brain dysfunction, dyslexia, developmental aphasia, etc. They do not include learning problems which are due primarily to visual, hearing or motor handicaps, to mental retardation, emotional disturbance, or to environmental disadvantage.

Ongoing pressure from parent organizations and professionals resulted in the Children with Specific Learning Disabilities Act of 1969. The Act authorized federal funds for teacher training, demonstration projects, and research; however, funds for educational services were not authorized. With the passage of Public Law 94–142, the Education for All Handicapped Children Act of 1975, special education services for learning-disabled children were federally mandated and funded. The Act also included a revised definition of a learning disability (*Federal Register*, 1977):

> "Specific learning disability" means a disorder in one or more of the basic psychological processes involved in understanding or in using language, spoken or written, which may manifest itself in an imperfect ability to listen, think, speak, read, write, spell, or to do mathematical calculations. The term includes such conditions as perceptual handicaps, brain injury, minimal brain dysfunction, dyslexia, and developmental aphasia. The term does not include children who have learning problems which are primarily the result of visual, hearing, or motor handicaps, of mental retardation, of emotional disturbance, or of environmental, cultural, or economic disadvantage.

This current definition of learning disabilities and identification criteria set forth by the act are broad in scope. Keough (1977) related that the definition and identification criteria (*Federal Register*, 1977) reflected (a) research from several disciplines, including medicine, psychology, education, and sociology, (b) multiple characteristics of learning disabilities, and (c) the need to conduct further research leading to operational definitions of etiology and intervention.

The federal definition, identification criteria, and intervention approaches have received particular and widespread criticism. Cruickshank (1976) compared the definition with that for the mentally retarded and claimed that this population manifests characteristics similar to the learning disabled. Kirk (1976) also noted that "exclusion clause children" are not understood or served appropriately. Sartain (1976) and Lovitt (1978) argued that school personnel identify slow learners as learning disabled, provide services to "special" children whose education would not otherwise be funded, and develop poorly conceptualized intervention programs as a result of liberal labeling. Similarly, the National Advisory Board of the Association for Children with Learning Disabilities (ACLD) has expressed frustration with the present federal definition, identification criteria, and intervention implications. The ACLD has proposed a new definition and educational recommendations. Another agency dissatisfied with Public Law 94–142 is the National Joint Committee for Learning Disabilities. It too has proposed a new definition, which applies not only to children but also to adolescents and adults (Hammill, Leigh, McNutt, & Larsen, 1981). Other concerns about the misrepresentation and vagueness of the current federal definition include intraindividual causation of learning disability and insufficient translation of theory into teaching methods. Collectively, the issues suggest that research in educational settings is needed to provide more precise operational definitions for etiology, characteristics, and educational programming for learning-disabled individuals.

Identification Practices

This section offers a brief discussion of practices for identification of preschool, elementary, and secondary level learning-disabled (LD) students. The reader is referred to work by researchers such as Lerner (1981), Bryan and Bryan (1978), Houck (1984), and Mann, Goodman, and Wiederholt (1978) for extensive descriptions of screening and referral procedures, assessment tools and administration, placement decisions and intervention strategies.

For preschool-age children, factors in child development such as reception, production, and functional use of language are the primary areas of concern for identification. The areas, in addition to motor skills, social adjustment, and attention to tasks are describable from observation data and certain standardized tools. However, school achievement criteria, in relation to the federal definition, are inappropriate for preschool children, and preschool screening measures are regarded with skepticism. Nevertheless, preschool test batteries are generally utilized to label handicapped children and thus qualify programs for Public Law 94–142 funding.

Elementary and secondary school students are identified as LD students if they demonstrate severe discrepancies between their potential and academic achievement in areas delineated by the federal definition of learning disabilities. What constitutes a severe discrepancy is not dictated by federal regulations. Therefore, consensus among the states and school districts is nonexistent. Each state regulates the quantification of a discrepancy between potential and achievement, and local school districts then determine statistical patterns and cutoffs. In this regard, school districts usually choose either achievement-grade level cutoffs or a percentage of discrepancy between achievement and potential. To facilitate determination of discrepancies with either method, numerous formulas are utilized (Myklebust, 1968; Salvia & Clark, 1973; Goodman & Mann, 1976; Cone & Wilson, 1981). Inherent in this key identification device are advantages and disadvantages for school districts and the students served. For example, since some formulas do not require a limited range of performance on intelligence measures, mentally re-tarded and gifted students could be served with a learning disabilities label. One weakness is illustrated when use of one formula indicates that a student qualifies for special services while use of another formula may disqualify the same student. Although these and other strengths and weaknesses of discrepancy formulas have been widely discussed (Bruininks, Glaman, & Clark, 1973; Macy, Baker, & Kosinski, 1979), they remain the typical means of identifying learning dis-abilities.

Medical Approach to Management of Learning Disabilities

During the period from 1930 to approximately 1960, the medical profession maintained a crucial role in the development of the field of learning disabilities. Specialists in pediatrics, neurology, ophthalmology, otology, psychiatry, and other areas held that brain function disorders precluded some children's learning. In order to determine the causes and nature of such disorders, collectively labeled "minimal brain dysfunction," medical specialists contributed research and par-ticipated in the diagnosis and treatment of learning disabilities. Controversy within the medical professions about the nature of learning disabilities and the inability of medical specialists to translate their findings into educational practices resulted in a diminished emphasis on minimal brain dysfunction as a cause of learning disabilities (Bateman, 1974; Lerner, 1981). Although there has been less input from the medical profession in general during recent years, contributions from a few medical specialties, such as otology, psychiatry, and pediatric neu-rology, continue to broaden the knowledge base of learning disabilities.

One medical approach to the treatment of learning disabilities should be noted. During the 1970s, drug therapy for LD students was quite prevalent. Various drugs were used to control or manage behavior such as hyperactivity, attention-span difficulties, impulsivity, and distractibility. However, apprehension and vehement criticism of physicians' apparently increasing and indiscrete use of drugs substantially reduced their readiness to issue prescriptions. Although major issues on the effectiveness of drugs on behavior and learning have not been re-solved, drug therapy is still utilized with some learning-disabled students. Cur-rently, public awareness of problems with drug use, including use of illegal sub-stances, chemical dependency, controversy surrounding legalization of certain drugs, and the availability of drugs to the student population, has invited greater caution and parental concern in administering drug therapy.

Educational Programs

Historically, the field of learning disabilities has advocated a variety of instruc-tional models. Schools of thought reflect the early beliefs, theoretical constructs, and intuitive wisdom of some beginning educators in the field. Particularly, models of instruction have focused on areas of human development—for example, motor development (Kephart, 1963; Getman, 1965; Delacato, 1966; Ayres, 1968); perceptual development (Gillingham & Stillman, 1966; Frostig, 1968; Wepman, 1968); cognitive development (Kirk, 1967; Ames, 1968; Koppitz, 1973); and language and learning (Myklebust & Johnson, 1967; McGrady, 1968; Wiig & Semel, 1976; Knott, 1979, 1980, 1981, 1983; Wallat & Butler, 1984). As indicated by recent contributions to the literature, dramatic shifts in educational perspectives and instructional methods have occurred during recent years. From a preoccupation with psychomotor and perceptual modality training (visual and auditory) to improve academic achievement, the field has come to recognize the vital importance of cognition and language in advancing LD students' knowledge across all academic areas. For examples of discussions of the shift in perspective, the reader is referred to Reid and Hresko (1981) and Houck (1984).

Prominent among educational plans that incorporate cognitive and linguistic viewpoints are developmental and information-processing models of instruction. In choosing either of the models, there is a growing recognition that the LD student is active in the instructional process. Therefore, consideration is given to other elements that affect student response. These elements include the teacher, the task, and the setting in which the learning activity occurs. Instruction becomes a student–teacher task-setting interaction. Although not all educators and researchers involved with learning disabilities have understood the nature of the shift in perspective or recognized the ineffectiveness of earlier educational approaches, efforts to effect change are progressing.

The New Concept of Learning-Disabled Gifted Students

The concept of a gifted student with a learning disability is relatively new. This concept is difficult to understand and accept because giftedness is generally viewed to include exceptional facility in processing information and learning at accelerated rates, including reading and written expression. As discussed earlier, many LD students manifest primary difficulties in verbal behavior, particularly reading and writing. It appears, therefore, that there is no logical basis for the concept of a person who is both intellectually gifted and learning disabled. However, an examination of the federal definition of giftedness illustrates the possibility of the coexistence of learning disabilities and giftedness. The Marland Report to Congress (1972) defined gifted and talented children as follows:

> Gifted and talented children are those identified by professionally quali-
> fied persons who by virtue of outstanding abilities are capable of high
> performance. These are children who require differentiated educational
> programs and services beyond those normally provided by the regular
> school program in order to realize their contribution to self and society.

Children capable of high performance include those with demonstrated achievement and/or potential ability in any of the following areas: general intellectual ability, specific academic aptitude, creative or productive thinking, leadership ability, and visual and performing arts.

Theoretical frameworks describing cognitive performance that have been generated over the past decade seem to have the potential of explaining some facets of learning-disabled gifted students' learning behavior and academic difficulties. One framework is a cognitive developmental approach based primarily on the work of Piaget. It suggests that some students, through their use of higher order reasoning strategies and problem solving skills, develop cognitive structures that enable understanding of abstract concepts and complex subject matter. While the student may demonstrate this outstanding comprehension, and derive principles for problem solving in one academic discipline with exceptional efficiency, similar ability may not be demonstrated in a different, or even similar, academic area. It is obvious that there are intra- and inter-individual differences among all learners, including those learning disabled and gifted. Therefore, not all learning-disabled gifted students will demonstrate the same or similar levels of ability across various areas of knowledge and kinds of complex cognitive tasks.

Heterogeneity within the learning-disabled gifted population is particularly understandable when group performance is viewed from the perspective of recent information processing models and constructs. One example is the model proposed by Bauer (1982), which depicts information processing as occurring serially in four stages: encoding, manipulation, response selection, and response execution. Bauer's model suggests that the specific behavior in each stage of cognitive operation involves underlying processes, such as processing rate, syntactic complexity, and memory. From investigations to date, it seems reasonable to hypothesize that learning-disabled gifted students may experience difficulties in any of the four stages of information processing as a function of specific alterations in the underlying cognitive processes involved. Similarly, in considering group characteristics, it seems evident that differences in neurological development and/or cognitive structures, for example, short- or long-term memory, or in experiential background, also may affect specific learning outcomes and patterns for a particular student and among members of a particular group.

These facts and theories indicate that there is a logical basis for the concept of an intellectually gifted individual who is learning disabled. While research on this group of students is limited, the emerging theoretical frameworks to explain intelligence and learning portend greater understanding of this phenomenon in the future. Current research is revealing significant variations and complex patterns of individual differences in cognitive functioning that challenge our tradition of viewing learning from limited information about normative behavior. Not only are there multiple kinds of intelligences but highly complex processes that allow for widely varying profiles of specific cognitive abilities. Accelerated investigation of this population is warranted to refine this new concept.

Indicators of Intellectual Giftedness

Although awareness of learning disabilities and efforts to identify students for special educational programming have rapidly developed over the last 20 years, a very high percentage of the LD population remains unidentified and underserved. Logic suggests that this failure to recognize and respond to the special needs created by the disability is most likely to occur with those LD students who are intellectually superior. Marcia's case illustrates the rationale for this assumption: creative strategies for coping with academic tasks and compensating for weaknesses obscured her difficulties and consistently resulted in her evaluation as a C student. In fact, since the process of identifying LD students has led in recent years to the discovery of significant numbers of those students who also qualify as gifted, objections have been raised in many states and school systems to denying special educational services to students unless they are performing below grade level. Fox (1984) explained one school practice that excludes many LD gifted students from special services. In many school districts, group tests of intelligence or achievement are administered to screen for gifted students. However, on such measures LD gifted students' performances may not be significantly below grade-level placement. Thus, deserving students are not considered qualified for special educational programming. There are other obstacles that impede accurate identification and recognition of the special educational needs of this subpopulation.

Obstacles to Identification

Principal obstacles to the identification of intellectually gifted students with specific learning disabilities are the *stereotypic expectations* that prevail regarding expectations for the classroom behavior of gifted students. Those stereotypes have been disseminated through popular and professional literature for nearly 50 years as a somewhat distorted representation of Terman's classic study of young gifted students who were recognized high achievers (Whitmore, 1981, 1982; Tannenbaum, 1983). Although the recent professional literature and, to a lesser extent, the popular literature have begun to focus attention on gifted students who are not high achievers in school, prevailing attitudes and practices in communities and schools suggest that inaccurate stereotypic expectations still interfere with the perception of giftedness in students who are not high achievers, especially in those who have some disabling condition.

Three categories of stereotypic expectations for gifted students impede the discovery of intellectual giftedness in LD students. First, there is the expectation that gifted students tend to exceed the norms in all developmental areas—socially, emotionally, physically, and intellectually. This expectation has centered on what might be called a "maturity" factor. Teachers assume that a gifted child will be diligent in following directions; will be well-organized (e.g., have correct paper and pencil in hand as expected); and will exhibit high levels of "task commitment" propelled by high motivation to excel in school. The gifted child is expected to be a mature, independent worker who strives to excel. Such expectations cause teachers not even to consider the possibility of giftedness in a child like Marcia, who frequently skipped school as early as second grade; who was dependent upon teacher restatements of directions to remove her confusion about how to proceed with learning activities; who became so fatigued by the intense struggle to perceive accurately, to remember how to write, and to read that work was left incomplete even after work periods were extended. It is expected that gifted children "catch on fast," produce at an accelerated pace, and do not require repetition and reminders. So the LD child does not evoke in the teacher the consideration of potential intellectual giftedness based on academic work behavior.

A related major obstacle to early identification of intellectually gifted students with learning disabilities is the assumption that reading ability not only is predictive of later academic achievement but also directly reflects the levels of intelligence. Thus, when a child is completely unresponsive to reading instruction, does not evidence satisfactory progress, and seems slow to comprehend word attack skills, elementary teachers tend to discount any possibility of giftedness and to regard the child as a "slow learner" with limited abilities. Similarly, when the child has difficulty in copying letters accurately (e.g., remembering which direction a "b" or "d" goes) and in completing writing exercises neatly in the time allowed, there is a tendency to assume the child is developmentally below the norm intellectually as well as physically. Although Marcia did not recall writing difficulties in particular, they commonly accompany learning disabilities.

As a consequence of new literature describing gifted students with learning disabilities, expectations are slowly changing. However, many teachers are too isolated from current experimentation and recent discoveries to be informed in order to alter their practices. LD students are now being discovered at the college level (Lerner, 1981), most of them having never been identified and appropriately served during their elementary and secondary years of education. They enter with mediocre academic records, particularly in states where admissions are open to high-school graduates seeking to attend state universities. It is through assistance with academic difficulties at that level that many young adults become aware of the fact that they have specific learning disabilities and can be helped to compensate more effectively.

The second category of obstacles to the recognition of giftedness in LD students is *the curriculum and the instructional process* used by the teachers in many classrooms. As discussed previously, traditional educational practice has been characterized by emphasis on psychomotor and perceptual modality training, rather than currently advocated interactive learning processes. Most inhibiting to the expression of intellectual giftedness in those areas of advanced ability is the "traditional" textbook-workbook or lecture-exercise-test mode of instruction that emphasizes lower levels of learning—that is, memorization of factual knowledge and some measure of comprehension. Apparently, Marcia had this type of instructional program, consequently the teachers were unaware of both the higher levels of comprehension she observed in herself and her superior capacity for analytical reasoning and creative problem solving.

The third category of obstacles to identification is related to the first two. As a consequence of stereotypic expectations and the restricted nature of curriculum and instruction in most classrooms today, teachers have *very limited information* about individual children. The lack of more complete information about individuals, accumulated through frequent teacher-pupil interaction in the learning process as well as through a variety of other sources, results in ignorance of a child's special characteristics and needs.

Teachers often do not observe exceptional intellectual abilities in LD students, not only because of the nature of the curriculum and instructional process commonly employed with "slow" learners but because the child often does not reveal knowledge and powerful thinking abilities through self-expression. In most classrooms there is very limited opportunity for a child to share with the teacher and peers personal knowledge or thought processes. More impeding, however, is the likelihood that the LD child has become reticent to speak out in class owing to fear of erring, of being ridiculed, or of eliciting expectations impossible to achieve because of the learning disability. Shyness is a common human response to feelings of inadequacy, which LD children possess. Those youngsters who become assertive, and perhaps rebellious, in response to school expectations are more likely to manifest their giftedness through verbal expression, ingenious manipulation, or obviously creative problem solving. Parents often can provide valuable insight regarding the exceptional intellectual abilities of their child, but all too often they are not invited to do so, or the right questions are not asked of them. Through guiding the parents to observe specific behaviors outside of school, important information can be gathered.

In summary, there are many understandable reasons that classroom teachers fail to recognize intellectual giftedness in LD students. The encouraging message is that all obstacles are removable through accurate information about the nature of giftedness and learning disabilities, through training teachers to elicit and observe higher cognitive abilities, and through allowing teachers time to gather accurate information about individual children with whom they work.

Early and Reliable Indicators of Giftedness

Giftedness will be revealed in the *oral language* of many LD students. As these children engage in self-expression, they often evidence a more advanced vocabulary than expected, more complex language structure and syntax, and perhaps fluency of ideas as well. It is through oral communication pertaining to student interests that advanced comprehension of concepts, relationships, and principles can be recognized. Exceptional analytical abilities and facility with logical reasoning, and superior capacities for creative production and problem solving may be observed. The student also may reveal exceptional perceptiveness or intuitive judgment about people and situations, insightfulness, and remarkable understanding. Language has always been a reliable indicator of intellectual giftedness used to assess how a child reasons, comprehends, and uses information to problemsolve. This group of characteristics manifested at home and school is the most reliable indicator of intellectual giftedness. The child not verbally gifted but exceptionally capable in mathematics and science may not manifest superior language so much as surprisingly advanced thought processes reflected in oral or written communication.

Memory tends to be a reliable indicator of giftedness in all persons with some form of disabling condition. It is important to note that it remains a reliable indicator in LD students even though specific deficits related to visual or auditory memory are typical. Perhaps a fair analogy here is with motor skills. A talented athlete with exceptional gross motor skills may have poor fine motor coordination, resulting in writing difficulties. Similarly, a gifted LD person may have superior memory for facts, general knowledge, concepts, principles, or events and yet manifest deficits related to memory for specific details such as letter or number sequences. As in Marcia's case, the individual may rely heavily on superior auditory memory skills and general knowledge to compensate for specific memory difficulties in reading—for example, remembering what was heard earlier from teachers or students, using knowledge to reason context clues. Too often educators may focus attention on the deficit ability and neglect to consider possible strengths in closely related abilities.

A third reliable indicator of superior intellectual abilities relates to *problemsolving skills*. This is a particularly good indicator with those students possessing exceptional scientific aptitude and given opportunity to engage in scientific problem solving in a classroom or laboratory. When asked to explain the line of reasoning used in the problem-solving process, such students reveal exceptional analytical ability, use of information and logic, and creative manipulation of alternatives and aspects of the problem. With other LD students, these exceptional abilities may be observed only in practical problem solving, as in how to complete a required task. In a young child it may be revealed in the "creative genius" used to figure out how to get what the child wants!

Related to problem-solving skills is a fourth category of reliable indicators of giftedness, *curiosity and drive to know*. This characteristic has an affective as well as an intellectual component, the intense drive to know and understand. Characteristically the child persists in wondering, mentally and physically exploring and experimenting, and asking questions. Cognitive superiority is most easily recognized in the advanced level of questions asked for the child's age, the progressively higher line of questioning the child pursues, and the complexity of the issues the child wants to explore. Parents describe these young children as never satisfied with a simple answer; they seem to always ask the next level of question and pursue the matter further. Marcia illustrated this characteristic in her persistent line of inquiry about animals and their biological and anatomical composition and functioning. It is in these areas of interest that the potential for exceptional task commitment, involving motivation to delay gratification in order to engage in sustained research or creative production, is most easily recognized.

The last indicator is less reliable and involves greater difficulty in assessing its expression: creativity. Although it has long been accepted that intellectually gifted individuals tend to be highly creative when that capacity is nurtured, creativity is the characteristic parents and teachers have most difficulty in judging. Assessing the creative abilities of a child is made difficult by the issues related to what is "exceptionally novel" and the extent to which the process and/or the product should be judged for expression of creativity. However, intellectual giftedness is almost certain in individuals who produce obviously unique ideas, generate creative solutions as a result of exceptional perception and manipulation of related ideas or elements, or are highly motivated to engage in complex and sustained creative activity, such as that required to write a novel or produce a drama. What is critical to the accuracy of the indicator is the emphasis on cognitive abilities employed in the creative process, as distinct from creativity expressed through talent in the arts—such as dance, painting, or voice—which is not necessarily accompanied by intellectual giftedness.

In sum, the reliable indicators of intellectual giftedness in LD students cut through the masking disability of difficulty in reading and/or writing, which lowers performance on standard academic tasks and tests, to reveal the cognitive abilities manifested through such activities as oral self-expression, problem solving, questioning, and creating. For these characteristics to become evident in school settings, the appropriately stimulating and nurturant environment must exist along with opportunity, time, and rewards for such behavior in school.

Implications for Standard Identification Procedures

Standard procedures for identifying gifted students for special educational programs rely on group-administered standardized tests of achievement and aptitude, students' grades, and teacher recommendations as the primary data base for decision making. When a student meets cutoff criteria on these measures, or meets a certain level determined by points assigned to each criterion, the district often administers an individual psychological test of mental ability (e.g., the Stanford-Binet or the Wechsler Intelligence Scale for Children–Revised [WISC–R]) to determine final selection (Fox, 1984). As noted in a previous section, the gifted student does not usually perform well on group-administered tests, and the overall or total score does not reflect superior intellectual potential. One implication for this situation is that scatter analyses can be performed to determine uneven performances across the content of standardized measures or across subtests, as has been done in reporting performance on the WISC–R. High scores in one area of aptitude or achievement may suggest additional testing to determine giftedness as well as learning difficulties.

With respect to teacher recommendations or nominations for gifted education, the more mature students who learn at an accelerated pace, students who read at advanced levels, and those who are motivated high achievers in school are those most often recommended. The likelihood of appropriate referral of LD students for psychological testing as possible candidates for gifted education seems very low. One implication for improving teacher recognition of superior ability among low-performing LD students is the need to develop more accurate checklists and to train regular and special education teachers to use them with students whose abilities and achievements are questioned.

In order to identify accurately LD gifted students, classroom teachers must be trained to observe student behaviors systematically. First, teachers must acquire a knowledge base of *what* behavior to observe and *how*. For example, many teachers need inservice education to improve their knowledge of recent advances in current understanding of communication development, including specific skills of receptive and productive oral and written language. Particularly, advances in knowledge of how children acquire, develop, and use oral communication point to elements that can be used as significant indicators of needed special services. Advances in knowledge of how children develop skills for written communication, even when they may be unresponsive to traditional classroom practices, also will guide teachers in making instructive observations.

Teacher reliance on test data to determine students' needs in classrooms should be challenged, and skill in conducting systematic observations of classrooms should be developed. The set of skills needed for accurate teacher observations is dependent on precise knowledge of how children learn—that is, how learning and nonlearning are represented in behavior in relation to what the student knows already, in relation to the requirements of the task, and in relation to what the student needs to learn. To illustrate the importance of accurate observations and the cautious use of tests, a child named Robert was referred for LD screening because of below-grade-level achievement. In the third grade, he was a nonreader, scoring about first-grade level on standardized achievement tests, and was estimated to have an IQ of about 89 based on a group-administered aptitude test. On the Stanford-Binet, administered as part of the assessment for special services, Robert scored 163 (Whitmore, 1980)! The classroom teacher's perception of Robert's abilities had been obscured by his disruptive classroom behavior and indifferent, arrogant manner, his inability or unwillingness to complete schoolwork, and his inability to read. She had not observed his advanced cognitive abilities evidenced in science, social studies, and arts activities. Teachers must be trained to elicit and evaluate accurately higher levels of cognitive ability through educational activities that encourage self-expression, problem solving, and creative production.

Potential Interaction between Giftedness and Learning Disabilities

Of all the categories of intellectually gifted persons with some handicapping condition, those with learning disabilities are most vulnerable to neglect and unintentional abuse. In early childhood, if any exceptional ability is noticed by family or friends it is most apt to be early and/or advanced language and problem-solving skills and perhaps exceptional memory. Any early signs of the learning disability are likely to be attributed to the child's age or immaturity. Therefore, parents are inclined to describe the youngster as bright and capable of learning rather easily. The learning problem usually has not become evident in preschool years because formal instruction in reading and writing has not yet begun. Consequently, parental expectations for the child are positive relative to school achievement. As a result of parent communications and interaction, the child goes off to kindergarten or first grade with positive, if not high, expectations for success in school and equipped with a generally positive self-concept for ability to learn, solve problems, and adapt.

During the first three or four years of schooling, the child formulates a self-concept for school achievement based on his or her perception and interpretation of responses from teachers and peers and on personal reactions to the sense of relative satisfaction or failure in academic activities. Teachers at this level of instruction tend to focus their attention on the development of basic skills of reading, writing, and arithmetic. To the extent that this focus crowds out time for informal and formal discussions, sharing of personal interests and knowledge, exploratory inquiry and problem-solving activity, and creative self-expression, so there is little opportunity for the teacher to recognize the child's giftedness. In a genuine concern about preparing the child for future academic success, the curriculum emphasis is usually on mastery of basic skills, and if progress is slow, as in the case of the LD child, more time is devoted to those activities. Consequently, it is the teacher who is most apt to recognize signs of learning problems, and who monitors closely the behaviors that can indicate needed referral for special education because of possible learning disabilities. The general feeling that the child develops, as a result of perceiving messages of failure to meet expectations on academic tasks, is a sense of not fitting in, being a problem, or being slow or "dumb," and the child becomes unhappy at school. Thus, intense psychological conflict arises between earlier self-expectations and the feedback received in school. The powerfully negative potential of the interaction between the child's giftedness and learning disabilities in the context of school experience clearly demonstrates the need for early identification and intervention to prevent serious emotional and behavioral problems or resignation to failure. Unfortunately, not all children respond with the determination of Marcia!

Positive Effects

The most obvious positive impact of the child's giftedness on the problems created by the specific learning disabilities is an ability to adapt by devising creative strategies to cope with the psychological conflict and the school demands. Without guidance from adults, the development of successful coping strategies to facilitate learning and achievement depends on the child's personality, creative genius, and luck. Recently an intellectually gifted college undergraduate student who also is ''dyslexic'' volunteered to participate in the authors' research on the subject. She was never identified as learning disabled or dyslexic while an elementary or secondary school student. After daring to tackle a college education to become a music teacher, she became aware of the precise nature of her years of struggle to learn and read, and subsequently sought professional help at the university. Her learning strategies as a college student well illustrate the potentially positive effects of giftedness:

1. Before understanding the nature of her difficulty, she learned to rely on other students for help, since teachers were not very responsive to her requests. She identified the ''sharpest'' students in each class and sat near them, befriended them, and asked to study with them often. She knew she learned best by hearing information restated, reviewing subject matter orally, and having someone check her errors.
2. She developed a variety of strategies for memorizing information for classes that involved oral repetition, imaging to remember, tape-recording her oral recitation and replaying it during relaxation periods, and using flashcards.
3. After seeking professional help from Disabled Student Services, she informed professors about her dyslexia and requested proctoring of examinations in a distraction-free environment.
4. She began to study her learning style more intentionally and to question the extent to which she was disabled or inappropriately instructed. She decided to review all spelling rules taught in the elementary grades to determine if she could improve her spelling ability through study. She experienced some improvement initially, perhaps more from repetition than comprehension.
5. She examined her study habits in terms of problems she had identified over the years. She experimented and found that studying in a dark room with a light turned on at her desk increased her ability to concentrate. She added headphones, thickly padded, to wear when studying to block out all sound (note: no music was playing through them!). She requested a change of

dorms and now resides in the Honors Dorm, in which quiet hours are enforced at all times.

6. She has become increasingly aware of the effect of fatigue on her performance. She has worked to improve her schedule in terms of balance between fatiguing study, physical exercise, and rest. She has found her highly disciplined activity as flag girl with the marching band helps to channel her energies and increases her ability to study. She feels as though the effort to memorize marching routines has benefited her academic work, but that is only an impression. When she is tired and must study, she has discovered that reading aloud to herself improves her comprehension and concentration. Working despite being tired is important, she believes, because employers expect their workers to produce well on the job even when exhausted. Her practice under those conditions is preparing her for those occasions, she says.

The strategies just described illustrate the tenacity and problem-solving skills of an LD student whose capacity for gaining insight and self-understanding also allows exceptional levels of self-modification. Just as disciplined practice in music or athletics can channel energies that might interfere with powers of concentration, other LD students establish personal rewards as incentives to reach goals in studying or class participation, self-correct counterproductive methods of learning, and modify their behavior to alter effectively the attitudes or willingness of teachers to cooperate with requests for special provisions. The ability to engage in self-modification seems to extend to the ability to control hyperactivity, distractibility, and supersensitivity—all characteristic vulnerabilities of LD students.

Perhaps the most significant attribute of gifted adults with learning disabilities who have succeeded educationally and professionally is that of perseverance or drive to succeed, as in the case of gifted persons with other handicapping conditions. Even though that characteristic is identified throughout the literature as an attribute of giftedness, it is difficult to ascertain accurately the extent to which its presence and strength is a function of intellectual ability as opposed to personality. That question must remain open until adequate research is completed to verify its presence in gifted persons who have not achieved such success educationally or professionally. Nonetheless, its effect in the lives of the successful LD adults studied warrants its inclusion here.

The rationale for attributing the perseverance to giftedness can be developed from the base of research indicating that gifted individuals possess tendencies toward perfectionism; high aspirations to achieve in some area(s) of interest; and an intense drive to know, master, and excel in some valued endeavor. The effect of that attribute can be seen in Marcia's persistence in trying to learn how to read until finally, somehow unknown to her, she became able to decode and comprehend in the ninth grade. Similarly, the college student whose learning strategies were described previously reported that she has always spent three times more time on homework than other students; all through elementary school she studied for hours each night, with amazing persistence and patience for her age.

Two final positive effects of giftedness in interaction with learning disabilities are exceptional memory and potential creativity. The earlier descriptions of Marcia's methods illustrated well her reliance on auditory memory. For other LD individuals the specific kind of memory skills may be somewhat different—for example, the need to physically move through the process in order to remember. Typically, however, the person's exceptional memory becomes a critical factor to academic success because of the reading and writing impairments. Similarly, expressions of creativity vary among LD gifted individuals, but exceptional creative ability seems to predictably have positive effects on their problem-solving needs.

To summarize, the LD person who is also intellectually gifted benefits from the positive effects of superior problem-solving skills for adaptation, greater capacity for gaining personal insight and self-understanding to facilitate self-modification for personal improvement, and exceptional drive to achieve or master a task or situation. Added to those positive effects are the benefits of strengths in memory which compensate for reading and writing difficulties, and superior creative potential which facilitates problem solving.

Negative Effects

A child can be pictured in the center of a field of forces all exerting pressure, from within and without, to shape a self-concept, self-esteem, and behavior. This dynamic has been described in detail elsewhere (Whitmore, 1980) as creating psychological conflict for every gifted child. In the case of a child who also has a learning disability, the psychological conflict is greatly intensified, producing severe stress and vulnerability to emotional and behavioral handicaps as a consequence.

Internal pressures influencing the child's perceptions of events and feelings about social interactions have been documented in studies of gifted underachievers (Whitmore, 1980). The characteristic tendency to be perfectionistic inclines the gifted child to perceive mistakes as failure, particularly on tasks that appear relatively simple, such as forming letters correctly on the paper or sounding out letters and words to read. Teacher and parent admonitions to the LD gifted child about being disorganized and producing messy work create additional feelings of failure over tasks that seem quite simple and certainly not intellectually demanding. Invidious comparisons of personal achievements with those of peers—a natural tendency of gifted children related to their exceptional ability to think critically and evaluatively—further intensifies the sense of failure and inadequacy as others are observed to complete the tasks easily.

When teachers and parents have observed the intellectual strengths of the child, they often try to be encouraging about "difficult" work: "You can do it if you just try! Don't give up!" A common response of the gifted child is to ask "How?"—as Marcia did—or to assume some personal intellectual deficit accounts for not knowing how to proceed. When confused over directions everyone else seems able to follow, except a few who seem very slow to understand everything, the child begins to believe even more that he or she must really be "dumb," rather than "smart" as it had seemed before entering school. If Marcia's classroom had not afforded her the opportunity to make comparisons with older peers, so that she became aware of her advanced comprehension abilities, her development in later childhood might have been drastically different as a result of perceived denial of her ability and resulting extremely low self-esteem. In addition to the sense of failure and inadequacy evoked by teacher and parent statements of intended encouragement, there often is guilt instilled in the child for being lazy in that a lack of effort is implied. In fact, "lazy" is the most frequently used descriptor in the academic records of young gifted children with learning disabilities. This is perhaps a natural assumption for adults who perceive average or superior abilities in other learning activities and do not understand the child's lack of sustained effort to complete work or its poor quality when the task appears simple.

These negative external forces that shape the child's self-concept for school achievement can be eliminated by adults who understand the specific nature of abilities, the possibility that highly gifted children may have significant difficulty achieving on certain tasks or may be very average in the use of some cognitive processes, and the psychological stress and pain created by the large gap between the gifted child's intellectual level of interest and the relatively low performance level affected by areas of weakness. Such understanding will lead to more appropriate expectations by teachers and parents, which will help them monitor the messages they send to the child verbally and nonverbally regarding the adequacy of effort and achievement. It also will equip the adults to guide the child toward more accurate self-understanding of personal abilities and disabilities in order to temper the negative effects of internal drives for perfection and high achievement.

Needed Modification of Educational Programs

The first and foremost need is for all educators, in regular classrooms as well as in resource or support services roles, to have a more accurate understanding of the characteristics and needs of this special population. With that understanding, and the development of appropriate skills, four conditions critical to the appropriate education of gifted students with learning disabilities can be achieved.

1. An appropriate curriculum must be provided that addresses both sets of special education needs—those related to specific intellectual giftedness and those related to specific learning disabilities.

Each student is entitled to receive instruction that seeks to balance strengths and difficulties in learning. Such instruction is based on a model suggesting ongoing assessment-intervention, clinical teaching, and decision making by teachers in relation to individual student needs rather than instruction guided solely by commercial products. A general framework for such a model is discussed elsewhere (Knott, 1980, 1981).

2. The student must be skillfully guided by a well-informed teacher to grow in accurate self-understanding.

The gifted student needs desperately to understand the nature of the learning disability as well as of the giftedness. It is important for the LD gifted student to understand the source of anger, frustration, lack of self-confidence, and periods of low motivation. The goal must be the shaping of a healthy, realistic self-concept that accepts personal strengths and weaknesses, with overall positive feelings about potential future contributions and happiness.

3. Wherever possible, groups of similar peers should be grouped together for at least a portion of the day.

Through sharing common difficulties, giving feedback to each other, and developing a sense of social acceptance within the group, the emotional support is provided that enables the individual to cope more effectively with social situations and personal struggles. For these students to be placed in self-contained LD classes is hazardous unless there is a cluster of LD gifted students and the teacher is able to meet their special needs for gifted education. Similarly, placement in a gifted education program is not necessarily beneficial if it means being grouped with highly accelerated achievers to work in areas that are affected by the student's specific learning disabilities. The setting in which special educational needs are supplied is not important so long as the program provides a suitable peer group and a complete, appropriate curriculum.

4. The LD gifted student must be provided with intentional and skillful guidance by the teacher in developing more effective strategies for coping with the personal consequences of both the intellectual giftedness and the specific learning disability.

The student needs an adult companion or mentor in the process of discovering what conditions or strategies will facilitate learning in areas of difficulty. The teacher's role should be to share ideas about what has worked for others, to suggest ways of experimenting with some alternative learning methods, and to guide the evaluation process. This assistance not only results in improved coping strategies but also mediates more positive feelings about self.

SPECIFIC GUIDELINES AND RECOMMENDATIONS

Family Members and Friends

First of all, it is most important that adults close to the child avoid hasty conclusions about potential for intellectual achievement based on observed difficulties in acquiring the basic skills of reading and writing, being organized, or following directions. Such "flaws" do not negate the possibility of superior intellectual abilities. Difficulty in completing work, poor performance on "simple tasks," or failure to carry out directions should not be interpreted as evidence of general intellectual "slowness" or mental deficiency. Furthermore, the manner of communication with the child should not convey such assumptions or expectations. Parents should not instill through responses to poor performance a sense of guilt in the child (e.g., "You could do it if you would only try!"). Realistic expectations for the child must be formulated in each independent area of ability, and overgeneralizations about intelligence based on specific abilities must be avoided.

The second recommendation is to approach the child's relative weaknesses or areas of disability as challenges in problem solving. The child should be engaged in reflection about the personal learning process, and a description of the particular difficulties experienced should be elicited. Together, parent and child can generate ideas of possible ways to approach the problem constructively, acknowledging the undesirable consequences of tendencies to avoid tackling it. Then, from the identified alternatives, one or more can be selected to use experimentally to diminish the difficulties and facilitate academic achievement.

In assisting the child to ameliorate the weaknesses, equal or greater attention must be given to the development of particular strengths. Certain hobbies, such as music, sports, building models, and the like, which require disciplined practice, perceptual-motor coordination, some degree of organization and precise following of directions, should be encouraged. The child should be informed that such hobbies have been found to improve the ability of other children with similar difficulties to achieve more success in schoolwork.

Parents have a very important role relative to the educational opportunities provided to the LD gifted child: careful observations of the child's various *specific* intellectual abilities must be made, and precise descriptions of exact behaviors must be written in a log, to share with school personnel. Parents should not reject the significance of any exceptional achievement, even if only a one-time occurrence, because it may be a clue to greater potential yet to be developed. Opportunities through conversation, educational games and activities, and assistance with personal interests should be provided for the child to reveal exceptional abilities to remember and use information, to problem-solve effectively, and to comprehend.

Parents' collected information about the child should be shared with school personnel, with emphasis on the child's special needs created by specific academic strengths and weaknesses. Parents should insist on appropriate assessment procedures and educational services in the school system and should seek a second, independent opinion regarding programming if necessary. This process should focus on the objective sharing of accurate information about the child and determining appropriate educational programming. Questions about past practices should be worded carefully to avoid making the school staff feel defensive. Parents should be positive advocates for the child and for others with similar needs.

At home, parents should not allow invidious comparisons among siblings to negatively influence the child's psychological development. For example, it is most difficult for an older LD child to have a younger sibling who reads and writes at a more advanced level. A lowering of self-esteem with regard to those specific abilities is inevitable in such a case. Genuine affirmation of individual differences, and recognition that each one has varying strengths and weaknesses, must be continually emphasized in the home to mitigate against the effects of invidious comparisons. Unhealthy levels of competition must not be encouraged, and ridicule or taunting about failures among siblings must be prohibited.

School Personnel

Teachers, administrators, school psychologists, and counselors must be informed about this subpopulation and must avoid unintentional discrimination against serving them appropriately. All the guidelines for parents essentially apply to the school setting also. Judgments about specific abilities must be only tentative, and evidence must be collected over a period of time before any conclusions can be drawn. The value of tests should be viewed in proper perspective, because intelligence tests do not provide evidence of all important intellectual abilities and do emphasize verbal skills.

School personnel should work as a team to piece together significant observations of the child's behavior that evidence cognitive potential and developed abilities. Inappropriate classroom behavior, immaturity, and/or failure to meet grade-level expectations in basic skills should not lead to a disregard for careful assessment of the child's observed aptitude for learning and achievement, particularly in the sciences and the arts. Be thorough in testing, observing, and collecting information from all school personnel, community professionals, and the parents, who know the child in a variety of settings. Even development across all areas is not to be expected, nor should any clue of exceptional potential be rejected.

The school must guarantee the child has a fair and thorough assessment, receives appropriate educational programming for particular strengths and weaknesses, and develops healthy self-acceptance that comes from understanding the nature of the learning difficulties as well as of gifts. Unkind teasing or ridicule among peers when mistakes are made or failure experienced must be prohibited, as must unhealthy levels of competition among the students. Class members should be helped to see the strengths in every child through providing opportunities for them to be manifested in group activities. Teachers and other personnel can create a partnership with the LD child, whose intellectual abilities can help create a more effective instructional program for the identified needs. All personnel should listen attentively to the LD child's reflection, analysis, and hypothesizing, which can lead to the discovery of a better alternative or a solution to a problem.

Parents and educators must intentionally guide the LD gifted child in the development of self-understanding and self-acceptance. This can be a slow, tedious process, but it is one that must continue throughout childhood. The child should be helped to avoid unrealistically low or high goals, tendencies to limit career possibilities, and unproductive or destructive coping strategies. Understanding and acceptance of the child's unique combination of characteristics are essential to effective guidance.

The puzzling paradox of the LD gifted child affects most the family members and school personnel. Medical and community service professionals are mentioned in the next section, but their direct involvement with the child on matters relevant to educational needs tends to be minimal. All those who live and/or work with one or more LD gifted persons should be familiar with identified strengths and vulnerabilities, their weaknesses and special needs, in order to facilitate the development of potential. Most of all, members of this subpopulation need to be identified so that they can be served appropriately!

CONCLUSIONS

Intellectually gifted individuals with specific learning disabilities are the most misjudged, misunderstood, and neglected segment of the student population and the community. Teachers, counselors, and others are inclined to overlook signs of intellectual giftedness and to focus attention on such deficits as poor spelling, reading, and writing. Expectations for academic achievement generally are inaccurate—either too high and unrealistically positive or too low and discouraging of high aspirations. Even employers are guilty often of eliminating strong candidates for positions because of minor deficit abilities and a reluctance to alter the job requirements to accommodate that individual. It is not uncommon for gifted students with learning disabilities to be told that college study is inappropriate for them, that professional careers will be unattainable, and that jobs requiring only mechanical or physical abilities are more fitting to their abilities. Without equal opportunity to try, these individuals may be denied access to appropriate educational and professional career opportunities.

To correct this situation, all informed professionals and parents must help disseminate accurate information to all educators and into the community to reach employers and policy makers. Medical professionals, researchers and practicing neurologists are needed to assist with the development of more accurate knowledge about brain functions and the neurological system that affect learning. Neurologists need to communicate more regularly with school personnel, and those most experienced with the educational problems of the LD gifted student should assist others in the medical field to interact more effectively with families and children, as well as school personnel, to alleviate the difficulties.

University administrators and professors particularly need to become more informed about this student population and to address their specific needs. Some recent studies have shown that university teachers hold negative academic expectations for LD students and are pessimistic about their ability or responsibility to teach them (Minner and Prater, 1984). Attention is now being directed by some educators to LD adults, with implicit concerns about those who are unrecognized as intellectually gifted. A recent review of existing research on the LD adult suggested that critical needs exist relative to educational and vocational opportunities, socialization problems, and need for continuing intervention to provide support and guidance (Kroll, 1984). Although educational opportunities may have been more accessible to the physically disabled as a result of the federal legislation in the mid-1970s, it appears that most institutions of higher education have not given serious consideration to the needs of LD students with superior cognitive abilities. The current conservative academic climate in higher education may result in denial of an appropriate college education to these gifted students because of their specific disabilities and consequent low test scores, slow reading, and inferior writing. This possibility poses a major issue to be debated in higher education in the years ahead.

The authors assert that the need for professional attention to this area of concern is urgent. Unless practices change significantly in the near future, society will have thwarted much giftedness and lost great contributions to benefit humanity. It is encouraging to consider the possibility that, in the process of educating others about the characteristics and needs of the intellectually gifted student with specific learning disabilities, persistent patterns of thinking about learning, teaching, and student potential may be altered; and changes in diagnostic and educational practices that will improve educational opportunities for *all* children may be implemented. This challenge may identify the extent to which school experience can exacerbate disability and interfere with intellectual growth and achievement.

Chapter Reaction

Anne Udall

For the past four years I have been a teacher of gifted learning-disabled students, and it is my experiences that form the background for this chapter reaction. As individuals, the gifted learning-disabled are remarkably different from each other. They display a wide range of characteristics due to the complex interaction of their giftedness with their learning disability. Yet as a group, my gifted learning-disabled (LD) students do share common characteristics, and with few exceptions Marcia's case study illustrates many of those. These common characteristics include the following:

- poor, sometimes nonexistent, organizational skills
- a lack of coordination in fine motor tasks, exhibited in poor handwriting
- high motivation only in areas of interest
- high degree of creativity, humor, and verbal skills
- poor self-concept
- a repertoire of compensatory strategies
- good memory on topics of interest
- superior higher-level thinking skills

In addition, the students tend to demonstrate these characteristics:

- a strong fear of taking risks
- disabilities primarily in the area of language arts, notably spelling

Severe reading disabilities are not common. Ninety percent of LD students are male; in my experience, gifted LD females are comparatively rare.

Marcia's intense motivation to succeed may be the one characteristic that differentiates between successful and unsuccessful gifted LD adults. I observe motivation and persistence in my students, but it is difficult to assess empirically or to predict future success. Yet all successful gifted handicapped individuals possess this drive to succeed. Case studies of successful people are helpful because they offer numerous insights into the transition from childhood to successful adulthood.

It was persistence that enabled Marcia to obtain many of her goals despite the educational system. Her observations of the educational system should be heeded by parents and educators. Individuals' attitudes were her biggest obstacles. Those same attitudes, which continue to exist today, convey certain messages: if a student is gifted he or she can't be learning disabled, and vice versa; teachers of the gifted don't need to talk to teachers in other areas of special education; giftedness means academic achievement; and curriculum modifications for special students are too difficult or unnecessary.

The educational system is changing, primarily owing to the growth of special education and the subsequent advent of federal legislation. Students with special needs are being offered a wide variety of services. Today children's chances of being identified as both gifted and learning disabled are considerably improved.

However, these students are usually identified as gifted LD because they are initially referred for learning problems. Teachers are quick to notice a student's difficulties in school but do not as easily notice giftedness. This is true for several very crucial reasons. School success is largely determined by a student's ability to complete written work within a specified period of time. Students who can do this successfully are the ones teachers are likely to notice as "gifted." Although gifted LD students excel in nonacademic areas, their failure to produce written work means that their strengths often are overlooked. Only when teachers are presented with empirical data, notably intelligence test scores, do they recollect other behavioral indicators of giftedness.

There may be a large group of students who will never be identified. Although Marcia and my students illustrate a typical profile of *identified* gifted LD students, it cannot be assumed that all gifted LD individuals possess such traits. For example, consider the gifted student who performs successfully at grade level but whose learning disability disguises the giftedness. So little research has been done on this population that identification may be limited by testing instruments and by lack of a sophisticated conceptualization of the interaction between learning disabilities and giftedness. It must not be assumed that the theories in either the LD or the gifted field can be applied to these students without either serious revision or the development of a new theoretical base. This present narrow perspective means that many students continue to "fall through the cracks."

If identified as gifted LD, these students frequently find themselves in LD resource rooms concentrating on their deficits. Often in the LD resource room the sense of failure, first enforced in the regular classroom, is reinforced by the strong deficit approach in learning disabilities. In addition, the gifted LD students' inability to produce written work within a set time period, combined with their lack of organizational skills, often prevents them from being successfully mainstreamed into available gifted programs.

When students are identified, *all* their needs must be met. It is not enough to focus on their disability. It is possible to provide these students with a curriculum that meets all their needs. However, the gifted curriculum must not be presented as a reward for completing other requirements. Too often I have observed this phenomenon, where the gifted needs of these students are seen as secondary. Gifted LD students need an equal opportunity to utilize their strengths.

There are some general areas which must be included in any curriculum for gifted LD students. Marcia developed numerous strategies for success, including working with other students, developing memory strategies, analyzing her learning style, developing study habits, and learning relaxation techniques. Gifted LD students can be taught these and other compensatory strategies in a systematic manner. Highest priority should be given to organizational and study skills.

The students should be involved in decisions concerning their education. They are often the best judges of their particular strengths and weaknesses. In addition, students should understand the phenomenon of being both gifted and learning disabled. All teachers working with these students should use areas of interest to motivate active participation, such as science, art, or social studies; should allow for alternative means of expression; should provide opportunities for students to meet others, both children and adults, like themselves; should employ cognitive modification techniques; and should utilize modern technology such as computers and tape recorders.

The primary responsibility facing both educators and parents is to alter the negative self-image these students possess. Perhaps this is key to instilling the persistence and motivation to succeed; my experience makes me believe there is a clear relationship between a positive self-concept and success. Students must have opportunities to succeed at an early age.

Marcia accomplished many of her goals without professional help. With a change in attitudes, a growing body of research, and the implementation of curriculum modifications, gifted LD students will have more opportunity than ever to realize their potential. I hope in the future, gifted LD students will achieve their goals not in spite of education professionals but with their help.

*   *   *   *   *

Anne Udall is the teacher of a special program for learning-disabled gifted elementary students in the Tucson public schools. She earned a master's degree and certification in the fields of both learning disability education and gifted education. Miss Udall also is a doctoral student in gifted education at The University of Arizona, Tucson.

Chapter Reaction

Nancy Wingenbach, Ph.D.

The case study of Marcia is representative of a specific dyslexic disability, which was reflected in her experienced difficulty with the communication skills of reading and writing. Other learning-disabled individuals may present quite different problems, for example, difficulty with arithmetic concepts or a lack of auditory memory. The similarity across the learning-disabled (LD) population is the difficulty evidenced in the receptive, productive, or pragmatic language areas; the specific weakness in communication skills may vary. These weaknesses in communication skills in Marcia's case involved reading and writing but also extended to her use of language to accomplish her specific personal goals. Marcia had the cognitive/linguistic capacity to structure adequate syntactic/semantic relations. However, she was unable to demonstrate the use of these elements to accomplish personal goals. For example, Marcia could use language instrumentally with her colleagues to accomplish her professional goals but was unable to use language socially either instrumentally or in a regulatory manner to establish rapport with others. Marcia apparently was not productive in her use of language because of her inability to use language in the pragmatic sense.

Although Marcia was disabled in the use of linguistic skills and the weakness was illustrated through her reading and writing performance, she apparently was not cognitively disabled as demonstrated by her comprehension of academic content and her ability to survive the academic schedule by relying on auditory memory. Marcia's teachers perceived the gap between her cognitive ability and linguistic performance, were aware that the interaction of the two was not resulting in the expected outcomes, and thus kept telling her "I know you can do better." Their expectation was that the language skills would rise to the level of Marcia's cognitive processing skills. This reflects a weakness in the teachers' abilities to perceive Marcia's unique needs. The positive, productive interaction of cognition and language was interrupted by Marcia's inability to control or prioritize information and produce it in an organized expression.

Marcia and other gifted LD individuals comprehend their difficulties and recognize the frustration and its source. This comprehension and recognition is indicative of a meta-awareness: a transcending awareness of the gestalt *and* the components. The gifted LD student, armed with this meta-awareness, then begins to engage in self-modification by developing coping strategies. Marcia, for example, used her exceptional auditory memory to complete successfully high school and college.

Gifted LD students ask "how" but are aware of not knowing and not being shown "how." This point is reflected in Durkin's study (1978–1979) of reading comprehension. The classroom instructor teaches about and identifies the strategies, such as context clue usage, but fails to model or show "how" to use or implement them. The strategies are intellectualized and verbalized but are not modeled, nor is the student's use of the strategy recognized. For example, Marcia's use of context clues to discern meaning in reading and her listening techniques that enabled her to make her book reports were not recognized by the teacher. Those specific strategies could, however, be taught to all students as strategy for learning, through the teacher's use of explanation, examples, and application.

The successful gifted LD student, in the drive to succeed, requires a meta-awareness, task analysis ability, and the incorporation of strengths to compensate for weaknesses, as in the development of coping strategies based on strengths. Marcia's use of her other skills, such as auditory memory to retain important information to be used later, her use of her ability to select important and critical bits of information to memorize for a test, and her use of prior knowledge and experience to obtain a high score on the Medical College Admissions Test during which she had to read, to remember, and to determine the appropriate responses are indicators of these requirements.

In summary, the LD gifted student typically possesses a meta-awareness of the requirements of the academic setting and a meta-awareness of specific abilities. Within that context, and as a result of this meta-awareness, coping strategies are developed according to the information-processing strengths that allow the individual to progress in the academic environment.

REFERENCE

Durkin, D. (1978–1979). What classroom observations reveal about reading comprehension instruction. *Reading Research Quarterly, 14*, 481–533.

*   *   *   *   *

Dr. Nancy Wingenbach is Coordinator of Gifted Education for Lorain County Schools in Ohio. Her doctoral program included advanced study in learning disabilities, giftedness, and reading skills. Nancy coordinated the pilot project for Intellectually Gifted Learning Disabled at Kent State University in 1984.

Part III

Implications and Recommendations

The purpose of this last section is to synthesize for the reader the implications and recommendations the authors have formulated from the case studies presented, the existing literature relevant to the subject of gifted persons with specific disabilities, and the authors' current research activity involving ongoing study of individual cases. Since the number of cases studied to date is relatively small and the field is in its infancy, in many instances only very tentative hypotheses can be offered that must be tested in more extensive and systematic research that particularly involves young subjects in early stages of development. Most of the recommendations for improved practices of parents and professionals are grounded in established theories of human development with logical implications drawn for the specific population of gifted individuals with disabling conditions.

The motivation of the authors in writing this book was to begin dialogue within professions and communities about tendencies to focus on the weaknesses or disabilities of individuals and to neglect their strengths and exceptional potentialities. A fundamental issue inherent in the authors' concern about this population is the question of the extent to which potential yet undeveloped can be identified. In some ways that is a false issue. There is no doubt that the quality of life for these individuals will be greatly improved if all persons carefully avoid setting unfounded limits on potential by communicating inappropriate expectations, which so adversely affect motivation. Furthermore, by intentionally requiring ourselves to be psychologically open to the possible presence of far greater potential for achievement than is evident in the current moment, we may become facilitative of the individual's natural desire to become more able and to develop fully all potential that is within. By developing an understanding of the particular needs of these persons, professionals and others can assist them in their struggle to discover their potential and to build a more fulfilling future. Individuals with special gifts to share should not be handicapped by the ignorance, neglect, or interfering ''help'' of others. The individuals in the case studies of this book believe they succeeded *despite* professionals generally and, in some cases, despite parental protection and discouragement. How many similar persons have not been so successful because of a lack of understanding support, acceptance, and opportunity?

Chapter 7 examines the special affective needs of intellectually gifted persons with specific disabilities as they impinge on the individual's motivational characteristics. Implications for parenting and teaching practices, in particular, are offered. Chapter 8 focuses on the cognitive and educational needs of gifted and disabled persons. Specific implications and recommendations for changes are supplied for three areas: (a) improved assessment procedures so that early identification of exceptional intellectual potential can be made, (b) more appropriate educational programming and rehabilitation services, and (c) improved community services and employment practices to make independent living and appropriate careers more accessible. In Chapter 9, the questions raised and the tentative answers found in this book are summarized, and conclusions are given to challenge parents and human services professionals.

Chapter 7

The Affective Needs of Intellectually Gifted Persons with Disabilities

Undoubtedly the reader has been impressed by the persistent motivation of the individuals in the case studies to achieve in spite of many obstructions in their lives. Certain questions naturally arise in response to hearing their stories: Why did they persevere so? Could another have done so well in their situation? How are they similar to or different from other gifted persons with those same disabling conditions? Will understanding by others of their experiences and characteristics lead to development of techniques and programs that allow similarly disabled persons to develop their potential and be more successful? Were they so successful because of their characteristics, or did the characteristics develop because of their success? After raising all those questions, one may be inclined to respond that at least it is definitely possible to use the understanding gained from their examples to work toward the elimination of obstructions and toward increased support for the desires and efforts of such individuals at all ages.

Although only limited conclusions can be drawn from a handful of case studies, particularly of successful adults reflecting on their childhoods, the information provides an excellent beginning and a guide to further investigation. In fact, perhaps some of the subjects will become inspired to conduct related research of their own! The information gathered from these case studies may stimulate research as productive as Maslow's study (1962) of self-actualized persons, the study by Goertzel and Goertzel (1962) of eminent geniuses, and others.

THE BASIS FOR ANALYSIS

The content of this chapter is not at all speculative, based only upon a few case studies. Using the case studies as vivid illustrations of the problem, the authors have synthesized established theories and research findings from existing literature to guide an analysis of the problem and the needs of this specific subpopulation of intellectually gifted persons with specific disabilities. The work of Maslow (1962) and others has shown that, regardless of the giftedness or the specific disability, all individuals share similar basic needs: physiological comfort; a sense of safety and security; a feeling of belonging and being valued as a member of a social community; a capability of achieving mastery and success, a sense of competence; a sense of efficacy in being able to positively influence one's own life; and a sense of one's exceptional potential ("gifts," "talents") for contribution and achievement as an adult. There is an extensive body of literature defining those needs and demonstrating their direct relationship to achievement behavior.

Thus the psychological literature on human development, especially theories and research pertaining to self-concept and motivation, provides a defensible base for the analysis presented here. Similarly, the literature on giftedness has identified specific characteristic attributes that significantly affect self-concept, motivation, and behavior (Whitmore, 1980; Roedell, 1984). The authors also draw from the literature pertaining to children with handicapping conditions that reports research on the impact of disabilities on self-concept and behavior. It is beyond the scope and purpose of this book to detail the research literature that supports this analysis, but key references are provided.

In the analysis, the existing research literature is applied to the commonalities of traits and needs indicated in all the case studies. Out of a critical analysis of accepted theory and research findings and the needs of gifted disabled persons indicated in the case studies, guidelines for parental, professional, and community practices can be hypothesized. The authors have identified ten commonalities across the case studies:

- intense drive to succeed in reaching goals; exceptional persistence
- the devising and flexible use of creative coping strategies for goal attainment
- recognition and use of strengths, often despite uncertainty about personal giftedness
- a somewhat fragile self-concept and constant struggle to maintain healthy self-esteem
- confusion about mixed messages received from others, especially in school, regarding abilities, differentness, acceptability
- strong desire to be understood and accepted by others and a constant need to work on self-acceptance
- powerful influence of the home providing motivating challenge through supportive encouragement or protective discouragement
- struggles with feelings of social discomfort, embarrassment, shame
- intense frustration and anger requiring a constructive channel of expression
- a need to vent or release pent-up energies through some rewarding activity

These characteristics of intellectually gifted persons who *succeeded* academically and socially may distinguish them from individuals who resigned themselves to failure and/or unfulfilled dreams. However, the long history of research on characteristics of gifted persons suggests that these factors are common to gifted individuals and that the attributes involved positively affect the person's ability to cope effectively with the disability.

This chapter first considers the needs of intellectually gifted individuals with disabilities in relation to self-concept formation and maintenance of healthy self-esteem. Then, the dynamics of motivation that shape behavior are applied to their life experiences, particularly in the home and at school. The chapter concludes with specific recommendations for parents, educators, and others to enhance the self-perceptions and motivation of these individuals relative to their exceptional potential.

SELF-CONCEPT FORMATION AND MAINTENANCE OF SELF-ESTEEM

For more than half a century, psychologists have been studying human behavior in an effort to identify critical factors that would account for some individuals evidencing high levels of perseverant motivation to achieve while others seemingly become indifferent to potential success and neglect the development or use of their abilities. The resulting body of literature has established an unquestionable link between self-concept and self-esteem and established patterns of behavior (Hollingworth, 1942; McClelland, 1958; Sears & Sherman, 1964; Purkey, 1970).

How Is the Self-Concept Formed and Self-Esteem Developed?

The self-concept is the mental picture or concept of self formed in the natural process of asking, "Who am I?" It has been described as the central developmental task of a young child, who builds a unique personality around an emerging self-concept that serves as the core and consequently becomes a primary determiner of behavior. As the child matures, the self-concept becomes a complex cognitive map that allows the individual to predict what will happen during interaction with the world. Self-esteem is the worth and related emotional feelings the individual associates with the self-concept.

A child formulates a self-concept through experiences that provide feedback regarding the unspoken question "Who am I?" Some experiences influence the child's self-image without feedback from other people; such experiences create feelings of relative success or failure, competence and independence, or incompetence and dependence, as the child acts on the environment—for example, tries to solve a puzzle, explores a broken toy to try to fix it, attempts to ride a bicycle, practices writing letters, or follows directions to build a model. The outcome of the child's effort, perceived as success or failure, in combination with outcomes of other efforts forms a pattern that creates a force shaping the developing self-image.

Perhaps even more influential on the concept being formed is feedback from others, particularly persons significant to the child. Adults and peers tend to interpret events to the child as relative success or failure; to affirm the child's ability to succeed or to convey reservations about an ability; and to communicate general feelings of affirmation, reservation, or rejection to the child. The more important the individual is to the child, the more influential the feedback, whether it is delivered intentionally or unintentionally or through verbal or nonverbal communication.

The self-concept becomes stabilized about the age of 9 or 10 years, according to research (Hamachek, 1965), when the child begins to consistently give the same kind of responses to questions about self. That self-concept is the product of interaction between the child's innate sense of self—of potentialities, dispositions, abilities—and the perceived messages from experiences and people. After it has become stabilized, the self-concept continues to be influenced by external forces; thus, it is always subject to change. Research has shown, however, that the self-concept becomes quite resistant to change, increasingly so over the years. Therefore, the older the individual, the more difficult it is to effect significant change in general self-perceptions, even though specific elements of the concept may change. It is rather easy to influence positively the self-concept during the formative years; the child is constantly taking in information and interpreting it for that purpose. Once the self-concept for school achievement, for example, becomes stabilized as generally positive or negative, contradictory messages or experiential evidence tends to be discounted or rejected by the individual, who finds it painfully dissonant with self-knowledge.

The self-concept is extremely complex. Although each individual has a general self-concept that predicts overall success, acceptance, and competence (or the reverse) in the sum total of roles and responsibilities, it also can be viewed as a constellation of specific concepts of self for various activities (e.g., tennis, singing, reading), situations (e.g., home, school, church, concert), and roles (e.g., son, student, friend, musician in the band). Each specific self-concept provides a basis for predicting what to expect during attempts to achieve success in an activity, situation, or role. Figure 7–1 portrays simply the most basic elements of a youngster's overall self-concept.

As has been stated, during the first eight to ten years of life, the child is constantly seeking to define the aspects of self through testing specific abilities, sensitively perceiving outcomes or consequences of behavior, and listening to feedback from others. The child comes to school with general perceptions of personal ability to learn, solve problems, relate to others, adapt, and so forth. It is

Figure 7–1 Elements of a Child's Self-Concept.

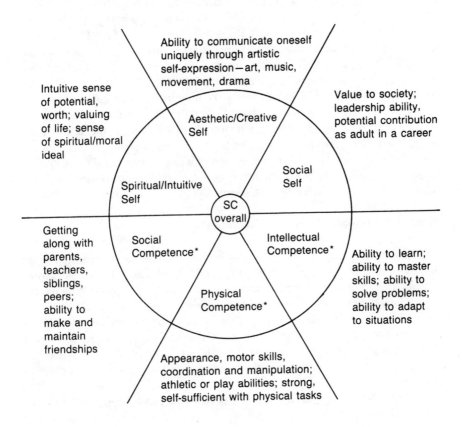

*Develop from earliest months of life; others develop somewhat later and more slowly.

during the first three to four years of school that a self-concept for school achievement is formulated. By middle childhood, when the self-concept for school achievement has become stabilized, most of the child's behavior is motivated by a desire to maintain or preserve that self-concept because it enables the prediction of outcomes; the child begins to behave consistently in keeping with the established self-image. From that point on, much of the child's behavior can be interpreted as defensive, protecting the integrity of the self-concept against threats.

When feedback (e.g., disappointment or higher expectations expressed) threatens the self-concept, the individual is compelled to find ways to cope with that dissonant information. Essentially, the information being received must be either devalued or changed, or the beliefs about self must be modified. Research has shown that it is human nature to tend to reject the information and to accept only compatible ideas once belief systems about self are formed. The individual also seeks out people, situations, and events that reinforce the self-image because the consistency of information about self is comfortable. When conflict between feedback and self-image occurs, the individual must alter the self-concept to accommodate the new information, withdraw from the source of the information, or aggressively counter the information to reaffirm the self as previously developed and identified. This coping behavior provides explanations for "problem" behavior in school and at home, such as noncommunication, no effort to try a task, fighting, "putting down" others, defiance.

What Is the Impact of Specific Disabilities?

It appears that there are no positive effects but only negative ones of specific disabilities on the individual's self-concept and self-esteem. When a child grows up with a disability, its impact seems more subtle and gradual, stemming mostly from a lack of opportunities that normally enhance self-esteem and through self-comparison with nondisabled peers. When the disability occurs through induced trauma in later years, as in John's case, its effect is immediately so destructive that the individual experiences a devastating loss of personal identity as well as feelings of self-worth and is forced to restructure a new self-image in order to survive.

Different disabilities affect different aspects of the self-concept, and the value placed on the affected portion of self determines the magnitude of effect on overall self-esteem. For example, whereas severe neurological injury for John and Herb resulted in extremely negative physical self-concepts, the effect tends to be much less severe for visually impaired persons such as Abe, who instead merely feel awkward and uncertain about their ability to negotiate motorically. Generally, visually impaired children are slower to develop the ability to conceptualize abstractly (Maker, 1976), which may adversely affect their self-concepts for academic achievement, depending upon the requirements of their school instruction. However, learning disabilities seem always to have severely negative impact on self-concept for intellectual competence, most often creating feelings of being "dumb."

All disabling conditions negatively affect self-concept and self-esteem because of the feelings of social discomfort or embarrassment created by the individual's differentness. Even Marcia was adversely affected by the feelings of awkwardness in social communication and embarrassment created by her sensitivity to being disorganized. Myron similarly experienced social discomfort caused by his inability to hear or "read" others communicating with him in the early years, but the impact was minimal compared with that reported by other hearing-impaired persons. Myron's ability to read lips well in later years of childhood and to speak quite clearly significantly diminished the potential negative impact of his disability. John and Herb have experienced social discomfort and thus adverse effects on self-concept for social relations, primarily because of the discomfort others seem to feel in dealing with the more severe physical disability. Persons with such disabilities report that many people seem tense and awkward around them, and that it is difficult not to feel the same way; consequently, interpersonal interaction may be very limited and inhibited.

The potential negative effects of disabilities on self-concept and self-esteem are rather obvious. The degree of effect is directly related to the severity of the disability, the social visibility of the handicap, and the value placed by the individual and others on the ability that is impaired. The effect is most devastating when the ability is needed for the individual to achieve highly valued personal goals, such as specific career options and development of talent, and when the condition is severely impairing.

What Is the Impact of Giftedness?

Intellectually gifted children have been found to be surprisingly vulnerable to low self-esteem (Whitmore, 1980; Roedell, 1984). Even high-achieving gifted students who have no disabilities identify negative feelings about various aspects of self that affect their perceptions of and feelings about themselves as well as others, school, and society (American Association for Gifted Children, 1978). The primary characteristics that make them vulnerable to lower self-esteem can be described as six clusters of traits that also are potentially positive influences on development:

1. *Supersensitivity*

   Cruickshank (1963) posited the theory that intelligence is a direct function of the sensitivity of the nervous system. Professional attention focused on application of that theory to education of slow learners, in whom learning was effectively improved by increasing stimulation. Initially the application to gifted students was overlooked, even though the tendency of gifted students to be high in energy—sometimes described as hyperactive and easily distracted—is well known. This physical energy can produce increased need for movement, high levels of stress, and excessive fatigue. Similarly, intellectually gifted children tend to be keenly perceptive and supersensitive to social communication. For example, parents and teachers often report tendencies of those youngsters to perceive nonverbal signs of disappointment or irritation, to react to criticism as rejection or failure, and to be overly sensitive to teasing or perceived injustice. The supersensitivity has negative impact on the gifted child's self-esteem to the extent that the increased need for movement evokes frequent disciplinary action or criticism, and that social feedback from adults and peers has often been perceived negatively by the child. The youngster's supersensitivity to social communication can foster superior social competence and leadership. It probably accounts for high levels of concern about moral issues and empathy often reported as more prevalent in the gifted population.

2. *Perfectionism*
Beginning with the early classical work of Terman (1925, 1947), studies of gifted individuals have indicated a tendency to be excessively self-critical and perfectionistic—to hold unrealistic self-expectations. This characteristic can be explained as a function of the discrepancy between mental and chronological age; the individual, particularly a young child, envisions a product similar to that expected of older children because of the ability to function intellectually at that higher level. The younger child has difficulty accepting the inability to perform at the higher level, even when explanations about undeveloped skills and readiness are supplied. The perfectionistic tendency also is manifested often in competitiveness and the habit of making critical comparisons, evaluating others as well as self constantly. On the positive side, this trait contributes to high achievement through tenacity to master knowledge and skills and to overcome obstacles. It seems to be this characteristic that accounts for the response by severely disabled individuals to the obstacles posed by their handicaps with exceptional determination to succeed and for John's expressed belief that he was highly motivated to develop his giftedness *because of* his severely disabling condition, not in spite of it!

3. *Desire for independence, self-management*
It seems that the trait of independence emerges early in childhood as the gifted preschooler enjoys becoming increasingly able to manage specific learning activities, exercising high levels of initiative. When a gifted child is encouraged to develop and use this particular ability, positive feelings and motivation to participate occur. When it is discouraged or forbidden, negative attitudes and behavior problems can develop. This trait becomes a negative influence on self-esteem only as a consequence of conflict generated by a restrictive setting. Generally it has positive impact on self-esteem because it contributes to the child's sense of competence and efficacy.

4. *Intense drives to satisfy curiosity and to communicate*
Gifted children exhibit intense desires to know and understand in areas of personal interest. There is an inner pressure to explore, question, and analyze until satisfied with personal comprehension. This is a positive

attribute that contributes to high achievement, unless the individual feels thwarted when questioning, feels excessively restricted in time allocated for exploration, and is actively discouraged from analyzing "too much." The intellectually gifted child also often feels an acute need for self-expression, for communication with others. The danger here is that parents and teachers often must curb the child's self-expression to accommodate group needs and schedules.

5. *Advanced problem-solving skills*
   The exceptional skills of gifted children for problem solving extend to the area of manipulating peers and adults in order to achieve their personal goals and desires. It is the gifted child's facility for successful problem solving that enhances the self-concept for intellectual competence and self-esteem. It can produce some negative effects created by social responses of individuals to being manipulated and by feelings of isolation and alienation when peers do not share similar abilities.

6. *Learning style*
   The natural learning style of young gifted children consists of self-directed inquiry, active exploration, scientific problem solving, and creative and critical thinking. Learning in this natural way is highly motivating to the gifted child. Conversely, the limited and restrictive nature of the traditional classroom or of the special education curriculum for disabled students is incompatible with the gifted child's natural learning style developed and enjoyed in preschool activities. The conflict between the child's desire to focus on higher-level thinking and learning and the school's emphasis on excessive repetition, memorization, and practice at the lowest levels of learning can produce negative attitudes and low motivation to participate.

All these traits are positive in their potential to motivate high achievement and to enhance self-esteem. All of them can also contribute to negative self-perceptions, such as feelings of not fitting in, not being valued socially, or being undesirably different. For a child highly valuing social acceptance, these traits are most apt to have significant negative impact on self-esteem. The response of school personnel to these traits in particular students, and the individual's ability to effectively channel and use them to personal benefit, will determine whether their effects on self-concept and self-esteem are enhancing or diminishing.

The Interactive Effects of Giftedness and Disabilities

It is obvious from the discussions of the potential impact of giftedness and disabling conditions on individuals that the person who is both gifted and disabled is extremely vulnerable to negative perceptions and feelings about self. Those negative expectations for self tend to result in low levels of aspiration, withdrawal

from risk and self-disclosure, hostile defensiveness, and/or achievement significantly below the level of which the individual is capable. It is also true that positive
attributes of giftedness may counterbalance negative effects of disabilities. Six
specific aspects of the potential interaction between giftedness and disabling
conditions are explored here.

Depressed Ability and Perfectionism

To the extent that areas of ability highly valued by the individual are depressed
by the disabling condition, the natural tendency to aspire to achieve some degree
of perfection in those activities generates intense psychological conflict requiring
the development of effective coping mechanisms. This interaction is most readily
seen in a case like John's. He had enjoyed his talent for artistic drawing and writing
poetry, but his accident left him unable to use his hands with any ease or to control
sufficiently his hands to make intended, well-formed marks. After years of
therapy, John's handwriting, with the help of a special prosthesis to give him more
control, remains very difficult to read, and there is no way he can write the words
of poetry or prose he creates as fluently as his mind generates them. The artist Joni
Erikson, however, upon becoming a quadriplegic, developed the ability to express
her talent in drawing through using her teeth to hold the pen and moving her head.
Her response to the disabling condition reflects a drive to create at a high level of
skill that motivated her to persevere in seeking a way to overcome the obstacle
created by her disability. That drive to perfect one's talent, to achieve mastery of
some valued skill(s), to perform generally at a recognizable superior level of
proficiency, enables persevering individuals to diminish significantly the negative
impact of the disability, because they are determined to devise creative strategies
to meet their needs and reach their goals.

Less obvious perhaps to most people is the painfully negative effect of the
interaction between specific learning disabilities and the perfectionistic tendencies
of young gifted children. The reader should recall the internal conflict Marcia
suffered when she felt confused about directions and when she could not seem to
learn to read. Young LD children often have great difficulty in learning to form
letters correctly, to spell words, and to read. The tasks appear very simple for
others, so the LD gifted child tends to assume he or she is "dumb."! Since the early
years of school focus most learning activities on development of the basic skills of
reading, writing, and arithmetic, the gifted child with specific learning disabilities
is extremely vulnerable to feelings of self-contempt when important tasks affected
by the disability cannot be achieved at age-level norms. In the process of trying to
master the skills, the child's perfectionistic bent tends to create impatience with
repeated errors, and a phobia regarding that aspect of the instructional program
may develop (Whitmore, 1980).

Frustration and Anger

The emotions precipitated by the painful struggle to master "simple" skills to a level of relative perfection and by repeated failure to achieve success are frustration and anger. The extent to which these emotions become impairments to mental health and achievement seems to be determined, at least in part, by personality factors as well as the nature and degree of the disability. Feelings of frustration and anger are commonly experienced by persons coping with disabling conditions, but with greater personal awareness of innate potential to achieve, to create, to contribute, and with a strong desire to excel in or perfect an ability, such feelings are intensified. Some individuals, such as Herb, John, and Marcia, are able to convert that emotion into energy for perseverance. Other persons may find the emotions crippling to their ability to cope, especially as the anger is turned inward toward self. The individual who directs anger and hostility toward the situation more than to self, and who expresses those feelings overtly, is more apt to be positively influenced by guidance and to achieve good mental health (Horney, 1945).

Desire for Independence and Feelings of Dependence

Even young gifted children are characterized by the high value they place on feeling relatively independent and self-sufficient. The desire for independence, for being able to manage well and achieve without being dependent on others for help, increases with age and the normal expectations for adolescents and adults. Disabling conditions increase dependency and decrease feelings of independence. Even LD students become dependent upon friends to repeat directions, to help them review for tests, and to explain confusing matters. The visually impaired individual must depend on a guide dog, cane, or another person to achieve mobility, as well as taped or braille reading materials. The hearing impaired person skilled in total communication is least dependent but still depends on others to signal danger (as when a siren or bell sounds) and to indicate that a phone out of sight is ringing. The extreme dependency on others that Herb and John must accept make every little way in which independence can be felt of extreme emotional value.

It seems as though the dependence forced upon the individual by a disability is most difficult for gifted persons to accept. The capacity to achieve higher levels of independence than expected for the condition and to be rigorously independent in thought, if nothing else, can alleviate the discomfort created by the imposed dependence. Thus giftedness can both intensify the negative effects of the disability and potentially assuage those effects by enabling higher levels of independence than expected and the pleasure of independent and productive thought.

High Aspirations and Low Expectations

Gifted persons tend to have a concept of the Ideal Self that inspires them to have higher aspirations than those of other people, to set higher goals for themselves. Relatively low expectations for success often accompany disabling conditions, causing the gifted individual to struggle with the nature of the Real Self in relation to the Ideal Self. As illustrated by the stories of Myron, Herb, and Marcia, often the drive to achieve higher goals mitigates negative messages from parents and/or teachers that reflect low expectations and a belief that personal goals are unattainable. It should be recognized that it requires a great deal of personal courage and energy to cope with the stress induced by the conflicting levels of personal aspirations and the expectations conveyed by others. Formulating a truly realistic self-concept is made more difficult when significant others hold inappropriately low expectations and/or when personal aspirations are unrealistically high.

Social Discomfort and Misperception

The fact that most people recognize a disability but are unaware of exceptional abilities in the affected person is the major source of social discomfort and cognitive dissonance for that person who has a more realistic self-concept based on awareness of exceptional intellectual abilities. If the feedback from others, particularly to the young child, consistently negates those feelings of worth based upon exceptional abilities, the tendency is to deny the giftedness and then to modify the self-concept according to social messages. This conflict between self-perceptions and social feedback seems to occur most intensely for more severely disabled persons.

More moderately disabled gifted individuals tend to have a different experience, particularly in cases in which the disability is not visible—for example, a learning disability or mild hearing loss. In such cases, adults may tend to set unrealistically high expectations because of other evidence of superior ability or general expectations for the age of the child. The potentially negative effect is then a product of the child's inability to understand the difficulty in meeting others' expectations, the adults' impatience with confusion and error, and the communication that the child is being lazy or intentionally "difficult." In either case, the discomfort of being misperceived and the resultant uncertainty or confusion over real abilities can be damaging to self-concept and self-esteem.

Inappropriate Educational Programming

In general, gifted disabled individuals are dealt with educationally more in terms of their deficit abilities than their giftedness. In fact, most often the giftedness has not been recognized until adulthood, as illustrated by the case studies. If the child is placed in a full-time program or school for students with the specific handicapping condition, the likelihood of receiving any appropriate curriculum and instruction for gifted intellectual abilities is negligible. The consequence to the forming self-concept can be very negative: the child structures the self-image only in terms of the disabilities and in fact denies the giftedness. Furthermore, children often experience a lowering of self-esteem as a result of being grouped with others identified by a pejorative label (Hobbs, 1975). This is particularly likely to occur if there are no intellectual peers in the classroom.

In a regular classroom the psychological effects can be negative if the child experiences little success, has inadequate assistance and inappropriate or insufficient modification of the instructional program, and experiences some social isolation as a result of being disabled. Similarly, placement in a gifted education program can be very positive, but it also can be negative if the curriculum requires advanced skills in areas affected by the child's disability, particularly when the peer group tends to be quite competitive. The educational experience *can* be positive in any situation with an appropriate teacher, modification of the instructional program, and a group of intellectual peers. Unfortunately, such conditions often are not provided for gifted children with disabilities.

A potentially positive outcome of the interaction between the individual's giftedness and the disabling condition is the possibility that strengths associated with the superior intellect will offset the negative impact of weaknesses created by the disability. The mentally healthy person accepts into consciousness knowledge of both strengths and weaknesses; having a degree of balance between the two seems most important. In other words, human nature can be quite resilient to impairing deficits if nourished by the satisfaction of achievement allowed by the specific giftedness/strengths. The critical factor is whether the complex interaction among all factors and forces shapes a positive self-image and realistic expectations that are grounded in self-understanding and self-acceptance.

MOTIVATIONAL DYNAMICS SHAPING BEHAVIOR AND ATTITUDES

As stated earlier, self-concept and self-esteem have been consistently identified by researchers as the most powerful determinants of human behavior (LaBenne & Green, 1969; Purkey, 1970; Felker, 1973). Just as the self-concept and feelings of relative worth are shaped by experiences and social feedback, so are the child's habits of thinking and behaving shaped. An understanding of a child's behavior in the school setting, specifically in terms of academic motivation and social interaction, requires an understanding of (a) the child's perceptions of messages from teachers and peers, and the resulting feelings about being in school, and (b) the child's perceptions and feelings about the educational tasks—that is, the curriculum and instructional process. It is the interaction between the child's personal attributes and the two forces of perceived social feedback and planned learning opportunities that produces a specific behavior pattern—such as that described as highly motivated to achieve, disinterested, compliant, or lazy. The dynamic is diagrammed simply in Figure 7–2.

Creation of conditions fostering high achievement motivation may require (a) manipulation of the social environment to convey positive invitations to the child to participate and be successful (Purkey, 1978) and (b) modification of the content, process, and expectations of product in the instructional program to maximize intrinsic and extrinsic rewards. To determine the changes necessary in order to shape more positive responses, or to prevent decline in achievement motivation, the unique combination of needs, feelings, abilities, interests and values of the individual or group must be carefully studied. Then appropriate educational settings for intellectually gifted students with specific disabilities can be selected or developed according to the information about their special needs.

Figure 7–2 The Child's Motivational System

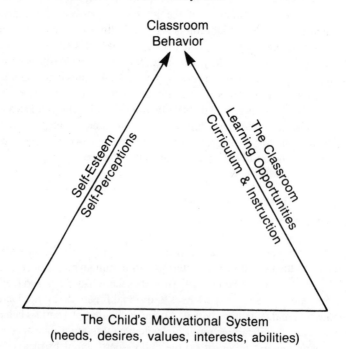

The Child's Motivational System
(needs, desires, values, interests, abilities)

Source: Reprinted with permission from *Giftedness, Conflict and Underachievement* by J.R. Whitmore. Boston: Allyn & Bacon, 1980, p. 214.

At least eight critical motivational factors can be identified for gifted persons with disabilities as a result of analysis of the interaction between attributes of giftedness and the consequences of the disabling condition:

1. *A perceived possibility of success in a learning experience that is challenging*
    The giftedness in the individual leads to selection of challenging tasks when the perfectionistic tendency is satisfied that there is a reasonable possibility of success. If the learning experience provided or required does not appear to be challenging, as is often the case with repetitious drill work, the child is apt to be motivated *not* to participate. If the task seems far too difficult for success to be possible, the child will not desire to try.

2. *Fear of failure*
    Although perfectionism creates anxiety about the possibility of failing, there is a quite different aspect of fear of failure that seems to operate with disabled persons: a fear of failing in activities associated with independence. For example, John feared failing to master certain skills (e.g., feeding himself) that he needed to decrease his dependence on others much more than he just feared failing when he tried. In other words, the only hope for increased independence was to risk again and again frustrating failure in the attempt to develop skills for more independent living. In a similar but different way, Marcia expressed her fear of failing to gain an education to equip her for a career that would make her self-sufficient as being the motivating force that overshadowed her fear of failure in the process of trying for years to learn to read and write. Undoubtedly, some persons with disabling conditions, perhaps even intellectually gifted, have resigned themselves to repeated failure and a dependent life style that perhaps feels safer and more comfortable than a constant struggle to achieve.

3. *The degree of match between the individual's desires and abilities and the nature of opportunities*
    The child is motivated to participate fully in learning experiences when the content often is related to personal interests and when the activities allow the child to enjoy using the higher cognitive abilities characteristic of the natural learning style. When the curriculum is composed of rote memorization and drill exercises, content that is intellectually unstimulating and uninteresting to the child, and demands for products that are difficult or impossible for the child to produce in the time allocated (e.g., amount of writing and/or reading necessary to complete the assignments), then the child naturally is motivated to avoid the learning experience and to divert energies elsewhere (e.g., to social interaction or daydreaming).

    In older individuals, the motivation to develop abilities can be significantly diminished by a perceived lack of opportunity to use them. For example, an individual's desire for a college education can be thwarted by a belief that appropriate employment will not be available upon completion of the degree program. With feelings of being doomed to endure employment in an occupation that is boring and perhaps insulting to the level of intelligence as well as unrewarding, motivation to achieve higher development of any special abilities is significantly diminished.

4. *Positive models*

Most persons with disabling conditions do not have models of similar individuals who have been successful and rewarded for their achievement. As John noted, during his rehabilitation treatment he was surrounded with negative images of what he could become or remain. Critical to his sustained motivation to achieve higher levels of habilitation was his relationship with the woman who later became his wife, who was in her tenth year of rehabilitation at the time and had been very successful. John still lacks models for succeeding in this chosen career of higher education administration; however, that need is perhaps offset by the meaningful relationship he has with professional colleagues with whom he works and studies in the college of education. When disabled persons achieve success in a career, they become inspiring models for others to emulate.

5. *A positive vision of what the individual can become*

The dream of achieving a goal, of being someone with certain valued attributes, can be a powerful motivator of behavior. The risk with disabled persons is that motivating visions of what they can become as persons are not cultivated, or they are destroyed by a belief that the disability makes the dream unattainable. A motivating vision blends elements of the person's ideal self with realistic goals that can be attained. Belief in personal ability to reach those goals supplies the motivation that others describe as remarkable perseverance.

6. *Accurate self-knowledge*

Motivation to achieve can be negatively affected by unrealistically high or low estimations of personal abilities and disabilities. The individual needs accurate knowledge of the possibilities created by particular strengths or gifts and of the limitations created by the specific disability. If the person dreams unrealistically, feelings of failure and personal disappointment, perhaps even self-contempt, will be intensified. Realistic visions of life goals, with full consideration and acceptance of the limiting disabilities, can heighten motivation to strive to develop all abilities. The base of self-knowledge must be rational and not governed by emotions that distort reality.

7. *Ability to control emotions*

In order for the disabled person to maintain high levels of motivation to achieve, that individual must be able to control the emotions that may be evoked in the process and tend to elicit negative responses from others. The person must develop a high tolerance for frustration, feelings of embarrassment, falling short of perfection, and enduring persons who are obstructive. Inability to curb such debilitating emotions, not merely their expression, to a healthy level will adversely affect attitudes and behavior. The result will be interference with the positive elements of the motivational dynamics, resulting in lower achievement.

8. *The energy factor*
   The disabled individual must have sufficient energy to cope with the strain and stress incurred by motivation to achieve and the process of achieving established goals. LD persons typically identify disciplined athletic or musical ability, for example, as both channeling energies in positive ways and reducing stress that enables greater concentration and effort in doing difficult tasks. Persons who are physically disabled, such as Herb and John, must find ways of coping with pent-up psychological as well as physical energies that may interfere with task commitment and completion. The disabled person requires great amounts of energy to cope successfully but also needs to channel excessive energies into constructive outlets so that they do not interfere.

These are some of the critical factors influencing the motivational characteristics or responses of intellectually gifted individuals with disabling conditions. The more positive factors exist within an individual and in the particular setting, the greater the chances of higher levels of motivation and a greater capacity for sustained effort. Negative factors tend to diminish motivational response and lower the ability to cope successfully and achieve, although all of the subjects in the case studies seemed to have increased motivation in response to negative, obstructive experiences. Perhaps the success of these individuals can be attributed most to their positive response of determination to overcome obstacles.

RECOMMENDATIONS FOR PARENTS, TEACHERS, AND OTHERS

This section begins with some guidelines for parents and teachers to enable them to create or contribute to the creation of optimal conditions that will facilitate the full development of the individual's abilities. Individual personality characteristics will create variance in the specific responses to conditions provided, but following these guidelines will eliminate or reduce common obstructions to growth and achievement and will enhance other facilitating factors.

1. *Keep perceptions of the individual's limitations open-ended.*
   All judgments about abilities and disabilities should be tentative; in particu-

lar, a low ceiling of expectations must never be placed on the child's potential achievement. Experiment, encourage the child to try, but caution against unrealistic self-expectations and interfering impatience. This is both the most fundamental and important guideline and the most difficult one for adults to enact. Parents and teachers often find it difficult to ascertain when a child has reached the current limit of ability and should be provided with an alternative or be discouraged from continuing. This recommendation is most important for the parents and teachers of the more severely disabled; the converse may tend to be true for more mildly and less visibly disabled children—that is, the expectations may be too high.

2. *Convey positive, realistic expectations.*

   The child should be encouraged to try; to accept failure as part of the learning process; to evaluate after erring and then to modify the strategy used, if necessary, and try again! This guidance will support the individual's natural perseverance and temper the necessary frustration with a matter-of-fact attitude about the "trials" necessary before success can be achieved. Parents and teachers should convey confidence in the child's general ability to succeed, without pushing him or her beyond the readiness/success level; this is particularly important when the child becomes discouraged and inclined to give up.

3. *Encourage the development of increasing levels of independence.*

   Parents and teachers should recognize the emotional significance to the child of feeling able to manage well alone and to become appropriately independent. This recommendation is most important for adults who tend to feel protective of the disabled child and unwittingly foster dependence. Without diminishing the undergirding support and technical assistance needed for the child to succeed, parents and teachers must intentionally encourage the child to become increasingly self-sufficient.

4. *Help the child to formulate a positive, attainable goal for the future.*

   Children are not born aware of possibilities for their lives as children, much less as adults. Parents and teachers must help children to explore alternative careers and life styles for adulthood that will help them discover their special abilities. The vision of a positive future outcome of all academic efforts, for instance, can help the child sustain greater motivation to master basic school subjects.

5. *Guide the child's development of self-understanding and constructive coping strategies.*

   First, during the developmental years, parents and teachers should continue to help the child understand the nature of specific difficulties and strengths. Literature and social interaction with similar peers can be used to convey the fact that such difficulties are not unique to the child. Then, alternative ways of coping constructively with the disability, or with negative effects of being intellectually gifted, can be suggested, with emphasis on strategies used by others. For example, the use of self-talk (Webb et al., 1982), to temper emotions by using reason, should be encouraged. Similarly the child should be helped to consider possible methods of self-modification and gaining self-control, and experimentation with whatever positive strategy the child believes might be effective should be encouraged. Parents should not allow self-pity to prevail; the child should be guided to accept as "normal" the feelings of frustration, anger, and self-pity that arise now and then. Teachers and parents should encourage patience, persistence, and an experimental approach to life that places high value on risk-taking behavior that is responsible, thoughtful, and informative about personal possibilities.

6. *Provide daily opportunities for the child to build inherent superior abilities and to enjoy feelings of success.*
    Parents can supply the child with educational toys and materials for hobbies that encourage the development of specific gifts and talents. Reading to the child and obtaining books and games that match the child's interests and abilities can be powerfully positive influences. Teachers need to provide daily opportunities for the child to experience satisfaction in his or her area of giftedness—for example, scientific inquiry, creative self-expression, or analytical problem solving.

7. *Advocate for appropriate educational opportunities to be provided.*
    Parents need to be assertive when necessary to obtain the appropriate educational placement for the child. More than for placement in a regular or special educational class, or for the formulation of an Individual Educational Plan (IEP), the parents must advocate for the child's right to appropriate teachers, curriculum, and peers in the classroom. For the gifted child with disabilities this requires teachers who can develop the strengths as well as remediate the weaknesses. It requires a curriculum or IEP that includes adequate attention to the giftedness as well as to the deficit skills. In addition, it requires a group of intellectual peers to share in the learning process. Parents need to be diplomatic but very firm advocates for their children in school.

    Teachers also are frequently needed to advocate within the school system for appropriate educational programming to be provided a child. They should attack restrictive policies, such as rules allowing a child to receive only one kind of special educational service. If the child is to be served in a regular classroom with support services, the teacher must have an accurate understanding of this type of child and the specific needs, as well as skills to provide appropriate instruction. Young children need advocates; while they are formulating their self-concepts for school, they tend to regard adults as unquestionable authorities, and after all, they have little or no knowledge of the alternatives that should be available to them.

8. *Pursue positive social experiences for the child.*
To minimize social discomfort and underdeveloped social competence, parents should seek good preschool programs for the child. It is most important that the young child not be hidden or protected from social situations but be placed in carefully selected social settings for early, positive social experiences, such as church school, preschool, or the homes of neighbors or friends of family. During the elementary school years, supplementary positive social experiences may be gained through scouting, clubs centered on hobbies, classes in the arts, and the like; both informal and more structured settings are valuable learning opportunities. Teachers also must seek to provide the child with opportunities to develop a sense of social acceptance and competence. A few special friendships sometimes develop at the initiation of the perceptive teacher who contrives opportunities for the children to become acquainted. Teachers who frequently have children complete tasks in pairs or small groups, and who provide time for more informal interaction among peers in the classroom, can easily facilitate the disabled child's social integration and growth. In addition, it is desirable for the teacher to use literature read orally to the group, sociodrama, social studies, science, and the arts to develop knowledge and understanding of self, others, and society. In those educational experiences the teacher can skillfully infuse information to shape desirable attitudes and values regarding cultural diversity, individual differences, giftedness, and disabilities.

Parents and teachers can powerfully influence the development of the disabled child who is intellectually gifted. This influence continues throughout life: at any age, a disabled person can be positively guided in various aspects of development by parents or teachers. However, the impact is greatest and most easily achieved during the early, formative years. Since the adult incurring severe disability must restructure the self-concept, those working with the disabled person during the rehabilitation process could be expected to have similarly profound impact on that person's adjustment and achievement.

Of course there are many persons besides parents and teachers who significantly influence the development and achievement of intellectually gifted individuals with specific disabilities. The authors have chosen to illustrate the kinds of implications that can be drawn by discussing three of the most common groups: medical professionals, counselors or psychologists, and employers.

Representatives of the medical profession, physicians and nurses, are among the first to begin to influence expectations and opportunities for the infant or the newly disabled person through the information and advice given to parents or to the disabled adult. There seems to be a tendency to set lower expectations to prevent disappointment, and to ignore the possibility of superior cognitive abilities. Often very limited information is provided and as a child matures there seldom is careful guidance by the physician(s) to develop more accurate self-understanding and expectations.

Much more complete information and accurate advice needs to be provided by the medical profession to schools as well as to families. Physicians, fearful of misleading the patient's family, may present the entire range of possibilities and then provide genuine encouragement regarding more optimistic outcomes with patient work toward that goal. Clearly, recommendations of automatic institutionalization for more severely disabled children is inconsistent with the purpose of Public Law 94-142, and medical professionals should be cautioned against giving such advice too soon. The fact that the ultimate achievement level of any person is not accurately predictable can leave hope in the hearts of the patient and family for greater improvement than may seem possible. At the same time, it prevents surprise if the hoped-for progress is not achieved.

Counselors or psychologists frequently are placed in a position of influence similar to that of the medical professionals. This influence perhaps is greatest with the rehabilitation counselors, who, as John described, may tend to focus on "survival" skills for "independent" living but fail to explore special abilities, which still could be developed through a new career that would increase life satisfaction for the disabled person. Counselors who work with families need to go beyond helping the parents and siblings cope with the disabling condition to helping them explore potential strengths to be nurtured. This more balanced approach can reduce feelings of pity and enable family members to find more positive ways of interacting within the family unit, including with the disabled child.

Employers are seldom discussed as having significant impact on the lives of disabled persons, except in circles of professionals sharing that concern. Community agencies must help to ensure that employers do not discriminate against disabled persons. Employers need to be helped to see how they may capitalize on the superior abilities of the intellectually gifted person who is disabled by adjusting slightly the job description to emphasize the individual's strengths. Disabled persons should be given adequate opportunity to test their ability to succeed on the job, with reasonable support given. If communities do not provide these persons with respectable employment opportunities appropriate for their giftedness, there will be great difficulty in inspiring young disabled students to maintain a positive vision of the future and to persevere toward their goals.

In summary, in this chapter the authors have attempted to consider briefly the critical factors that influence the gifted disabled individual's motivation to try to develop fully innate potential as an intellectually gifted person. The authors have used their understanding of how the individual's self-concept and self-esteem are shaped by social feedback and experiences of relative success or failure, and the parallel effect on the development of behavior patterns, to develop the recommendations presented to guide parents, teachers, and others so that they may be more facilitative and less obstructive of the individual's development.

Chapter 8

The Intellectual Needs of Gifted Persons with Disabilities

This chapter begins with a discussion of a research study from which much of the information presented here was derived. Following that discussion, the chapter focuses on knowledge and skills necessary to provide needed educational strategies and programs to develop the intellectual potential of gifted students who have disabilities. Three areas of need that significantly affect cognitive development and intellectual achievement can be addressed by everyone in all settings: (a) the need to develop expectations based on realistic perceptions of strengths and weaknesses; (b) the need for gifted, impaired individuals to acquire specific strategies for learning and for coping with the disability; and (c) the need for successful role models.

First, more generally applicable guidelines and specific techniques for meeting the intellectual and educational needs of disabled persons are presented for families and friends, educators, and community agencies and institutions. Then specific guidelines for educators are delineated relative to more technical concerns: identification and assessment of disabled students who are intellectually gifted and the development of appropriate educational programs for this population. Finally in this chapter, cooperative programs for families, educators, and agencies are discussed.

The authors have been interested in and concerned with the education of "special populations" of gifted students for at least 15 years and were involved in the first efforts to identify and serve gifted children and adults with handicapping conditions. Collectively, they have created and implemented a special program for highly gifted underachievers; developed or assisted in the development and implementation of programs for gifted students who are learning disabled, deaf or hard of hearing, or blind or visually impaired; and assisted in the development of preschool programs for gifted children who have a variety of handicapping conditions. In their professional activities they have interviewed and worked with numerous gifted people who have mild to severe disabilities. Files of notes and other records have been maintained as part of their ongoing inquiry into the special needs of this population in an effort to formulate a knowledge base to guide practices derived from the analysis of many individual cases.

The content of this chapter, as well as the remainder of the book, has been integrated from four major sources: the available literature, a synthesis of information gleaned from the authors' case studies, the authors' professional experiences and reflections, and a study of successful handicapped scientists conducted with the cooperation of the American Association for the Advancement of Science (AAAS) from which three subjects were selected for inclusion as case studies in this book.

Prior to the discussion of guidelines and recommendations that are the focus of this chapter, a somewhat brief but detailed explanation of the study of handicapped scientists is provided to illustrate the research methodology employed. The purpose of injecting this description is to give the reader a more complete basis for understanding and evaluating the recommendations and conclusions offered and for recognizing the value and limitations of the research base from which much of this chapter's content has been derived.

A STUDY OF SUCCESSFUL HANDICAPPED SCIENTISTS

After interviewing 30 individuals with disabilities for a book commissioned by the Council for Exceptional Children (CEC) (Maker, 1977), June Maker became convinced of the value of interviews in the understanding of a relatively new field and requested that people contact her if they were gifted and disabled or knew of those who were. Martha Ross Redden, who was involved in a project on handicapped scientists for AAAS, heard of this interest and suggested that many individuals in her project were gifted. Together, Maker and Redden conceptualized a research project that would gather and synthesize data about significant life experiences and coping or learning strategies employed by individuals who had been successful in overcoming the handicaps placed on them by society and the limitations imposed by their disability. It was believed that the information so derived could then be used in a variety of ways.

Design of the Study

The study (Maker et al., 1978) consisted of three major foci: first, collection of information about events perceived by the interviewees as significant in the development of their potential (in either a positive or a negative way); second, the individuals' beliefs about the causes and effects of their success or failure in achievement-related events; and third, the collection of other data regarding the interviewees' backgrounds and experiences, including their perceptions of successful coping strategies and recommendations for dealing with others who have similar disabilities. Individuals interviewed were selected from a pool of over 900 successful scientists with disabilities who had contacted the AAAS in response to an announcement in *Science* magazine. Selection of subjects was based on four criteria: (a) a handicapping condition that was documented at birth or incurred before age 14 years (while the subject was still in elementary or junior high school); (b) the subject's completion of at least a college degree program; (c) the subject's employment in a position commensurate with educational level, in the specific area of training; and (d) possession of a disability in one of the four areas being studied. An attempt was made to interview the same number of individuals in each of the following categories: legally blind, legally deaf, cerebral palsied, and mobility impaired.

Approximately 140 individuals (data from 120 were included in the final sample) were interviewed using Flanagan's (1962) Critical Incident Technique. According to Flanagan, an "incident" is any human activity that is observable and complete enough in itself for inferences and predictions to be made about the persons involved. In order to be "critical," an incident must leave little doubt in the observer's mind about its effects or consequences. The Critical Incident Technique has as its basis the assumption that if an observer can recall and describe fully a specific incident, then this event had an effect on the observer. Not only are the critical behaviors specified, but the antecedents leading up to and the consequences resulting from the behavior also are reported. Reporting of the same type of incidents by several observers assures a certain amount of objectivity.

The subjects were asked to describe the three events in their lives that were the most significant in helping them realize their potential. The events could be those having either a positive or a negative effect and could involve any period or aspect of their life. When an incident was given, the interviewer asked certain probing questions to obtain as much detail as possible regarding the actual event, the circumstances leading up to the event, the people involved, the outcome, and the immediate as well as long-range effects. The interviewee also was asked to state why that event was significant. The second part of the interview was more structured and was designed to obtain specific information about the handicapping condition, family background, education, present career, successful coping and learning strategies, and recommendations for dealing with others who have a similar disability.

An open-ended but structured interview approach such as this seemed particularly appropriate in the investigation of personal perception of behaviors in self or in others. The types of incidents reported, as well as the personal beliefs about the significance of the events, the behaviors observed and the causes and effects of events and behavior were of interest. Such a method precluded the description of influences on success in abstract or general terms. Instead, these significant events were easily visualized. Since the approach was open-ended, the particular biases of the interviewer were effectively eliminated (e.g., the subject was not given a checklist or questionnaire on which to record responses). Subjects chose events they perceived as significant in their development and described their perception of actions, causes, and effects.

All interviews were tape-recorded and later transcribed verbatim. Critical events were examined and classified independently by two objective raters according to a general frame of reference developed by a group of handicapped scientists. The final system was judged satisfactory, since raters disagreed on the classification of less than 10 percent of the events, coping or learning strategies, and causes and effects of achievement-related events.

Several aspects of the Critical Incident Technique offered advantages for this investigation. The following list presents those aspects and a short discussion of their advantages in the study:

1. *Only those events perceived important by the individual were studied further.* The types of events selected as important were themselves of interest in the study of self-perception. In addition, the behavior of others was studied in the context of events perceived important by the subject rather than those perceived important by the experimenter.

2. *The individual was required to specify personal reasons for selecting the event.* This permitted the analysis of criteria used by different individuals in selecting events as significant.

3. *Specific details of significant events were given.* This made clear the context of the situation, the circumstances leading up to the event, and the exact behaviors of the subject and of other people (as seen by the subject). Such detail permitted the description of a handicapped individual's perceptions in specific rather than general terms. Inferences and predictions were then tied to a more concrete base.

4. *Individuals gave their perceptions of causes and effects of the significant events.* This permitted the study of perceptions of causes and effects in relation to specific events regarded as critical to the individual's development.

5. *The approach was open-ended but structured.* Experimenter bias in selecting the exact situations to be studied was eliminated, and the same *type* of information was obtained from each interview.

6. *The technique has been used in numerous and varied situations and has been refined by its developers.* The procedures were clear and easily applied to these situations.

Limitations of the Study

Although the Critical Incident Technique offers the advantages just outlined, it does have certain limitations that should be recognized. First of all, some influences on success that are long-term may have been lost in the attempt to identify critical events. Emphasis on incidents may have obscured the cumulative effect of several influences. In an attempt to overcome this limitation, interviewers allowed individuals to describe what they felt were long-term influences. When these were given, the interviewer asked the individual to describe an event that was an *example* of that long-term influence. A second limitation inherent in any retrospective method was the subject's recall. Some individuals were unable to recall specific events or the details of events. Flanagan would probably argue that events that cannot be recalled are not significant, but the fact remains that some people have a better memory than others, so that those with poor memories are not represented accurately in the data analyzed. A third limitation is inherent in any open-ended approach. The bias of the interviewer may have influenced the number and kind of probing questions asked about each event. Attempts to overcome this limitation included specifying the questions to be asked as well as training and retraining of the interviewers. Procedures devised to overcome these limitations may not have been completely successful. However, the advantages recommended the method in spite of its limitations.

A limitation of both the foregoing research project and most of the literature on the subject of this book was mentioned earlier but deserves mention again in this context: because the subjects were adults who have become successful, it is not possible to determine whether the events reported caused success or whether the individuals' success influenced their perceptions of the effects of events and techniques. In fact, what they perceived as causes *of* their success may have been caused *by* this success. It is the authors' opinion that too often educators confuse the concepts of *success* and *ability*. Many individuals with high ability have not been successful. Studies of only those who have achieved at a high level must necessarily be limited in value because such studies do not yield information about how or whether those with ability who have not achieved success are different from those who have. Longitudinal studies of gifted disabled individuals from early childhood through adulthood are needed to address these limitations. In the meantime, these case studies provide a wealth of ideas to guide further investigation and experimental efforts to improve professional and parenting practices.

The following section applies the relevant research base to needs affecting the cognitive development of gifted youngsters with handicapping conditions. First, the overall effect of attitudes and stereotypes on achievement is explained in the context of the well-known construct of "self-fulfilling prophecies." Next, suggestions are presented to assist parents, teachers, and others in recognizing and modifying the behaviors that successful adults with disabilities have identified as indicators of lowered expectations and negative stereotypes. Emphasis in the subsequent section is on techniques the individual with a disability can employ successfully in overcoming or changing these low expectations or minimizing their effect on intellectual performance; the strategies described by successful scientists with handicapping conditions are presented as examples.

Finally, individual attitudes, specifically, personal beliefs about the causes of success or failure in achievement-related situations, are explored. The reader should note that there is a very direct relationship between attributions (beliefs about the causes) for success or failure and motivation to achieve. This motivation or willingness to exert the effort needed to overcome negative stereotypes and perceptions also appears to be directly related to development and use of appropriate coping and learning strategies.

MEETING THE INTELLECTUAL NEEDS OF DISABLED PERSONS

Understanding Attitudinal Influences on Achievement

One of the most significant barriers to the achievement of gifted individuals with handicapping conditions is negative perceptions and stereotypes regarding their abilities. Every individual included in the case studies presented in this book discussed these attitudes and gave numerous examples of stereotypic expectations, such as exclusion from advanced classes, inaccurate assessment of ability to learn a particular subject or pursue a particular career, or placement in unchallenging, restricting situations. In the study of successful disabled scientists, the majority of events that were reported as significant to their development, either positively or negatively, involved the attitudes of others toward their ability. Numerous studies also have shown that attitudes of the public, teachers, and other students toward persons with disabilities tend to be unfavorable (Maker et al., 1978). A number of issues can be addressed on this subject, but negative stereotypes become most important when lowered expectations become self-fulfilling prophecies—that is, "when they produce the very conditions or behaviors erroneously assumed to exist" (Mitchell, 1976, p. 309).

Research, as well as practical experience, shows that expectations do not always become self-fulfilling prophecies. Indeed, if they always had that effect, the majority of handicapped individuals would not achieve any measure of success in occupations since so many studies show the overwhelming negative attitudes of others. Good and Brophy (1973) reviewed the research on expectancy effects and conducted several studies of the process by which expectations can become self-fulfilling prophecies. They have outlined five steps that seemingly must occur if teacher expectations are to function as self-fulfilling prophecies (Good & Brophy, 1973, p. 75):

1. The teacher expects specific behavior and achievement from specific students.

2. Because of these different expectations, the teacher behaves differently toward different students.
3. This teacher treatment tells each student what behavior and achievement the teacher expects from him and affects his self-concept, achievement motivation, and levels of aspiration.
4. If this teacher treatment is consistent over time and if the student does not actively resist or change it in some way, it will tend to shape his achievement and behavior. High expectation students will be left to achieve at high levels, while the achievement of low expectation students will decline.
5. With time, the student's achievement and behavior will conform more and more closely to that originally expected of him.

Although the work of Good and Brophy is only concerned with the effect of *teacher* expectations, there is evidence to indicate that the behavior of other individuals (especially significant others such as parents) can function in the same way.

Only a brief summary of research on this five-step process as it relates to individuals with disabilities is presented here (see Maker et al., 1978 for a more complete review):

1. Studies show that teachers do have lowered expectations for the achievement of persons with disabilities.
2. There are specific identifiable behaviors that communicate these lowered expectations to the individuals.
3. Even though child behavior strongly contradicts a teacher's perceptions, the original perceptions often are retained.
4. Often such variables as contact with disabled individuals, information about their capabilities, and experience working with them will cause a teacher, parent, or another individual to revise these expectations so that they more nearly conform to reality.
5. There is evidence that the behavior of teachers and significant others does have a long-range effect on the achievement of a disabled individual.

Review of these considerations and their application to education of handicapped students suggest that a definite problem exists, but that attitudes and stereotypes *can* be changed. Although outside influences can have a positive impact, the principal actors in the process of change are the disabled person and the individual interacting with the disabled person. Both can share in the responsibility for making changes. Teachers, parents, and others who work with a disabled individual must first be aware of the general tendency to underestimate ability, must recognize the behaviors that can communicate expectations, and then must continually work to modify their own behavior so that realistic expectations are communicated. They also must be open to the *possibility* that the disabled individual's abilities are unlimited. Only repeated demonstration of limits should cause revision of these expectations. The disabled individual, on the other hand, must be an advocate for himself or herself and must use active strategies to change or modify unrealistic expectations. The individuals studied in this book and in the research cited have probably been successful in overcoming or changing the lowered expectations others have for them. At the very least, they have prevented these low expectations from becoming self-fulfilling prophecies.

The following discussion focuses on methods of modifying expectations in three general areas: behaviors perceived by gifted disabled students as evidence of others' expectations for their success; coping and learning strategies used to change or overcome low expectations; and techniques for outside agencies, teacher training programs, counselors, and others to use in facilitating change in interactions with individuals who are disabled.

Modifying Behaviors to Convey Positive Expectations

Often people are not aware of the full impact of their behavior on others. Many parents and teachers can recall discussions with children in which the children were told that their behavior was perceived in a way that was unintended. There is obviously no way to avoid occasional problems like this, but an awareness of the behaviors that generally are interpreted in a certain way can reduce misperceptions.

Behaviors that indicate low expectations for achievement have been identified in all the case study chapters. The authors offer as a supplement the following list of behaviors characterized by low expectations derived from interviews with other competent disabled individuals:

- directing a conversation or giving instructions to others rather than to the disabled person
- avoiding intellectual discussions
- accepting one failure as proof that a task cannot be accomplished
- excluding a student with mild cerebral palsy from a laboratory course because he would be a ''hazard''
- telling a deaf person that he or she cannot have an apartment alone
- giving higher grades for lower performance in relation to others
- accepting and/or giving excessive praise for inferior-quality work
- responding to children's questions about what a disabled person can do by describing only a cafeteria worker, factory worker, or laborer rather than a professional

- telling a deaf daughter that all a deaf woman will be able to do is become a librarian
- using simple words and sentences in discussions with individuals who have cerebral palsy or a hearing impairment because their speech is difficult to understand
- attempting to put a disabled person into a vocational program even if that person is eligible for and is more interested in a college preparatory program
- sending a coauthor rather than the disabled person to present a paper at a conference
- calling for an interpreter rather than attempting to communicate with a deaf individual
- putting disabled children in their own subgroups within organizations such as the Boy Scouts or Girl Scouts
- not allowing a student with cerebral palsy to practice math skills at the chalkboard because he or she has difficulty walking
- excusing a child with a disability from doing chores that other siblings are required to do
- prohibiting a blind child from going anywhere in the neighborhood alone because of the possibility of injury or of getting lost (even though the child had "run away" several times and had found the way back home)

Teachers, parents, and others should be aware of the potential effect of such behaviors and modify them so that they do not reflect a *generalized*, negative perception of what a disabled person can or cannot do but instead reflect a *specific*, positive perception of one disabled person's strengths and weaknesses. For example, in an incident described by a deaf woman, in which she was told that her best choice of careers would be in library science, her parents could have discussed several career options by describing their advantages and disadvantages. Her communication difficulties could be described either as barriers to be overcome in pursuing a particular career or as barriers to be avoided by pursuing a different career.

With regard to household chores, parents should expect disabled children to perform their share but can select with the child those that are possible. Obviously, no one wants children with disabilities to get hurt or lost. However, even children without disabilities get hurt and lost. There is no way they can be protected at all times without severe restrictions. In the case of the blind child who was not allowed to go anywhere in the neighborhood alone, his parents could demonstrate both their concern and an expectation that he was capable of learning by teaching him about the neighborhood and how to get around in it (like Abe's parents did), and then let him go short distances alone to test his ability to get around. When he demonstrated this ability, he could be allowed and encouraged to explore on his own.

With regard to academic settings, the example of communicating at a low level (e.g., using simple words and sentences) illustrates a common problem. Educators have a tendency to assume that intelligence and expressive ability are equivalent, when in fact the child's level of understanding may be considerably higher than the capacity for self-expression. A severely impaired individual with cerebral palsy and no speech at all may be highly intelligent. When the child learns to use communication aids or devices, the expressive ability may more nearly match the ability to comprehend. To develop a realistic view of the individual's ability to understand ideas, the teacher and student can devise methods for checking to see that concepts or instructions are understood rather than assuming that a lower conceptual level is needed.

Another frequent behavior in an academic setting is to assign to disabled children only those tasks that are *certain* to be completed successfully, and to lower expectations for the child's performance after only one failure or to continually provide only those learning experiences at a "safe" level. The only way to test the student's cognitive limits is to provide a challenge and then to examine closely the performance, even if the child fails. Challenges can be presented as such, and the child should be told that the teacher wants to see "how far" he or she can go in this area. Challenges should be presented often, not just occasionally. With frequent experiences in challenging tasks requiring improved skills, students may begin to accomplish what the teacher was certain initially could not be done.

In summary, parents, educators, and others need to be aware of their behaviors that can communicate low expectations for the performance of gifted children with disabilities. Once aware, they must strive to change their behaviors so that they do not reflect a generalized, negative perception of the limitations of a particular disability but instead reflect a specific, positive perception of the set of strengths and limitations in the child, so that realistic, appropriate expectations can be formulated.

Developing Coping and Learning Strategies

In the past, emphasis has been placed solely on the responsibility of persons interacting with disabled individuals, rather than considering the responsibility of the disabled individual. The person with a disability was essentially viewed as a victim, or a passive recipient of negative treatment. Data collected from individuals who have been successful in academic settings and in their careers suggest that many techniques can be employed to alter significantly how their abilities are perceived by others. These strategies can be learned by disabled individuals on their own or can be taught to them by parents, teachers, or others. Older individuals who have been successful can serve as role models and can be extremely helpful in guiding a younger person to discover or develop effective techniques.

The specific coping and learning strategies reported by successful disabled scientists were classified according to the same general categories used to classify reported beliefs about the causes of success (Maker et al., 1978). The general categories and subcategories are presented in Exhibit 8–1.

It is important to note here the relationship between the coping and learning strategies used by individuals and their attributions or beliefs about the causes of their success. Most individuals tended to report coping strategies that corresponded directly to their attributions. For example, if an individual attributed personal success to *ability*, most of the coping strategies reported involved the use or development of ability. If *other people* were perceived as the major cause, most of the strategies reported involved soliciting the help of other people.

Since the handicapped scientists perceived the causes of their success as ability, other people, effort, intent, luck, stable effort (persistence), personality characteristics, and task difficulty, these general categories were chosen as a frame of reference for classifying the specific coping strategies reported. Within each of these general categories, subcategories were developed inductively by the methods recommended by Flanagan (1962). Examples of the strategies in each category follow.

Category I: Strategies Involving the Use or Development of Ability

General Learning Strategies. Most strategies in this category emphasized a broadening of academic background, especially through reading textbooks and extra materials. Most subjects reported learning to read and developing an interest in reading at an early age. One deaf individual reported attempting to grasp the particular style and method of expression of each author he read, whereas another reported efforts to see the correlation between an abstract idea in calculus and the more concrete and easily observable ideas of chemistry and physics. A blind individual reported looking for the "big ideas" or "big picture" so he could make the mental leap of understanding and then sit down and absorb the details.

Specific Skill Development. Strategies in this category included the development of a range of skills, from athletics to writing. Many felt that the development of a problem-solving approach was a corequisite with this skill development, "thinking of where I might find answers rather than always running to others to see if they have the answers." One person felt that by writing and developing mathematics workshops for other children, he simultaneously developed a higher-level understanding of mathematics. Another reported becoming an expert in an area that is very specialized so that fellow workers must depend on him to help with their statistical problems. Most responses could be summed up by the attitude expressed by one blind individual: "creating your own resources to overcome

Exhibit 8–1 Coping and Learning Strategies Reported by Successful Scientists with Disabilities

I. Strategies Involving Use or Development of Ability
   A. General Learning Strategies
   B. Specific Skill Development
   C. Strategies to Convince Others
   D. Development of Personal Attitudes
      1. Self-confidence
      2. Competitiveness
      3. Proving self

II. Strategies Involving Extra Effort
   A. Working Harder than Others (General)
   B. Working Hard in Academics
      1. Requesting outside help from teachers
      2. Spending more time on homework
      3. Practicing
      4. Preparing courses
      5. Extra reading
   C. Working Hard to Make Social Contacts

III. Strategies Involving Persistence or Stable Effort
   A. Attitude toward Giving Up
   B. Specific Examples of Persistence

IV. Strategies to Reduce the Difficulty of the Task
   A. General Strategies
   B. Use of Mechanical and Technical Aids
   C. Requesting and Using Assistance from Others
   D. Choosing Activities Where Influence of Handicap is Minimized

V. Strategies Involving Other People
   A. Role Models
   B. Counseling and Therapy
   C. Religion
   D. Requesting and Accepting Specific Assistance from
      1. Family
      2. Friends
      3. Classmates and teachers
      4. Others

VI. Strategies Involving the Intent to Succeed (Mental State)
   A. Philosophical Attitudes
   B. Personal Attitudes
   C. Strategies for Developing and Demonstrating Intent

Exhibit 8–1 continued

VII. Strategies Involving Personality Characteristics
    (Other than Intent to Succeed)
    A. General Attitudes
    B. Attitudes toward Self
       1. Self-concept and self-image
       2. Attitudes toward disability
          a. Accepting
          b. Denying
    C. Risk Taking

Source: Adapted from *The Self-perceptions of Successful Handicapped Scientists* (p. 64) by C.J. Maker et al., 1978, Albuquerque, N.M.: The department of Special Education, University of New Mexico.

barriers rather than trying to get someone else to do it" is the most positive and practical strategy for skill development.

Strategies to Convince Others of Capabilities. Most individuals felt it necessary to "go out and show people that you can do something." Demonstration of capabilities seems to be the most effective strategy for modifying attitudes and gaining opportunities. The majority of responses indicated vigorous attempts to show others that they were capable of a broad range of activities. Several individuals reported volunteering to work part time without pay so that employers could see that they were capable of doing the work required by the job. Another individual took courses even though she could have been exempt from them because of blindness, and a mobility impaired woman convinced a potential employer to allow her to work for a full day to show the work she could produce. Others reported having ready and informative answers to questions (whether asked or not) about how handicapped persons solve certain everyday problems.

Development of Personal Attitudes. Many felt that the development of certain attitudes (e.g., self-confidence, competitiveness, proving self) was essential to their success. The development of self-confidence was mentioned specifically by many individuals and was expressed particularly well by one: "I was as capable as most and more capable than some." The need for competitiveness was seen as a positive attitude, "competitiveness kept me going; [by] competing with myself and trying to adjust and keep going." Another saw competitiveness as a method for measurement of growth by "functioning competitively with someone who is not disabled." Some expressed the belief that it was necessary to prove to themselves that they could do what others believed they could not do. One individual believed that his intelligence allowed him to be successful; another stated that "the belief that I can solve problems takes me half way toward solving those problems."

Category II: Strategies Involving Extra Effort to Achieve Goals

Generally Working Harder than Others. Most expressed the belief that a disabled person must work a lot harder and be better than someone without a disability to achieve the same amount of success. Several responses indicated that the disabled person must be willing to put a tremendous amount of time and effort into activities—perhaps even more effort than the situation should require. One individual indicated that he worked hard in academics to compensate for the lack of social life in college and elsewhere.

Working Hard in Academics. This category of responses included several kinds of activities: requesting additional help from teachers in the classroom, spending more time on homework, practicing all activities, repeating courses, doing extra reading, getting outside help from teachers in the evening or after class, and arranging regular weekly conferences to discuss assignments and topics. Spending time on homework included additional work not required of others, such as making "copious braille notes from readings by others." Practice of any and all skills seemed to be important, including writing out presentations in full and practicing them in front of different groups of colleagues before presenting at a symposium.

Category III: Strategies Involving Persistence or "Stable Effort"

Persistence or stable effort refers to long-term tendencies to exert the effort needed to accomplish a goal. The essence of the "strategy" seems to be the attitude of not giving up, rather than simply "hard work" as in the previous category. The majority of the statements in this group included the word "stubborn," "determined," or "persistent." Most interviewees expressed their *resistance* to doing what they were told to do, to believing they were not capable, or to allowing themselves to be psychologically defeated. Two specific examples of such persistence were given. In one case, after being turned down by a medical school, the subject applied to 50 schools until one finally accepted him. In another case, a woman "wouldn't give [her] parents any peace" until they enrolled her in the educational program she wanted. Some subjects mentioned involvement in lawsuits to fight discrimination in admission policies.

Category IV: Strategies to Reduce the Difficulty of Tasks

General Strategies. Deaf individuals reported such techniques as arranging small group meetings with three or fewer people, being relaxed to allow better voice control, taking withdrawals in college courses to avoid a bad grade (and then taking the course the next semester), and taking one course at a time or doing research with one professor. Some persons with mobility impairments reported going to school half days instead of full days; taking reduced loads; holding clinics in the office instead of outlying buildings; having two sets of books, one at home and one at school; and lowering the laboratory working area. One blind person reported that it is more efficient to jaywalk than to walk in crosswalks because then there is no worry about cars coming from *four* directions!

Use of Mechanical and Technical Aids. The greatest number of task difficulty reductions seem to result from the use of mechanical or technical aids. Some
of these aids include a braille computer terminal; talking books; closed-circuit TV;
reader/writer services; sonic guides; tape recorders; dictation machines; visual
aids, such as charts and graphs; amplified telephones; raised line drawings; a van
equipped with a chair lift and hand controls; a light sensor for mechanical
experiments; and braille or audible meters to measure color or pH or to display
readings. Several deaf individuals report the use of finger-spelling or a combination of manual and oral communication methods so that nothing is missed.

Choosing Activities Where Influence of Handicap Is Minimized. A very
practical type of strategy reported by several individuals was to choose a course of
study, type of athletic activity, or methods of learning in which the influence of
their disability would be minimal. Specific examples include going to a small
college, where the student is able to get to know faculty and other students well;
going into laboratory science because of better ability in working with the hands
than in talking (deaf person); using a team teaching approach as a teacher (blind);
and selecting a university as employer in which there was not a "publish or
perish" philosophy. One blind person chose athletic activities including an
obstacle course, water skiing, canoeing, and track events in which he could run
anywhere on the track because sight did not make as much difference in these
events. A deaf individual reported giving and attending poster sessions at scientific
conferences because these sessions encourage and require interaction on an
individual or small-group basis and allow use of visual aids.

Category V: Strategies Involving Other People

The category of strategies involving assistance from other people included a few
instances of others serving as role models, counseling and therapy sessions, and
religious groups. The majority of strategies, however, were those involving
specific assistance from family, friends, classmates, teachers, and others. Some
people mentioned participation in organizations for the handicapped as a way to
identify role models. Some specific examples of assistance requested include the
following: (a) having parents and sister point out mistakes in grammar, (b) having
family members point out pronunciation errors in speech, (c) having other students "describe what I wish to see and can't," (d) helping others with schoolwork
as a way to get to know them socially, (e) having a friend as a laboratory partner,
and (f) having a friend go over a presentation and make suggestions for improvement.

Category VI: Strategies Involving Intent to Succeed

Although the category "Intent to Succeed" contains a relatively small number
of strategies, the mental state of intending to succeed is one that was implied by the

strategies employed by all individuals in all categories. Indeed, throughout the interviews, a common characteristic of the successful scientists was a very strong intent to be successful in academics as well as in their careers. Most of the "strategies" included in this narrow category are philosophical and personal attitude statements, with a few examples of strategies for developing and demonstrating personal intent to succeed. One example of a philosophical statement was "willingness to sacrifice a short-term goal for a long-term one." Personal attitude statements included "need to excel," "determined to succeed," "great desire to prove that I can do a lot of things," "determination to never accept second best," and belief in the philosophy that "if you really want to do something, you can." Strategies for developing and demonstrating intent most involved setting a goal and not changing that goal even though others might encourage lowering of aspirations because of a handicapping condition.

Category VII: Strategies Involving Personality Characteristics

Strategies classified as those involving personality characteristics excluded attitudes related to intent to succeed, as just described. These strategies included mainly general attitudes and attitudes toward self, so these two subcategories are considered separately here. A few strategies were classified as risk taking since they involved situations in which the individual did such things as "moving from a dead-end job to something with more promise, but unknown consequences."

General Attitudes. This subcategory included such "strategies" as thinking of the environment as a challenge rather than as an enemy, learning to ask for help, "making the most of what you have," not demanding "your own way" all the time, and not blaming failures on someone or something else.

Attitudes toward Self. This subcategory included both attitudes concerning general self-image and those concerning the handicap specifically. Items in the general self-image category were those in which the individual "did a lot of positive thinking about myself," learned to rely on himself or herself, maintaining self-confidence and communication of this feeling to others, having the attitude "I can do anything you can do, as well, if not better," becoming less supersensitive, and responding to others' who conveyed low expectations not with anger but by quietly "showing them you can do it."

The majority of strategies in this category were those involving accepting or denying the handicap. Denial strategies were cited almost twice as often as accepting strategies. Acceptance of the handicap included such responses as "being open about a hearing loss" and asking people to speak more slowly, "being open about the fact that there are conditions with which you can't cope," being realistic about career opportunities, and accepting a handicap as "part of the package" together with "being short, fat, or whatever." Denial strategies included such responses as avoiding association with other disabled people, a conscious realization that the disabled person is just as good as someone without a handicap, and setting personal norms to those of nonhandicapped rather than handicapped persons. Several individuals reported elaborate strategies to avoid the appearance of being blind or deaf because "people who initially accept someone will have a difficult time rejecting them later." Examples of these strategies are practicing with a friend on the appearance of "eye contact" (blind), doing things more slowly to avoid "banging around" and appearing clumsy, and intentionally practicing things that contradict "what people might think about my handicap."

In summary, the purpose of this section has been to suggest that gifted individuals with disabilities can take an active role in changing negative perceptions and low expectations for their performance. Coping and learning strategies found successful by others with a similar disability can be developed, either through self-instruction or through instruction by parents or educators.

A fundamental requirement for success in such an approach, however, is the disabled individual's beliefs about the causes of personal success in achievement-related situations. Also, as noted earlier, the individual's beliefs about the causes of success may influence greatly the choice of a particular coping or learning strategy or whether such strategies are developed. Attribution theory is reviewed briefly in the following section as a framework for understanding how a person's attributions of causality influence performance and achievement motivation, and how they may be used to help the individual choose and develop strategies for learning and for overcoming the negative stereotypes or attitudes of others. This theoretical framework is very valuable in influencing the motivation of disabled persons to achieve and in understanding lower levels of motivation.

Understanding the Influence of Attributions of Causality

Attribution theory is essentially a cognitive approach to understanding motivation. It suggests that self-perceptions and beliefs may have a greater influence on the individual's subsequent behavior than do the actual causes of behavior, such as intellectual abilities or handicaps. In other words, causal attributions may be more important predictors of future behavior than other factors related to ability.

Weiner (1972, 1974) has been influential in the application of general attribution theory to academic contexts in which achievement-related behaviors occur. According to his model, individuals attribute the causes for their success or failure to one or more of the following factors: ability, effort, task difficulty, and luck. These four factors vary on the dimensions of stability (stable versus unstable) and locus of control (internal versus external). Table 8–1 presents a classification of these factors. Theoretically, an individual assigns value to these elements and ascribes the outcome or consequence of behavior differentially to the four sources.

Table 8–1 Classification Scheme for the Perceived Determinants of Achievement Behavior

| | Locus of Control | |
Stability	Internal	External
Stable	Ability	Task difficulty
Unstable	Effort	Luck

Source: From *Cognitive Views of Human Motivation* (p. 52) by B. Weiner, 1974, Orlando, Fla.: Academic Press.

An individual, in making an attribution regarding the cause of an outcome, combines the elements either conjunctively (e.g., task difficulty *and* luck) or disjunctively (e.g., task difficulty *or* luck). Certain information about the person, the situation, and the performance of others in similar situations is used to reach conclusions about which of the four elements caused success or failure. Research has demonstrated that this information can include personal history, such as performance at this and other similar tasks, the pattern of prior reinforcement (random versus systematic), the situational characteristics or demands of the tasks, and the performance of others at this and similar tasks.

The consequences of an event, including resulting pride or shame and expectancy of future success, will be different depending on the cause to which it is attributed. The tendency to approach or avoid achievement-related events can be explained by both the attributed causes and the frequency or pattern of successes and failures at similar tasks. In general, an individual may react differently according to the dimension that is relevant in a particular situation. For example, Weiner (1972, 1974) has argued that the stability of a perceived cause rather than its locus of control determines shifts in expectation of success after success or failure. If the conditions are expected to remain the same (level of ability or the difficulty of the task), then the outcome experienced on past occasions will be expected to recur. A success should produce anticipation of future success, and a failure should strengthen the belief that there will be subsequent failures. On the other hand, if the causal conditions are perceived as likely to change (such as the amount of effort expended or the luck encountered), then the present outcomes may not be expected to be repeated in the future. A success should thus yield relatively small increments or perhaps decrements in the expectancy of future success, whereas a failure may not intensify the belief that there will be future failures.

Validation and Refinement of Weiner's Model

Hypotheses derived from Weiner's model have received considerable empirical support. This support has been both direct (through testing the theory in experimental learning situations) and indirect (through reinterpretation of the locus of control and achievement motivation literature (cf. Weiner & Kukla, 1970; Weiner, 1972, 1974; Weiner, Frieze, Kukla, Reed, Rest, & Rosenbaum, 1972; Weiner, Nierenberg, & Goldstein, 1976). Some studies have compared the hypotheses derived from social learning theory or the achievement motivation literature and have found that, in general, the attributional interpretations have provided better explanations for the results (Weiner & Potepan, 1970; Cohen, Reid, & Boothroyd, 1973; Schultz & Pomerantz, 1976), although the findings related to failure attributions are somewhat confusing (Weiner & Kukla, 1970; Schultz & Pomerantz, 1976).

Some studies also have suggested extensions or modifications of the theory. Only one investigation, conducted by Frieze (1976), has been identified that attempted to examine the validity of the categories of causes and the information people utilize in making references about causes. Using an open-ended format, Frieze presented a variety of academic and nonacademic achievement-related events and asked subjects to state why each event occurred and what information would help them better know why the event occurred. Categories were developed and responses classified into the categories. As expected, she found that the categories of causes and the types of information needed are the same as those theoretically derived. However, she also found that two other categories should be included: mood and other people.

Only one extension of attribution theory to gifted individuals without disabilities is known to the authors. In a study not yet completed, Maker (in progress) has found that the general categories of causes are appropriate for explaining the attributions of those who are gifted, and that gifted high achievers usually attribute their success to ability and effort and their failure to the difficulty of the task or bad luck. This is consistent with attributions made by high achievers who may not be gifted.

Unfortunately, except for the study of disabled scientists no research has been identified in which attribution theory is applied to overall or long-range success in either a disabled or a nondisabled population. In that study, when interviewees described a critical incident that involved success or failure in an achievement-related event, they were asked to explain what they believed to be the cause(s) for their success or failure. Very few failures were described, so only the causes of events involving success were analyzed.

A majority of the successful handicapped adults reported a belief that their success, in achievement-related events perceived to have been significant in their development, has been caused by the internal stable factor of abilities. Other important causes were facilitative: people, effort, intent, persistence, and specific personality characteristics. Internal causes were cited more frequently than were external causes. Some key words and phrases that are examples of the responses included in each category are the following: *ability*—intelligence, skills, past experience, education, and self-confidence; *effort*—striving, hard work, practice;

persistence—stubbornness, "wouldn't quit"; *intent*—wanting to "do it so badly," determined to succeed, determined to "make it," "hepped up" to succeed; *personality characteristics*—assertiveness, attitude toward the disability; *task difficulty*—"I did some research; there was no difficulty in that"; *luck*—good breaks, "in the right place at the right time"; and *other people*—"my mother's determination," "the teacher's encouragement," "my friend's help."

An individual's beliefs about the causes of personal success or failure will influence behavior in a way that will facilitate or inhibit performance in achievement situations, will affect the individual's choice or use of coping and learning strategies, and will directly influence success or failure in achievement situations. In other populations, research has shown that those who assume personal responsibility for their success (i.e., attribute their success to high ability and effort), in comparison with those who attribute their success to external sources, will tend to (a) approach achievement activities, owing in part to their heightened reward or pride in accomplishment (Weiner & Kukla, 1970; Weiner & Potepan, 1970; Weiner et al., 1972); (b) reward themselves more for achievement performance (Weiner et al., 1972); (c) perform with relatively great vigor, mediated by the belief that outcome is determined by effort (Weiner et al., 1972); and (c) persist longer in the face of failure (Weiner, 1972; Weiner et al., 1972). Research has also shown that individuals who believe their success is caused by high ability will actually perform better in achievement tasks (Weiner & Potepan, 1970; Schultz & Pomerantz, 1976; Weiner & Kukla, 1970).

In the majority of situations reported, the successful handicapped adults in this study believed that their success was caused by their own ability or effort. They also perceived that success experiences caused an increase in their intent to succeed by heightening their aspirations, increasing the available paths for reaching the goal, and increasing their effort. Thus, they seemed to approach achievement activities with confidence in themselves and with high motivation to succeed. Since they believed themselves capable of succeeding and also perceived effort as a cause of their success, it could be tentatively concluded that they performed with relatively great vigor. It also could be concluded that these individuals persisted in the face of failure, since they reported one or a series of failures as circumstances leading up to an event in which they succeeded. They also believed that their persistence, effort, and intent were causes of their success in situations involving negative environmental forces (e.g., attitudes of others). Since they have been successful in achievement situations (both academically and in their careers), there is support for a link between causal attributions to internal factors (particularly ability) and success in achievement situations.

Successful people, whether handicapped or not, seem to have similar characteristics. Cox (1926), for example, concluded that the three most outstanding traits of the eminent people whose lives she examined were persistence (of motive and efforts), self-confidence, and strength or force of character. The successful handicapped scientists interviewed for this study believe they are persistent even when environmental conditions are negative. They believe their success is caused by their own ability, and they see themselves as refusing to let the attitudes or beliefs of others change what they believe about themselves. Terman and Oden (1947) also identified similar characteristics in the most successful as opposed to least successful group in his longitudinal study of gifted individuals.

These successful individuals also developed strategies based on their perception of the causes of their success and failure that would facilitate their success. Although they generally believed that they were responsible for their own success (and developed techniques for increasing their ability and its effect), if they also believed in the influence of other people on their success, they developed techniques to enlist the assistance of others or to convince others of their ability.

To summarize, attribution theory can be useful in understanding how gifted individuals with disabilities view their achievement-related performance. Theory and research on its application also suggest that the development of attributions can be an extremely important factor in an individual's subsequent performance. Families and educators must exercise care in their discussions of the reasons for a child's success or failure so that children do not develop the belief that their successes, for example, are due mainly to luck. Since luck is unpredictable, the child would not know whether or not to attempt a task and expend the amount of effort needed to accomplish it. Although less is known about the impact of attributions for failure, it is certainly essential that gifted children with disabilities not develop the belief that their failure is due to lack of ability. Particularly important in the education of gifted disabled children is to avoid the development of the belief that their success is caused by the fact that the tasks they are asked to do are easy; instead, they should be encouraged to develop strategies that reduce the difficulty of challenging tasks. Thus, they can perceive themselves as responsible for their success. Gifted individuals must be presented with tasks they find challenging intellectually, and if disabled they must be provided with the support, modifications, or learning strategies that will enable them to succeed. Then they must be helped to believe (over time, and in specific situations) that their high ability and effort caused their overall success.

The most important message from attribution theory is that children must not only experience success in academic situations but also believe that they are responsible for their own success. Thus, they will be likely to attempt challenging tasks and to expend the effort necessary to succeed and will not be discouraged by occasional failures. A reasonable hypothesis, based on the theoretical framework and relevant research just presented, is that the related characteristics of the subjects significantly contributed to their success. Conversely, a reasonable speculation is that less successful or unsuccessful disabled persons with gifted potential have a tendency toward perceiving success as caused by unstable and external causes.

IDENTIFICATION AND ASSESSMENT

One of the most difficult tasks educators may face in providing programs for gifted children with disabilities is to locate and recognize them! Recognizing giftedness in disabled adults who have made significant contributions through high achievement, and who have described childhood events and characteristics that were early indicators of giftedness, is much easier than recognizing giftedness in children who have not yet learned the coping strategies or skills that enable the full expression of superior abilities. In essence, educators must look for traits that are indicators or signs of high intellectual ability. If only a few equivocal signs are present, the child should continue to be observed, and educators should remain open to the possibility that higher ability can be expressed as skills are acquired.

Three "stages" or levels of the identification/assessment process are discussed here, and specific recommendations for referral, screening, and identification are supplied. Since general issues regarding identification and assessment have been discussed in Chapter 1, and specific issues related to each type of disability have been discussed in relation to the case studies, this section focuses on the presentation of alternatives, options, and guidelines.

Referral

Referral is the process by which a pool of children is identified as possibly gifted. These children then are observed and/or tests are administered to determine whether special services are needed. Three guidelines for the referral process follow.

1. *Develop awareness in referral sources.*
   The first and most important part of the identification/assessment process is to develop an accurate awareness of the characteristics of gifted children as well as their needs for special services. Information about specific observable behaviors that can indicate giftedness, as well as ways these behaviors can be masked or inhibited by a disability, should be provided to all individuals who are potential sources of referrals: parents, regular classroom teachers, teachers of the handicapped, counselors, speech therapists, administrators, other educational personnel, staff members in community service agencies, and nurses, pediatricians, and other medical personnel. The best method for disseminating this information is through inservice training provided for various groups.

   A project designed to identify and serve preschool gifted students with disabilities (Leonard, 1978) included an excellent example of the type of inservice recommended by the authors. Project staff members provided workshops for teachers that included an overview of the project (e.g., its goals, philosophy, and criteria for providing services) and training for participation in the referral process. In discussing the program, it was emphasized that many children possess outstanding abilities that are never recognized because of focused attention on the handicaps. A slide-tape presentation, "The Identification of Giftedness in Young Children," explained the project, gave information about giftedness, and provided case studies of gifted handicapped preschoolers. These case studies were presented in detail and provided actual observable behavior. The trainers emphasized the idea that the children identified as gifted seen in the slides were not necessarily teacher-pleasers, and many of them had behavior problems. A second slide-tape, "Audrey: A Case Study," was a detailed case study of a gifted handicapped child. This tape, along with detailed written case studies, was used in the training exercise. The trainees filled out a checklist of gifted characteristics for the child observed. They were encouraged to provide specific examples of the characteristics they checked and were encouraged to add characteristics to the list that seemed to reflect giftedness. A sample of items from this checklist is presented in Exhibit 8–2.

General community awareness activities also are needed. They serve a dual purpose in that they not only increase the number of accurate referrals but also sensitize the general public to the fact that people with disabilities can be intellectually gifted. Community awareness can be developed through visits to potential referral sources and agencies; distribution of brochures, fact sheets, and letters; writing newspaper articles; appearing on television shows; and arranging radio public service announcements or television news spots. Announcements or letters can be sent home with children who are in school.

2. *Request referrals from a variety of sources.*

Many individuals in different relationships to children can refer individuals for possible identification services, and the larger the number of sources included in the process, the greater the likelihood that children will not be overlooked. These varied sources usually will provide different information about the child, or information about different areas of functioning. This can provide a good data base for beginning the more formal steps of the assessment process. All schools, community agencies, parent groups, medical service agencies, and other organizations that provide services to parents and children should be contacted. If possible, inservice training should be provided for the professional and support staffs of these organizations.

3. *Provide specific forms for referral that are adapted for the population being identified.*

All potential referral sources, in staff training sessions or in written materials, should be provided with checklists of specific, observable behaviors. They should be encouraged to use these checklists in their observations of

Exhibit 8–2 Checklist of Characteristics of the Gifted

Instructions

When filling out this checklist on a child, check the items that you have seen the child demonstrate, and write brief descriptions of specifically how those items were demonstrated.

I. Aptitude

ITEM	BRIEF DESCRIPTION
_____ Unusually advanced vocabulary for age (e.g., 4-year-old using words such as anticipate, perish, etc., appropriately).	
_____ May excel and become absorbed in one topic or subject.	

II. General Intellectual Ability

_____ Learns rapidly, easily, and efficiently.	
_____ Retains what is heard or read without much drill.	
_____ Asks many questions.	
_____ Interested in a wide range of things.	
_____ Is alert.	
_____ Keenly observant.	
_____ Responds quickly.	
_____ Has capacity to use knowledge and information other than memorizing.	

Source: Adapted from *Chapel Hill Services to the Gifted/Handicapped* by J. Leonard, 1978, Chapel Hill, N.C.

---

children and asked to fill them out when they refer a child. General checklists used for identifying children without disabilities should not be used unless referral sources have a clear understanding of how these traits could be masked by a disability or the alternative ways "gifted" characteristics can be observed in a child with a specific disability. A more appropriate procedure would be to develop a checklist that focuses on behaviors indicative of giftedness and the alternative ways these abilities can be expressed in

Exhibit 8–3 Identifying Characteristics of Gifted Students

Primary Identifiers

Learns quickly and easily *when interested*

Exceptional cognitive power for learning, retaining, and using knowledge/information

Advanced problem-solving skills—challenged by problems to solve; uses acquired knowledge and superior reasoning skills to attack, and often solve, complex problems of both a practical and theoretical nature

Oral language incorporates an advanced vocabulary used appropriately and complex language structure

Unusual comprehension of complex, abstract ideas—develops or elaborates ideas at a level not expected

High level of inquiry—the qualitative nature of questions raised and the subjects that arouse interest and sustained curiosity

Exceptional quality of thought as revealed through language and problem solving—remarkable manipulation of abstract symbols and ideas, including perceiving and manipulating relationships between ideas, events, people; formulates principles and generalizations through transfer of learning across settings or events; reflects and reasons to gain insights and to generate solutions

Secondary Identifiers

Highly creative behavior in production of ideas, things, solutions; can be noticeably creative and inventive (originality); fascinated by "idea play"

A wide interest range; basically very curious

A profound, sometimes consuming interest in one or more areas of intellectual investigation

An intense desire to know and understand, to master skills and problems of interest to him/her

Shows initiative in pursuing "outside projects" and may have elaborate hobbies of his/her own choice; manifests resourcefulness and an unusual capacity for self-directed learning, though possibly only in out-of-school activities

Enjoys self-expression, especially through discussion but also often through the arts

Exhibits independence in thought, a tendency toward nonconformity

Demands a reason or explanation for requirements, limits, undesired events

Tends to be perfectionistic, severely self-critical, and aspiring to high standards of achievement; desire to excel and produce

Evidences greater sensitivity and awareness regarding self, others, world problems, moral issues; may be intolerant of human weaknesses

Source: From *The Psychology of Gifted Children* by J. Freeman, 1985, Chichester, England: John Wiley and Sons, Inc. Copyright 1985 by John Wiley and Sons, Inc. Reprinted by permission. (From a chapter written by J.R. Whitmore.)

an individual with a particular disability. Exhibit 8–3 provides a listing of characteristics that can be useful in the development of such a checklist. Table 8–2 outlines possible clues to the presence of intellectual giftedness in various disabling conditions.

Screening

Screening is a process for adding candidates to a pool of potentially gifted students. Usually these measures are used with the entire population of a school district, referrals to an agency, or children served by a certain intervention project. Generally the measures used can be administered individually or to groups of children but require little time. Children whose scores are in a certain range, indicating they may be gifted or may possess a particular disability, are added to the pool of children referred to the program. The screening process also adds information about children who already have been referred.

The most commonly used screening measures for gifted programs are group achievement tests. Sometimes group intelligence tests are included. Children who demonstrate high achievement in one or more areas measured by the test or who score above 115 or 120 on an intelligence test are often included in the pool. Even though these measures are appropriate screening procedures for many gifted children, they are not adequate means for locating gifted children with disabilities. As noted in discussions of the case studies, many children with disabilities achieve at a lower level on tests than their peers without disabilities, even though their intelligence is comparable or superior. The problem is that the tests may be inappropriate or contain items that are inappropriate for use with an individual with a particular disability (e.g., a written achievement test used with a learning-disabled student who cannot read, or an item requesting information about color given to a blind child). To minimize the effects of such problems, and to use appropriately the information gained from these tests, the performance of children with disabilities should be compared with the performance of others with similar disabilities. If the screening procedures are designed to locate the top 5 percent of children, for example, the top 5 percent of children with a particular disability should be included separately, even though the criterion score for the disabled group may be lower in some areas than the scores for children without disabilities.

Other, more appropriate, procedures should be used in addition to traditional methods. Screening procedures developed specifically for detecting handicaps often can provide information about superior intellectual abilities. An example of such a screening procedure is that used by the RAPYHT Project for gifted handicapped preschoolers (Karnes & Bertschi, 1978). This assessment technique, the *Comprehensive Identification Process* (CIP) (Zehrbach, 1975), uses a scale to detect behavior indicating developmental delays in one or more of eight areas: cognitive, speech and language, fine motor, gross motor, vision, hearing, medical history, and socioaffective. Such a procedure also can indicate areas of advanced development and superior potential.

Other procedures that can be used to identify gifted handicapped students are observations of children in classroom, play, or testing situations; parent interviews; peer referral; teacher interviews; and diagnostic teaching with skilled

Table 8–2 Gifted Students with Specific Handicaps

Obstacles to Identification	Key Observations
Little or no productivity in school Cannot read, write, spell easily or accurately ("learning disabled") Poor motor skills, coordination—writing is painfully slow, messy; often child is easily distracted from tasks and described as inattentive (neurologically impaired, "minimal cerebral dysfunction," developmental delay in motor area)	Superiority in oral language—vocabulary, fluency, structure Memory for facts and events Exceptional comprehension Analytical and creative problem-solving abilities Markedly advanced interests, impressive knowledge Keen perception and humor
Absence of oral communication skills (e.g., cerebral palsy, deaf)	Drive to communicate through alternative modes—visual, nonverbal, body language Superior memory and problem-solving ability Exceptional interest and drive in response to challenge
Behavior is "disordered"—aggressive, disruptive, off-task frequently extremely withdrawn, noncommunicative	Superior verbal skill, oral language Exceptional capacity to devise ways to manipulate people and to solve "problems" Superior memory, general knowledge The most difficult one to identify—the only key is response to stimulation of higher mental abilities unless superior written work is produced
Sensory deficits producing developmental delay—specifically, does not evidence superior language and thought, has difficulty conceptualizing and dealing with abstractions (blind, deaf, and children with mild to moderate hearing and visual impairments)	Exceptionally rapid response to stimulation and special education compared to others with similar handicaps Superior memory, knowledge, problem-solving skills Notable drive to know or master

Source: From "Gifted Children with Handicapping Conditions: A New Frontier" by J.R. Whitmore, 1981, *Exceptional Children, 48,* pp. 106–114. Copyright 1981 by Council for Exceptional Children. Adapted by permission.

observations. The following discussion provides a brief description of each of these methods. Readers should note that these same procedures can be used in the identification process as well. Regardless of whether they are employed early or late in the assessment process, they can provide useful information about the abilities of children with disabilities.

Observations

An individual familiar with giftedness and how it can be expressed in children with particular disabilities can make skillful observations of children in a variety of settings. Observers should use a form such as that developed in the Chapel Hill project for the gifted handicapped (Leonard, 1978), or a form developed from the characteristics listed in Exhibit 8–3 and Table 8–2. More useful information can be obtained from observations if the following conditions are met: (a) the observer is well trained; (b) observations are made consistently over a period of time; (c) children are observed in a variety of settings; (d) particular characteristics guide the observations; (e) the observer remains open to expressions of ability other than those listed on a form; and (f) anecdotal notes are made as children are being observed.

Parent Interviews

Many school districts routinely conduct interviews with parents of children entering school, both at the kindergarten level and when transferring into the district. These interviews can be modified to include questions related to specific attributes of giftedness and/or disabilities. For example,

- What special talents or skills does your child have? Give examples of behavior that illustrates these abilities.
- What special interests does your child have?
- What kind of stories does your child like?

Parents of children suspected of being gifted can be interviewed separately and asked more questions. If parents indicate that they believe their child is gifted, they should be asked to describe specific behaviors that substantiate their beliefs.

Peer Referral

Effective peer referral meets the following conditions: First, it must be conducted on an individual basis by interviewing each child and asking specific questions. By interviewing children individually rather than asking for nominations in a group setting, peer referral does not become a popularity contest. Second, it should contain specific questions pertaining to the talent area(s) being considered and should consist of questions about behaviors children can observe. Some sample peer referral questions follow (Maker, Morris, & James, 1981):

- Who in your class thinks of the most unusual, wild, or fantastic ideas?
- Who thinks of the most good ideas?

- Which boys or girls are the first to explain to others in your class how games are played or things are done?
- Which boys or girls are usually the first to suggest new games to play or things to do?
- Who would you ask for help with your classwork?

Teacher Interviews

Interviews with teachers regarding the specific behaviors and talents of the children in their classes are more effective than soliciting information about children through written forms (Maker, Morris, & James, 1981). Forms developed for referral based on lists such as the one in Exhibit 8–3 can be used to guide the interview process and to determine specific information needed about particular children. Interviews provide a setting in which teachers can ask questions about characteristics of giftedness and interviewers can request specific information about children's behavior.

Diagnostic Teaching with Observation

Diagnostic teaching with observation is very seldom used in programs for the gifted but is more frequently found in programs for the handicapped. Various formats for diagnostic observations are used, including placement of children in a special diagnostic classroom for several weeks or several months, special activities conducted on a regular basis by a trained teacher and observer in a regular classroom setting, and special activities conducted by a teacher and observer in a setting outside the classroom. When children are taken out of their classrooms for diagnostic assessment, it is usually because of the teacher's recognition of some indication of a need for special services, but diagnostic teaching within the classroom is usually designed to identify children with special needs that may not be recognized by the regular classroom teacher. In diagnostic teaching, learning activities appropriate for gifted students—that elicit higher levels of thinking, creative expression, and expression of talents—should be included. Children's exceptional participation and responses are observed. This technique is actually an extension of observation and a less extreme form of a technique often used to determine how a child fits into a particular program—trial placement. It allows children to experience a short trial placement without the risk of embarrassment if it is determined that the child does not need special services.

Student Interviews

Students should be asked to provide information about their perceived areas of strength and weakness, if at all possible. They can be asked to describe a project or activity in which they were very proud of their performance and to share the reasons for their pride. Other questions can pertain to their intellectual interests and to their perceptions of how challenging or appropriate their current educational placement has been. They should be asked to provide reasons and specific examples to support their statements. Student interviews also can be used in conjunction with assessment of products. They can be asked to discuss the merits of a product they have developed and the process they used.

Product Assessment

The creative products developed by students should be examined to determine their level of sophistication. The effect of a specific disability on the ability to develop a "polished" product should be considered in this assessment, and more attention focused on the sophistication of ideas than on appearance. Poems, essays, experiments, displays, drawing, illustrations, computer programs, inventions, and a variety of products are possibilities. Students should be allowed to select the medium or format. Criteria for assessment should include originality, sophistication of ideas, evidence of synthesis, use of critical and higher levels of thinking, and evidence of understanding of important principles related to the content area represented by the product.

Guidelines for Screening

Regardless of the procedures used, certain principles should guide the screening process:

1. A variety of information should be collected regarding children's performance.
2. Information should be gathered from a variety of sources.
3. Individuals collecting or providing the information should be knowledgeable about giftedness and specific disabilities.
4. Checklists or observation forms should be adapted for the specific population.
5. Children's performance should be compared with that of others with a particular disability as well as those without disabilities. Performance superior to that of others with a similar disability should be considered a strong indicator of giftedness.
6. *Specific examples* of children's characteristics should be elicited from teachers, parents, or others who are interviewed and should be recorded during observations.
7. Decisions about whether a child should receive further assessment or observation should be made on the basis of a compilation of information rather than on the basis of information from only one source.

Identification

Identification is the final stage in the process of making a decision about which students are intellectually gifted and need special services to receive appropriate educational opportunities. The most extensive individualized and personalized assessment procedures are used at this stage. As noted in the previous section, many of the methods described as screening procedures can be used for identification. Indeed, they *should* be employed at this stage if not used in screening. In addition to these methods, the identification process should include individualized tests of intelligence, problem solving, and creative and/or critical thinking. This discussion is divided into two general sections: general guidelines for identification and guidelines for testing. Specific tests are included in the discussion of guidelines for testing.

General Guidelines

Guidelines presented in the screening section apply to the identification process as well. Since these were not explained earlier, they are briefly described in this section.

1. *Information should be collected about the child's performance in a variety of areas.*
   This enables the development of a complete profile of strengths and weaknesses and thus better judgments about the child's giftedness and/or needs for special services. A broad view of intelligence, such as that presented by Guilford (1959, 1967), should guide the assessment process. Guilford's Structure of Intellect model, for example, suggests that there are three dimensions of intelligence: content, operations, and products. Each dimension has separate types of abilities. The operations dimension, for example, includes memory, convergent production, divergent production, and evaluation. These abilities are demonstrated in performance on very different types of tasks. Guilford's model is quite complicated: the reader is referred to his articles and books, as well as Meeker's (1969) book.
   A more simplistic model for looking at tests and procedures is described by Hokanson and Jospe (1976). They present dimensions for analysis of tasks used for testing that can be applied also to any activities of the child. These dimensions serve as guidelines for looking at the abilities required for task completion in order to isolate the specific areas of strengths and weaknesses. If, for example, a child does well on tasks at one end of the continuum, poorly at the other end, and average in the middle, this dimension can be used to describe and explain or predict the child's performance on tasks in which a specific ability is involved. The value of this system over others is that it recognizes and takes into account the fact that many different

abilities are required for every task. The dimensions are given in the following list (Maker, 1976, p. 32):

- Is the task a verbal (auditory) input or a visual (sight) input?
- Do the stimuli involve symbolic material (words, pictures of real things) or nonsymbolic material (such as shapes or nonsense words)?
- Is the task one [that] involves concrete or abstract thinking?
- Does the task provide structure or not?
- How much verbal formulation and verbal expression are required?
- How much context is employed or how much does the information stand by itself?
- How specific, detailed, and differentiated is the material one is considering, or how general is it?
- Are any numbers or number concepts involved (time, distance, quantity)?
- How much motor planning and responding is involved?
- How much passive rote memory is involved, or how much thinking is involved?
- How much do sequential operations apply to the tasks, or how much is the information able to be done in several ways?
- How much do the tasks involve showing what the child has learned via memory and modeling (imitation), or how much do they involve him discovering his own solution?

The principle of collecting information about performance in a variety of areas is illustrated by the use of achievement tests, creativity tests, intelligence tests, and measures of critical thinking to assess intellectual ability. This principle also suggests the use of intelligence tests that assess a variety of abilities.

2. *Information should be collected from a variety of sources.*
   This guideline is closely related to the first but requires that performance be evaluated in a variety of situations—for example, in the regular classroom, in a special classroom, at home, and in extracurricular activities. Individuals who have the opportunity to observe and teach the child in these different situations should be interviewed or asked to serve on a selection and placement team.

3. *Individuals collecting and providing the information should be knowledgeable about the interaction of giftedness and specific disabilities.*

This guideline relates to teachers who are being asked to provide observational data or referrals, examiners who are testing children, diagnostic teachers, and other professionals or individuals from the community who are being asked to supply data. It does not necessarily apply to parents or the students themselves at this point. After a positive decision about giftedness has been made, however, such information should be provided. When experienced or knowledgeable individuals cannot be located, inservice training should be provided.

4. *Checklists or observation forms should be adapted for the specific populations.*

   Since this guideline has already been discussed in the referral section, it need not be explained here.

5. *Specific examples of children's characteristics should be elicited from individuals supplying information.*

   Actual behavior should be described rather than inferences about behavior. This enables those who are making decisions to obtain a complete picture of the child's performance, rather than to rely too heavily on the interpretations or inferences made by observers. All checklists or forms, for example, should require that specific behaviors be listed as support for overall ratings of performance. During interviews, if parents, for instance, indicate that their child is "interested in a variety of topics," they need to be asked for examples of things the child does or has done that show this interest.

6. *Decisions about giftedness and/or the most appropriate placement should be made on the basis of all information collected and should be the responsibility of a committee that makes such decisions.*

   In programs for the gifted, placement decisions are sometimes made by one individual on the basis of scores on intelligence or achievement tests. Another common practice is to compile several scores, assign weights to them, and add these weighted scores to obtain a total index of ability. This is called a matrix and has been recommended as an alternative to the use of either a score on one test or as a more objective alternative to the use of a case study approach. Although a matrix is useful in compiling information from a variety of sources in situations involving decisions about large numbers of students, it is not recommended for use in decision making about giftedness in individuals with disabilities. Since every disability is different, and the degree of disability also is a factor, developing a matrix to fit all cases would be impossible.

   A case study approach, with decisions made by a group of individuals knowledgeable about the area (gifted students with specific disabilities) and the child, is the most appropriate method of identification. The committee should review all information to address such questions as the following:

- What is the child's pattern of strengths and weaknesses?
- Are the strengths high enough and in appropriate areas to justify the label of "gifted"?
- Are the weaknesses low enough and in appropriate areas to justify a label of "handicapped"?
- To what extent are the child's needs being met in the current placement?
- What modifications should be made in the educational program or placement to meet more effectively the child's needs relative to both the disability and the giftedness?

Guidelines for Testing

As noted in several chapters, very few tests have been developed specifically for use with children who have disabilities. For this reason, when these children are being assessed, the tests, the diagnostic tasks, the use of scores, the use of norms, and the testing situation must be modified appropriately. It is impossible to review all the possible problems related to testing or the adaptations that can be made for each type of disability. Readers are referred to Berdine (in press) for a more extensive discussion of each area. In this section only general guidelines related to the assessment of giftedness in the disabled are reviewed.

1. *Intelligence testing should be designed to determine patterns of ability rather than one overall "level" of ability as reflected by an IQ score.*
   Maker (1976) has discussed this idea in depth and has suggested that there are three basic reasons for the recommendation: First, a handicap has a different effect in both quantity and quality on different areas of functioning, causing unique ability patterns or clusters that are not reflected in an average score. Second, this average score gives neither an accurate picture of the general and specific ability patterns nor the magnitude of each strength and weakness. Third, this average score does not reflect the importance of certain areas of functioning, which may be more valid indicators of potential ability in individuals with certain handicaps. It is necessary to study individual areas of functioning and to look for specific skills or clusters of ability that may be indicative of a generalized area of superiority. If varied areas are assessed and considered separately, either a legitimately depressed area or an ability that is hard to measure would not lower the superior area by combining all subscores into an average. High abilities in specific areas indicate true intellectual superiority in those areas; the impact of handicaps makes overall superiority unlikely in children with disabilities.

2. *Test norms should not be used literally. Scores should be interpreted by considering factors within the child and the test.*
   Most tests do not have norms or data regarding the performance of children

with a particular disability. When this is true, a child's score should be compared with the scores of others with a similar disability in order to determine whether that performance is superior, average, or below average. These scores should also be compared with those of nondisabled to determine the degree of discrepancy and the areas of strength and weakness. This practice enables the examiner to consider whether a weakness may be due to a disability or whether it suggests that a child may not be gifted.

Some test norms may be appropriately used to interpret scores. In order to determine the usefulness of norms, the following factors should be considered: the number of children with a particular disability included in the norming sample; the extent to which abilities required to do the tasks could be impaired by the child's disability; and the extent to which the experience needed to complete a task or to answer an item could be limited by the disability. In making decisions about the appropriateness of tests, evaluators must exercise caution and seek information about the performance of others with a similar disability because it is difficult to know the effect of a disability in limiting experience and cognitive development.

Maker (1976) has provided three other reasons for making comparisons with the performance of others who have a similar disability. First of all, the general effect of a handicap seems to be that of slowing the rate of cognitive development. Since intelligence testing is based on the assumption that a gifted child or a child possessing a greater capacity to learn will develop at a faster rate, if handicapped children develop more slowly they will appear less intelligent when compared with their nonhandicapped peers. When they are compared with others having a similar handicap, the prediction of potential is much more accurate. Second, the rate of development may be different for different areas of functioning. Finally, certain skills and abilities may be more important as predictors of success for persons with a particular kind of handicap than for persons who are not handicapped. In using test results to make placement decisions, however, comparisons with children who do not have disabilities may be necessary. The child's performance should be compared with that of the children with whom he or she will be placed. A hearing-impaired child with low language facility who reads at a below-average level should not be placed with a group of highly verbal gifted students for language arts activities even if the child achieves a superior score on a test of nonverbal reasoning.

3. *The testing situation and the response mode may need to be modified.*
   The most important guideline to remember when altering the test situation is that "the purpose is not to make the task easier, but to make it possible" (Maker, 1976, p. 35). Changes such as pantomiming or translating test instructions into sign language do not impair the validity of a test but do make it possible for a deaf child to understand how to do a task. If a severely

impaired child with cerebral palsy does not have the muscle control to point to a correct picture, a response system devised to enable the child to indicate when the examiner has pointed to the correct picture does not interfere with the test's validity but makes the task possible.

In summary, identification of giftedness in children with disabilities is not an easy task. There must be a knowledgeable staff, a willingness to provide extensive inservices for those involved in the identification process, openness to the use of extensively individualized procedures, a willingness to consider a variety of sources of information about performance and potential, and a willingness to make judgments based on subjective information. Most important, all persons involved in the process must remain open to differing expressions of ability and must be aware of the ways abilities can be masked by disabilities.

EDUCATIONAL PROGRAMS

When a child is identified as intellectually gifted or as having high cognitive abilities that may indicate giftedness, the educational program must then be examined to determine what changes, if any, need to be made to facilitate the child's growth to the fullest extent. The educational program consists of an environment in which learning occurs through a curriculum, a systematically planned series of learning experiences. Materials, equipment, and support services are made available to enhance the learning. Each of these areas is examined briefly in relation to the education of gifted students with disabilities. Options and guidelines for making choices are also presented.

Determining the Learning Environment and Support Services

Usually a range of options is available for the delivery of needed services. Exceptional children can be educated appropriately in the regular classroom, in a regular classroom and resource room, in a special classroom, in a special school, or in a program that combines several environments. One of the most difficult decisions facing educators is determining what type of placement or provision of services is most appropriate for a gifted student with a specific disability. The child can be placed in a class or school with other gifted students, in a class or school with other disabled students, or in the regular classroom with resource room experiences with other gifted students and/or disabled students. A child's program also can combine one or more of these options. For instance, placement can be in a class or school for gifted students, with an hour each day spent in a resource room with students who have a similar disability.

There obviously is no generalization that can be made about the most appropriate placement, since each student and each situation is different to some degree. However, some guidelines or criteria for judging the appropriateness of an educational plan can be offered: (a) the plan must provide an environment with sufficient intellectual challenge from teachers, other students, materials, and the curriculum; (b) it must be flexible enough to enable the development of both strengths and weaknesses yet have stability and consistency; (c) it must make available the services necessary for development of coping and learning strategies and for skills in using specialized equipment and materials; and (d) it must provide a teacher who possesses the skills, knowledge, and attitudes that will enable the teacher to provide a stimulating environment while developing the child's areas of weakness.

Intellectual Challenge

The child needs to be placed in a setting in which there are high expectations for intellectual performance. These high expectations must come not only from the teacher but also from other students. Classmates need to have high expectations for themselves and others and need to be able to interact with the gifted student at a high intellectual level. Discussions, projects, and committee work will not be intellectually demanding for a gifted student if he or she is always the leader, the one who thinks of different solutions, or the one who understands a concept long before anyone else. Lectures will be boring if extensive explanations have to be provided to the class and they are not needed by the gifted student.

The case study subjects discussed the disadvantages of special schools in this context. Herb, for example, felt that the teachers at his school, with the exception of the two who were handicapped, had very low expectations for disabled students. In fact, the whole environment was seen as fostering low expectations and providing little challenge. However, it also must be questioned whether students as severely disabled as Herb could be given the support services they need to function in the mainstream setting of a "regular" school. It is realistic to expect educational institutions to provide an attendant or aide for a small group of severely disabled children, but unrealistic to expect them to be able to afford an attendant for each child to enable them to attend regular classrooms.

Flexibility with Consistency

The program certainly must be flexible to accommodate individual needs. Students must be allowed to attend classes or participate in learning experiences that challenge their intelligence. On the other hand, they must be able to receive instruction and participate in experiences that will help them overcome their weaknesses. However, it is equally important that the program not be fragmented or lack continuity. A highly gifted boy with learning disabilities was placed in a regular classroom and attended resource rooms for learning disabilities and for giftedness. His week consisted of three days in the regular classroom, one day in the LD resource room, and one day in the resource room for the gifted! Even though the teachers worked hard to develop a consistent, well-coordinated program, the fact was that he did not feel that he belonged anywhere. Even though this situation provided flexibility for his development, stability was lacking. His parents finally decided to move so that he could be placed in a full-time program for the gifted with pull-out into a resource room for learning disabilities.

Availability of Support Services

Placement options also must have services available that are necessary for the development of coping and learning strategies and skills for using materials or equipment that minimize the effect of a disability or enable learning in spite of a severe disability. As discussed in the case studies, many things learned naturally by individuals without disabilities must be taught to handicapped children. For example, hearing children learn language naturally by listening and imitating what they hear, but deaf children must be taught. Children who see can find their way from place to place on their own, but blind children need orientation and mobility training. Children with disabilities also need to be taught how to use specialized materials and equipment that can enhance their learning. For a blind child, this might include use of an Optacon, a Kurzweil Reader, or writing and reading braille. For a deaf child, it might mean extensive instruction in speechreading and/ or sign language. A child with a severe motor impairment might need to use a whisper typewriter (one that is activated by a puff of air), whereas a learning disabled child might need to have books taped. Regular classroom or public school settings may not have these extensive services or training available to the child, or they may be difficult to obtain. Thus, the extent of the child's need for them should be a major consideration in placement decisions. After a child has learned certain skills, however, changes can be made in the placement.

The Teacher

Very seldom is the teacher a primary consideration in the placement of a child. However, research shows that the teacher is the single most important influence in the classroom (Dunkin & Biddle, 1974; Gage & Berliner, 1979). In the decision about the most appropriate environment for a child, the teacher's attitudes and knowledge related to giftedness and the specific disability should be considered. If the teacher is not knowledgeable in these areas, then an attitude of desire and willingness to learn becomes the critical factor along with the resources for training.

A second area to consider is the teacher's skills in relation to the student's specific needs. If the teacher's strengths include use of a multisensory approach to teaching, then a blind or deaf child may need very little modification of the basic instructional approach. A teaching method emphasizing a structured, task-analytical approach to instruction may be appropriate for a learning-disabled child so long as the structure permits challenge, creativity, flexibility and open-endedness. Finally, and perhaps most important, the teacher's attitude toward gifted students and/or students with disabilities should be considered. If negative perceptions or stereotypes are evident, then, regardless of the teacher's skills, a different placement may be necessary. Attitudes toward the idea of having a gifted or a disabled child in the classroom should be considered carefully.

Various program options are available for serving gifted students with disabilities. When placement decisions are made, the four general guidelines in this section should be considered, with particular emphasis on matching the child's strengths and weaknesses to the appropriate option. Above all else, however, no placement should ever be considered permanent. Children's needs change over time. The ideal placement for a specific second-grader, for instance, may become very restrictive by sixth grade when the child has learned to use equipment or has developed skills to overcome the difficulties created by a disability.

Providing Appropriate Curriculum

A child's placement in a learning environment only serves an enabling function. If the curriculum is not appropriate or does not provide for intellectual challenge and development, the type or form of placement makes no difference. Curricula for the development of intellectual abilities have been described elsewhere (Gallagher, 1975; Whitmore, 1980; Maker, 1982a, 1982b), as have curricula for development of skills in those with disabilities. There are, however, certain guidelines that should be followed in the development of curricula for gifted children with disabilities, owing to the specific interactions between giftedness and disabling conditions. These include a balance of emphasis on strengths and weaknesses, planned experiences for cognitive development, and use of a creative problem-solving approach.

Balance of Emphasis on Strengths and Weaknesses

Educators have a strong tendency to focus on remediation, on the development of areas in which a child's skills are weak or lacking. This fact is especially true of those who work with handicapped children, but it also applies to many who work with gifted students. Certainly, it is important to provide learning experiences that teach missing skills or develop areas of weakness. However, missing skills often are overemphasized to the point that students are not allowed or encouraged to express or develop their advanced cognitive abilities. Activities designed for practice of weak skills need to be balanced by activities allowing the expression or development of strengths in which weaknesses are not a factor. For example, a blind child certainly needs to practice braille reading and writing skills, but if his or her verbal skills are very high, the child also should be allowed (and encouraged) to tape-record stories, essays, or reports. Similarly, a learning-disabled child with high oral language skills and difficulties in written expression needs to engage in some activities in which oral reports, dictated stories, or taped essays are substituted for written assignments. This allows expression of the ability or strength without the frustration generated by interference of the disability. Certainly, the student should engage as well in a reasonable amount of practice in developing written language skills.

Related to the need for balance of emphasis between strengths and weaknesses is the issue of time spent on a learning activity and the effectiveness of the teaching. In other words, it may be impossible to develop certain skills to a high level, so rather than spend a great deal of time in these areas, the teacher should emphasize areas where maximum growth can occur. Indeed, these areas of strength may enable the child to overcome the areas of weakness or may even preclude the need for skills in the weak areas. Handwriting is one example: it may be more time-effective to teach a learning-disabled or motor-impaired child to type than to try to improve skills in handwriting. Another example is speechreading by deaf children. A student who is having extreme difficulties in developing a significant degree of proficiency in speechreading but is proficient in the use of sign language may need to concentrate on developing greater fluency in sign language.

Support for the guideline of balanced emphasis comes from two sources: research on the instructional development of strengths and weakness and self-concept development. With regard to the development of strengths, Maker (1979) has reviewed studies showing that when strengths were the focus of instruction, areas of weakness improved even though there was no attempt at remediation! Such research seems to demonstrate the powerful influence of learning experiences on self-concept. If children continually practice skills in areas in which they see little or no progress or success, they begin to perceive themselves as failures and then lower their levels of self-esteem. If they are given opportunities to develop and demonstrate their abilities, they develop perceptions of themselves as capable. Balanced emphases will produce more realistic self-perceptions.

Planned Experiences for Cognitive Development

A second guideline for the planning of educational programs for gifted students with disabilities is to plan experiences designed to raise the level of cognitive development. Research cited in the case study chapters shows that the cognitive development of handicapped children tends to be slower than that of their nonhandicapped peers. This slower development usually is seen not as a direct consequence of the disability itself but rather as the result of a lack of experience caused by the disability. Cognitive growth occurs through *active* interactions with the environment. Children with a sensory disability, such as blindness, lack these active interactions in two ways: first, they cannot interact visually with the environment, and second, since their movement is limited by a lack of vision, they also have fewer tactile interactions. Children with severe motor impairments lack tactile and other *active* interactions at the sensory motor stage. Planned experiences for cognitive development, then, should include more tactile and auditory experiences or stimulation for blind children, more visual and tactile experiences for deaf children, and more visual and auditory stimulation experiences for those with severe motor impairments. Cognitive development activities also should include extensive experiences with concrete objects or manipulatives prior to activities intended to foster development of abstract concepts. For instance, if a blind child is being asked to discuss or understand the concept of buoyancy (i.e., sinking and floating), that child first should be given the opportunity to test several items in a sink or a water table. Use of teaching techniques such as the Hilda Taba teaching strategies (Maker, 1982b) may be valuable since such techniques are designed to foster children's cognitive development through teacher questioning techniques. The concept development strategy is especially effective with this gifted handicapped population.

Use of a Creative Problem-Solving Approach

Teaching gifted disabled children the attitudes and skills involved in a creative problem-solving approach will benefit them both intellectually and personally. Inherent in a creative problem-solving approach (Parnes, 1966, 1975; Maker, 1982b) is the viewing of problem situations in a positive way; defining problems in a way that enables the student to devise innovative solutions; "brainstorming" many possible solutions, especially new and unique ideas; developing criteria for evaluating these possible solutions to select the most promising; and devising plans to carry out the chosen solution(s). All too often, people tend to rely on only one resolution of the problem or an answer proved to have been successful before, rather than to view each situation differently and to devise a solution that fits the situation. Perhaps the most important element in this process is a positive attitude toward problem solving and the ability to develop unique alternatives.

When the necessary attitudes and skills are developed, students can use a creative problem-solving approach in academic settings as well as in personal situations. In an academic setting, students are often presented with a problem situation in which they are asked individually or as a group to devise a solution. For example, perhaps students are asked to describe a situation involving pollution in a local river or lake. Students then gather facts about the situation, about the pollutants, and about methods for eliminating the pollution. They next restate the problem in a way allowing creative resolution, "brainstorm" as many solutions as possible, develop criteria for choosing a solution and select the most promising one, and finally create a plan for implementing a solution. With regard to personal situations, students can apply the same methods to such problems as how to accomplish daily living skills, how to prove to a teacher or parent that they are capable of accomplishing a task, or other situations related to their disability. With practice in methods such as these, students become more creative and develop a repertoire of successful strategies. Students also develop confidence in themselves and in their ability to solve their own problems.

In summary, the educational curriculum should follow the guidelines developed in this section. Within these guidelines attention must be paid to the following areas: (a) the use of teaching behaviors that do not communicate low expectations; (b) development of effective coping and learning strategies through instruction, use of role models, balanced emphases on strengths and weaknesses, and use of a creative problem-solving approach; and (c) development of appropriate attributions for success and failure experiences that emphasize the role of internal factors in causing success (ability and effort), the role of internal and unstable factors in failure (effort), and external factors as causes of failure (luck or task difficulty).

Many options exist for service delivery. The option chosen for a particular student should reflect careful consideration of intellectual challenge, flexibility with consistency, availability of needed support services, and the qualifications of the teacher. Regardless of the option chosen, placements should be re-evaluated on a regular schedule and whenever a needed change might be indicated. The curriculum must be designed to achieve balanced emphases on strengths and weaknesses, to include experiences for cognitive development, and to use a creative problem-solving approach. The curriculum will be more effective if it also is planned and executed in cooperation with parents and the community.

CONCLUSION: THE NEED FOR COOPERATIVE PROGRAMMING

A child with a disability usually will be served by a variety of agencies and individuals. If the educational program is to achieve maximum effectiveness, all agencies and individuals should be working together to achieve common goals. To this end, meetings, discussions, cooperative planning sessions, and continuous feedback are necessary. Parents need to provide information about the child's behavior at home as well as ask for information about school performance. They should ask how to supplement the educational program at home and then to follow through on the suggestions made. Medical personnel need to provide data on treatment procedures being used as well as on the medical progress of the child. They also need to solicit information about the student's educational progress from parents and school personnel as well as to provide information regarding ways the medical treatment can be supplemented at home and in school. Educators must obtain information about medical treatment, ways to supplement it, and the child's progress in physical and academic areas at home. They also should request suggestions from parents regarding the educational program and provide continuous feedback on the student's behavior and progress in school. The following brief case study illustrates this needed cooperation.

Joe, a severely disabled child with cerebral palsy, was being treated by a physician and physical therapist because he needed to develop more muscle control and flexibility. The therapist had devised exercises for him. In trying to help him with his exercises, his parents were frustrated by his lack of interest in the activities. Joe was more interested in reading and playing computer games with his close friends. His parents were becoming concerned that he was becoming too dependent on adults, that he had only a few friends, and that he was becoming too isolated from other people. The teacher also was concerned that he was afraid or unwilling to attempt simple motor tasks and that he was isolating himself from many of the children in the classroom.

At a conference about Joe that was attended by the physical therapist, his mother, and his teacher, several plans were developed. His mother enrolled him in a swimming class at the YMCA with a group of children whom he knew but who were not his close friends. The counselor and swimming teacher discussed Joe's disability with the other children and enlisted their help in making him feel comfortable and a part of the group. They agreed to use a creative problem-solving process with the group because Joe enjoyed this kind of discussion in school and was creative in his development of solutions. In school, the teacher decided to focus on the value of physical fitness and exercise in social studies and health classes, with particular attention to the influence of early muscle development on later performance. She continued to use creative problem solving as they focused on the creation of unique solutions for social and academic problem situations. Joe's parents, teacher, and therapist discussed with him his perceptions of the causes of his success and failure in situations involving physical skills in an attempt to get him to discover that his reluctance to attempt all tasks involving motor skills was inhibiting his overall success.

The group agreed to meet again in a month to discuss the results of this cooperative program and to decide what revisions needed to be made. They also agreed to discuss his progress with each other whenever possible. At the end of the month, the teacher reported that he enjoyed the intellectual discussions about causes of success, and that he was beginning to put more effort into activities involving motor skills. The therapist was pleased with his physical progress, and his mother reported that he had learned to swim! She was even more pleased that he enjoyed the classes and had made friends with a group of children who liked to swim and enjoyed physical activity. He was certainly not the best swimmer in the class, but he was not embarrassed or afraid to try. His mother even reported that he had asked her to leave while he took his lessons because the other parents did not stay with their children. She was pleased with these beginnings of independence.

In Joe's case, the cooperation of several individuals resulted in positive growth and the development of healthy attitudes toward a disability.

Sometimes, meetings seem impossible to arrange. Cooperative programs, although facilitated by group discussions, can be accomplished without meetings of those concerned. Teachers can send home notes or exercises to practice, and parents can send notes or make telephone calls to report progress or suggest a solution. Constant communication is the essential element.

In conclusion, parents, educators, and others influencing the intellectual development of gifted children with disabilities need to be aware of their behaviors that communicate expectations for success or failure. They need to change their behavior so that it reflects realistic expectations. All these individuals need to plan experiences that facilitate the development of effective strategies for overcoming or coping with the disability and for maximizing intellectual development. They need to discuss beliefs about the causes of success and failure with an emphasis on developing in the disabled individual a belief in the ability to influence his or her own destiny. In deciding what programs to provide, an extensive assessment process should be initiated first, focusing on a variety of abilities, and then decisions about placement options should be made according to the guidelines presented. The curriculum should be individualized to meet specific needs and should follow the guidelines presented earlier. Finally, all individuals should cooperate in the provision of a program designed to challenge intellectual abilities while teaching skills and attitudes that facilitate the full development of intellectual potential in the gifted person with a specific disability.

Chapter 9

Summary and Conclusions

A SUMMARY OF WHAT WE KNOW

The Case Study Approach to Inquiry

Despite the limitations we have acknowledged with the case study approach to inquiry, we have found the methodology to yield invaluable results in the search to understand the special needs of intellectually gifted persons with disabilities. We are confident that the in-depth, open-ended study of individual cases is the best mode of investigation to answer the types of questions in this book. For example, do intellectually gifted persons with specific disabilities really constitute a special subpopulation for which a new field of professional research and practice is needed? Is this a specific population that can be identified accurately? What is the nature of the interaction between intellectual giftedness and a specific disability? How appropriately have professionals rendered services to members of this subpopulation? How have their parents and families been supported and assisted? How responsive have communities been to their special needs? Is there a need for professional leadership to create awareness, more accurate understanding, and changes in living conditions and professional practices?

From the responses of the subjects of the case studies, we have been able to formulate answers to key questions that we believe accurately reflect the experiences and needs of human beings in diverse places, stages of life, and roles. Although these cases comprise a relatively small sample, the experiences reported and the conclusions drawn are significant even if they are unique to the cases described. Their stories can sensitize each one of us to similar persons around us whose needs may be unrecognized, and can motivate us to respond more appropriately as friends or professionals. An important and unexpected benefit for almost all of the subjects, reported at the conclusion of the process of self-disclosure, was the profoundly positive emotional impact of being guided in reflection, so that deep feelings could be expressed, together with a sense of contribution to the improvement of life for others as a consequence of sharing their personal stories.

Some researchers may criticize the case study approach as insufficiently rigorous in controls, objectivity, and sampling size. We would argue that more systematic, large-scale studies cannot be designed until some fundamental questions are answered and the problems are well defined. The self-reported feelings, perceptions, and personal experiences of our subjects have face validity as responses to specific questions. From their responses some answers can be formulated, based on patterns of response that we are confident can guide our further inquiry. We also feel more equipped to meet our goal of facilitating through our work the provision of optimal conditions for the growth, achievement, personal satisfaction, and positive mental health of disabled gifted persons.

Answers to Our Questions

The pattern of consistency in responses among subjects and the congruity between the response patterns and our theoretical and/or experiential understandings suggest that there are some defensible answers to key questions about this emerging field of study. The following discussion offers answers that provide a knowledge base on which to structure research and professional practices in the future. We believe that these answers and conclusions, summarized succinctly here, are substantiated by the specific, more detailed content of preceding chapters.

Is This a Legitimate Field of Professional Inquiry and Practice? Is There a Distinct Population of Gifted Disabled Persons with Special Needs?

The interactive effects of specific characteristics associated with intellectual giftedness and with disabilities definitely produce psychological and educational needs distinctly different from those of other populations. This fact perhaps is most clearly illustrated in the learning-disabled gifted population: in this group, standard definitions often are not applicable, and placement in programs specifically for the learning disabled or the gifted is not always appropriate. The interactive effects produce implications for substantial changes in professional practices, which must be based on a more accurate understanding of the needs of gifted specific subpopulation and on a more accurate understanding of the needs of gifted disabled persons in general. Therefore, the field of inquiry is legitimized by the need for systematic research and scholarship to inform practitioners and improve services to disabled gifted persons.

Has This Population of Gifted Disabled Individuals Been Identified? Are They Easily and Accurately Identifiable?

Generally members of this population have not been officially identified and labeled as intellectually gifted, although perceptive and informed professionals and family members often have recognized the individual's superior abilities and potential for achievement. Learning-disabled gifted children tend to escape identification either as handicapped or gifted because of a rather "average" academic record. Although there were early, recognizable indicators of superior mental abilities in every case study presented, generally they were ignored by the disabled child, the family, and professionals because of a focus on the disability and stereotypic expectations associated with the condition. Typically, in these cases psychometrists or school psychologists conducting an assessment to determine educational needs did not find evidence of giftedness when standard measures and norms were used, and sometimes did not even attempt to assess intellectual potential because of a focus on physical and sensory handicaps.

Giftedness has been identified in disabled persons when they have distinguished themselves by high levels of success attributed to superior intelligence. When young children are placed in educational programs designed to ameliorate the handicapping condition, it seems unlikely that behavioral indicators of giftedness will be elicited. However, with proper, comprehensive assessment procedures that include the use of appropriately modified tests of intellectual ability and skilled observations of behavior in stimulating educational settings, reliable identification can be made. This population has not been dependably identified for appropriate services, but such recognition is possible with improved referral and assessment procedures.

What Are the Unique Effects of Interaction between Giftedness and Disabilities?

All cases we studied clearly evidenced both positive and negative consequences of specific attributes associated with giftedness interacting with aspects of disabling conditions. The positive effects can be regarded as strengths that allow such individuals to overcome their disabilities and achieve goals of success not attained by nongifted persons similarly disabled. Apparently, a strong desire to be independent, tendencies toward perfectionism and high aspirations for contributing to society, and intense drives to attain knowledge, to gain understanding, and to master skills and problems all nourish an exceptional capacity for perseverance and unrelenting motivation to attain goals. The case study subjects applied their analytical and creative intellectual powers to solve problems that enabled them to cope with undesirable limitations imposed by their disabilities and to adapt effectively by devising new ways to accomplish their objectives and to satisfy their needs.

Those same positive attributes of giftedness also make disabled persons very vulnerable to poor mental health resulting from low feelings of self-esteem and lowered expectations for success. Drives to achieve and high aspirations create extremely acute frustration that is difficult to tolerate. Unrelenting perseverance and determination to solve a problem or reach a goal can cause a disabled person to extend him or herself beyond the limits of available energy often, if not continuously. The extensive use of adaptive methods and devices to accomplish that which is not usually attempted or expected also tends to deplete mental and physical energy below critical levels.

Gifted persons seem naturally to desire higher levels of social interaction and access to educational opportunities (e.g., facilities, programs, events) than those sufficient for most nongifted persons, so disabled individuals with sensory or motor impairments are vulnerable to acute feelings of isolation and exclusion. All these vulnerabilities, plus the tension created by a very active mind, create a somewhat greater need for not only emotional support but also social and educational opportunities. The last particular vulnerability identified is related to career aspirations. Since these persons tend to aspire to careers that will appropriately challenge and satisfy their intellectual giftedness, they often are "charting new courses." In other words, they do not seek employment typical of persons with their disability so prospective employers frequently must be educated regarding their special abilities and ways the disabling condition can be accommodated to minimize interference with job performance. Obtaining suitable employment often is a most stressful, frustrating, and discouraging process requiring continued perseverance and creative problem solving.

Overall it seems that the benefits of giftedness in enabling the individual to adapt and achieve outweigh the liabilities created by negative consequences. With appropriate support services from well-informed and trained professionals, the negative consequences of intense frustration, feelings of isolation, insufficient energy, and difficulty in gaining career opportunities can be significantly reduced. Then disabled persons will find it unequivocally a great advantage and compensatory satisfaction to be intellectually gifted.

Have the Needs of This Special Population Been Served by Various Professionals?

It is evident from the case studies that too often professionals have failed to recognize and address the individual's giftedness and related specific needs. It is not unusual for disabled persons to view individual professionals, institutions of learning or rehabilitation, and government agencies as definitely having been obstructive in relation to personal goals. The obstruction appears to emanate from stereotypic expectations held for the disabling condition and a narrow view of the person—that is, a failure to assess the total attributes and needs of the individual and to design a holistic approach to treatment.

Appropriate educational opportunities often have been withheld from disabled children. Typically, such children are placed in programs of intervention for the handicapped and either are not considered for or are excluded from programs for gifted students. When the disability is not noticeable owing to the child's superior adaptive skills or the invisible nature of the handicap (e.g., learning disabilities), no special educational service may be provided. It seems quite common for special educators as well as regular classroom teachers to teach all handicapped children as though they were intellectually slow or even mentally handicapped. Consequently, these children frequently are systematically excluded from learning environments in which their superior intellectual abilities can be stimulated and developed.

Similarly, school psychologists have tended to conduct assessments with an exclusive focus on the "problem area" or disability, not even exploring the possibility of giftedness. Medical and rehabilitation professionals have tended to focus also on the areas of weakness associated with the disability and, when they are unaware of the possible presence of exceptional intelligence and the potential implications for treatment, have often communicated inappropriately low expectations, with no encouragement that higher aspirations may be attainable. Treatments have been rendered in a traditional manner, predetermined to a great extent by the classification of the disability and without regard for other patient characteristics.

Certainly, it could be argued that the individuals described in the case studies lived in an era in which special educational services, teaching methods, and assessment procedures were much less sophisticated than they are now. However, the authors' experiences indicate that, in too many instances, very little change has occurred with respect to the development and assessment of giftedness in individuals with disabilities.

Have Parents Been Assisted in Providing Appropriate Support and Guidance?

Although some professionals have given excellent support and counsel to parents of disabled children and families of disabled adults, communication has tended to be very limited in frequency and scope. Generally, specialists address only the specific concern that is within their area of expertise, but their responses to requests for advice regarding other related areas, such as educational or career aspirations, tend to be inaccurate because of stereotypic thinking. It also is common for parents to be confused by differing perspectives and prognoses among various professionals, such as teachers, physicians, family counselors, and rehabilitation therapists.

Parents appear to have little help in raising a disabled child, insufficient and often inaccurate information about alternative possibilities, and little or no information about the possibility of the child being intellectually gifted. Clearly there is a need for more accurate information to be made available to parents through prepared literature, individual professionals, and agencies. Literature disseminated by advocacy groups or networks of disabled persons and their families should include the fact that *no* disability, other than severe brain damage affecting cognitive functioning or a general mental handicap, automatically excludes any possibility of the presence of exceptional intellectual abilities. Parents should be given information to guide their observations, because precise reports of the child's behavior may reveal superior cognitive characteristics that can be capitalized upon to facilitate growth and adaptation to the disability.

Are Communities Providing Appropriate Support and Opportunities to This Population?

Certainly progress has been made in the elimination of physical barriers to facilities, and provisions are increasingly being made for hearing impaired persons at community levels. However, there seems to be much yet to be done to eliminate all barriers, psychological as well as physical, and to move beyond access to active encouragement of participation by disabled persons. Through the dissemination of more accurate information about disabilities, heightening awareness of unintended discrimination and the potential giftedness of some handicapped individuals, perhaps all obstacles to the full integration and participation of disabled persons in society can be eliminated. Community agencies definitely must enforce policies of equal employment opportunity and must make resources available— funds, technological devices, modified facilities, and so on—to encourage the participation of disabled persons.

In summary, with these findings in response to the key questions, defensible conclusions can be formulated to guide the development of the field of education of gifted disabled students. The need for continued study of the problems, development of a more complete and accurate knowledge base, and research to inform decision makers and improve professional practices is clearly evident.

CONCLUSIONS: THE WORK AHEAD

The goals of the field, identified in Chapter 1, seem appropriate in light of the needs established by our study and analyses. What needs to be done to address those goals and to meet the needs that have been identified can be divided into three arenas of activity: (a) research and development, (b) preparation of professionals, and (c) direct services and assistance to disabled persons.

Research and Development

The needs we have identified relative to the gifted disabled population are directly related to many current research and development activities in the broader fields of psychology and education. For example, researchers studying cognitive functioning can investigate the characteristics and needs of this special population. Brain research may lead to improvement in methods of assessing and developing cognitive potential, in rehabilitation and educational interventions, and in understanding of the interaction between superior cognitive abilities and disabling conditions. Longitudinal studies, comparable to Terman's classic work in scope and depth, need to be conducted on sizable subpopulations of persons with specific handicaps and various types of intellectual giftedness. Such studies should include systematic evaluations of the relative effectiveness over time of alternative rehabilitation treatments and educational programs. Additional research comparing the relative effectiveness of alternative educational and rehabilitation models currently being used is needed also to inform decision makers selecting or developing programs.

Three areas of development are needed to address the needs of this population: improved tests and other assessment tools, instructional technology and curriculum materials, and technological aids to student learning and communication. First, standard tests of specific intellectual aptitudes must be developed, experimentally used, and validated for specific subpopulations. Tests modified to accommodate specific disabilities must be normed appropriately and compared to information gained from adapted use of other standard measures. So, in addition to the development of new tests, more commonly available standardized tests must be normed for handicapped populations and the results compared with those obtained on adapted measures.

The second area of needed developmental activity pertains to instructional technology and curriculum materials. For example, how should curriculum materials and instructional methods be altered from standard practice with learning-disabled students for use in the intellectually gifted subpopulation? Instructional guides to modifying methods and materials, based on research findings, must be developed and disseminated to teachers of learning-disabled gifted students in regular and special education classrooms. Besides developing such "technical assistance" guides and resources for teachers of individuals in each subpopulation of gifted disabled students, a need for similar assistance exists for rehabilitation therapists and counselors. Given John's story, how should rehabilitation practices be altered for such individuals? How can professionals design educational and rehabilitation processes to appropriately utilize the strengths derived from traits as well as to accommodate the needs created by the disabling condition? Practitioners must be provided with clear, specific guidelines and with necessary tools and instructional materials; otherwise, the response to an identified need will never move beyond rhetoric among professionals to significant improvement in services to disabled gifted persons.

The third area of development is the one that is most advanced now, technological aids to student learning and communication. Particularly with recent advances in computer technology, remarkable aids have been and are being developed for use by persons with hearing, visual, motor, and language impairment. The Optacon, the Kurzweil Reader, new improved hearing aids that overcome nerve damage, and various adapted computers and electronic communicators exemplify these advances. Continued development of such enabling devices is needed, and they must become more accessible to all persons who would benefit from them. Without proper dissemination of information about new resources and widespread accessibility of innovative devices, developmental activities fail to achieve their ultimate purpose of improving the lives of disabled persons.

Preparation of Professionals

Substantial changes need to occur in the initial and continuing preparation of all professionals who work with disabled persons and their families. Major changes across all programs must be directed toward increasing the competence and collaborative efforts of teachers, school psychologists, counselors of families and children, and medical and rehabilitation professionals. Systematic programs of inservice training and continuing education of practicing professionals in each field must be developed, and improvements in the quality of preservice programs must occur. Otherwise, existing practices in schools, hospitals, and agencies will continue, and changes that benefit disabled gifted persons will not occur.

Available preservice programs and continuing education offerings for professionals in all roles need to be restructured in curriculum content and instructional methods to develop accurate knowledge of the nature of giftedness and its potential presence and influence on the growth of abilities in disabled persons. Through case studies read and directly experienced, professionals must become aware of inappropriate stereotypes and rigid expectations that place low ceilings on the possible achievements of disabled gifted persons. Those professionals responsible for facilitating the growth and/or rehabilitation of handicapped persons must become more skilled in (a) recognizing and nurturing attributes of intellectual giftedness, (b) capitalizing on those strengths to facilitate overall growth and to mitigate the effects of the disability, and (c) guiding the individual to cope effectively with the negative consequences of the interaction between the giftedness and the disability. All professionals need to become more skillful in eliciting behavior that allows an accurate assessment of intellectual ability and in judging the extent to which a handicapping condition will permanently interfere with specific abilities. Those skills will enable professionals to provide more helpful and realistic counsel. In particular, a range of positive outcomes of treatment and factors that may increase success can be determined; in turn, more appropriate decisions regarding medical treatment programs, home therapy, educational placements and program design, and recommendations for career and life style goals can be made. All programs of professional preparation can also do more to develop communication skills for collaborative work with professional colleagues and for working with parents and patients or students.

Some specific changes can be recommended for each professional group. First, teachers in regular classrooms must become knowledgeable about the characteristics and needs of gifted students with handicapping conditions so that they can be referred for identification and special education services. Although this need has been recognized for almost a decade, most teacher education programs still reflect little development of skills for identifying and modifying instruction for handicapped students in regular classrooms; even less, if any, attention is given to information about intellectually gifted children. Furthermore, programs preparing special educators of handicapped students seldom train students to look for indicators of giftedness and to make further modifications of educational programs for disabled pupils who are gifted. Similarly, teachers of gifted children are not prepared to adapt their programs to the needs of disabled students; they do not develop the knowledge and skills needed for working with the range of potential disabilities in gifted education programs. And unfortunately, teacher education students in all these programs are not prepared to work together collaboratively in behalf of children; there is as yet no recognition of a shared responsibility and of the need to combine their expertise and articulate their efforts. Instead, unless they are majoring in two certification areas, students preparing to teach are kept in compartments called "departments" that socialize them into a profession that lacks collaborative teamwork and articulated programming. All teachers should be skilled in modifying curriculum and instruction for individual differences and special needs. They should be comfortable with the use of adaptive skills and devices necessary to the success of disabled students and should specifically work toward providing the most normal, integrated school experience possible for each child.

School psychologists could be expected to be most knowledgeable about identifying and providing for individual differences, particularly those in "exceptional" students. However, relatively few school psychology programs adequately prepare professionals to understand the nature and needs of gifted students. The curriculum does not sensitize them to the possibility that a disabled student may be intellectually gifted nor train them through clinical experiences to modify assessment procedures to identify giftedness in disabled students. School psychologists also receive minimal preparation in most programs for providing leadership in the multidisciplinary team's efforts—determining the appropriate placement for a handicapped child who is gifted, selecting or designing an appropriate program for a gifted student with or without a disability, and articulating all service components of an individual educational plan. Yet that responsibility tends to be given to the school psychologist, who consequently has a powerful influence on a student's educational opportunities.

Counselors of families and children regrettably are little prepared to deal with the complexities of such conditions as those presented by a child who is both disabled and gifted. It is important that programs for family counselors include information about handicaps and giftedness and about appropriate referrals for educational programming. Similarly, medical and rehabilitation professionals must become more accurately informed about the positive and negative effects of giftedness on disabling conditions and be aware of tendencies to underestimate potential and the possible achievements of the gifted disabled population. They should be taught to advise parents to seek the advice of appropriately skilled educators regarding educational and career alternatives as well as to work collaboratively with educators to develop appropriate plans for the child.

In summary, it must be recognized that every community needs a staff of professionals who are well informed about the characteristics and needs of disabled gifted students; who work together with the family to provide appropriate services to the individual; and who are committed to eliminating inaccurate stereotypes, expectations, and assessments of ability. It probably will be easier to effect needed changes in preservice programs through accreditation agencies than to stimulate support for a systematic program of continuing education required of all practicing professionals. However, both programs are needed.

There are two conditions within professional preparation programs in higher education that also should be encouraged: (a) the acceptance and encouragement of disabled individuals to enter the human services professions and (b) the interdisciplinary integration of professional preparation programs, faculties, and students. Even though federal legislation has prohibited the discriminatory practice of excluding handicapped persons from educational programs, disabled students frequently are advised not to seek professional training because of their disabilities, and certainly they are not recruited or encouraged to apply for admission to professional preparation programs. The reader should take serious note of the significance of role models of success, such as were provided by handicapped teachers in Herb's case. Such models for disabled students likewise can be provided by competent teachers who happen to have specific disabilities. Certification and licensure requirements need to be re-examined in this light. We remember with pain the fellow student in high school who was impaired by cerebral palsy, and who was highly motivated to become a teacher. His father was superintendent of schools. After completing his education through a master's degree level, he was denied certification to teach because of his writing and speech impairments. In desperation, he volunteered for experimental brain surgery to attempt to increase his motor control. The surgery was unsuccessful and left him less able and more dependent on his parents for care than before.

One of our most instructive experiences was with a college student, majoring in teacher education, who was totally deaf and almost totally blind. She could communicate only through signing, which required the use of her remaining peripheral vision. She was one of the most academically competent students in the program and became a successful teacher! In another case not yet resolved, a "dyslexic" gifted student in an elementary education program is struggling to obtain certification to teach at this level. Faculty members do not believe that an LD adult can effectively teach elementary children.

Teacher educators must become more fairly discriminating in screening students, more accurate in their assessment of potential for a teaching role, and better prepared to assist disabled persons to pursue professional preparation programs. More fair and accurate methods of assessing qualifications for teaching are essential at the entry and graduation levels of professional preparation programs. The criteria must be carefully evaluated and validated; such methods as the use of newly developed standardized tests of basic skills and professional knowledge may be unfairly discriminating against certain populations. Actual performance in classrooms and the effects of teaching behavior on student learning should be most influential in the evaluation process.

A related recommendation is that professors from various disciplines and departments be integrated as the faculty of professional preparation programs. Instead of segregated units with no interaction among faculty members across programs, settings should be created through field work and clinical practice to bring together the expertise from the various disciplines for the most effective training of professionals. Projects of research and development should bring together faculty members of different disciplines with professional colleagues in the public schools to design better services of intervention and counseling programs for various subpopulations. Collaborative teamwork must be intentionally fostered in higher education if it is to spread throughout the field of human services.

Direct Services and Assistance to Disabled Persons

From the study of successful adults and general knowledge of educational and rehabilitation services available to disabled children, we have concluded that much more continuous effort must be directed toward better preparing the handicapped child or young adult for adulthood. From their early years, all children, disabled or not, need the skillful guidance of adults to grow in their ability to assess accurately their strengths and weaknesses in relation to possible careers and adult life styles. In later childhood and early adolescence, disabled students need to be gradually encouraged and helped to become effective advocates for their needs. When confident of the ability to succeed in a task or to pursue an educational or vocational direction, the disabled young person should be encouraged to be assertive in expressing positive beliefs about self and persisting in efforts to gain access to appropriate opportunities—as did Myron, Abe, Herb, and Marcia.

It seems that traditional educational and rehabilitation practices have tended to foster dependence on professionals for judgment about inherent abilities and potential adult life styles. As the case study subjects indicated, few people responded supportively when they fought for their rights to pursue opportunities to develop their special abilities and interests. Professionals tended to speak authoritatively about the limits imposed by disabling conditions and to respond to individuals as representatives of categories of handicap with predetermined limitations and possibilities. Individuals, like those in our research, have begun to erode stereotypes and to challenge professionals to regard the disabled individual as a responsible source of valuable information needed to make the wisest decisions relative to treatments, educational programs, and career options so that the chance of developing a satisfying adult life style will be increased.

Each disabled gifted individual should become an effective advocate for personal and group rights and needs. Furthermore, it is very important that specific subpopulations form networks among themselves to provide emotional support, to disseminate valuable information about available resources, and to create more powerful advocacy for community and government assistance. Some networking for gifted persons who want increased opportunities may occur within existing organizations for handicapped individuals, such as the Association for Children with Learning Disabilities (ACLD), which currently is disseminating through film, literature, and speakers accurate information about the ability of gifted students with learning disabilities to successfully complete a college education and to pursue a professional career. An example of an association with a very specific focus is the National Association of Blind Teachers, which is an affiliate of the American Council of the Blind. Through films, newsletters, directory of blind teachers, and other resources this association is greatly facilitating the successful pursuit of teaching careers by visually impaired individuals.

Communities must assist individuals and advocacy groups by actively seeking to facilitate their success. Instead of waiting for disabled persons to initiate communication and to advocate for change, members of the community should invite them to provide information about their needs through such channels as meetings of government officials, community agencies, church groups, and educational institutions. Then community members should respond to the disabled persons by (a) listening carefully with an openness to change, (b) assisting with the dissemination throughout the community of accurate information about needed changes, and (c) establishing appropriate policies to facilitate changes. The effective use of public media to create awareness of needed changes in attitudes, expectations, and practices will open the doors to change, but without enabling policies and changed procedures, sustained response to the identified needs will not occur.

Such community response to identified needs occurred in Nashville, Tennessee, in the 1970s. First, the mayor recognized the need and committed resources to increase opportunities in the community for disabled persons. Next, a position was created in the mayor's office to supervise the enforcement of local policies guaranteeing fair employment practices, access to community facilities and events, social opportunities for handicapped children and youth, and favorable public awareness and attitudes. Supplemental funding was then secured from various sources, including federal and state governments, to establish specific projects, such as a teen club for severely disabled youth. The local newspapers and television channels supported the efforts by highlighting in feature stories accurate information about needs, the accomplishments of individuals and groups, and special projects.

Community support as demonstrated in Nashville is critical to successful elimination of unfair discrimination against disabled persons seeking employment. Even the human services professions of medicine, rehabilitation, counseling, and education discourage or prevent highly intelligent and otherwise qualified individuals from entering their fields of professional practice. The experiences of Myron and Abe are examples of this discrimination. The National Association of Blind Teachers has been organized in part because of unfair discrimination in the employment of teachers. We have personally known highly intelligent graduates of teacher education programs, with scholastic honors, who were unable to gain or sustain employment as teachers because of being legally blind and having mild neurological impairment that produced somewhat rigid, awkward movement. The reasons given for nonemployment were the need to hold papers and books close to the face to read them, inability to effectively supervise children in the play area at recess, and slow movement suggesting the possibility of being "accident prone." The employing administrators also were uncertain that the mildly disabled individuals had sufficient energy to keep up with active, young children.

Discrimination in employment practices still occurs for all major types of disabilities, even within the education profession, though the legislation of the 1970s produced some constraints on it and substantially increased the employment of disabled persons. For example, the National Association of Blind Teachers reports that in the United States there are over 2000 successful blind teachers at all levels of instruction. However, communities should be cautioned against complacency. Community awareness, values, and policies must be evaluated continually and progress assured. As John, in Chapter 5, stated so well

In the community there is a need for awareness of the barriers to access that exist, architectural barriers preventing physical access to buildings and barriers preventing access to the opportunities for participation in community activities. The latter category includes failure to encourage the participation of disabled persons. In some communities it is assumed that the community responsibility ends with eliminating physical barriers; too often there is a total lack of encouragement of or opportunity for participation by disabled individuals in community events.

THE CHALLENGE

It is evident from our study that the social success and high professional achievements of gifted persons with specific disabilities have occurred primarily because of their characteristic motivating drive and persistence, with the facilitating assistance of a few persons. Unquestionably these disabled high achievers have excelled in their respective fields because of their personal attributes and in spite of repeated confrontations with discouragement, resistance, and rejection by individuals and institutions or agencies. We need to fight to eliminate negative stereotypes and restrictive practices that stem from inaccurate and incomplete information. We need to fight for the enforcement of policies and changes in practices that will protect the rights of disabled persons to explore their potential giftedness, to test their limits, and to pursue their goals of high levels of productivity, significant social contribution, and independent life style.

The high achievements and obvious exceptional abilities of the subjects of the case studies are clear indicators of giftedness. However, there unquestionably are many other disabled persons with exceptional intellectual potential or more fully developed abilities who have not overcome the psychological barriers of discouragement and frustration, and the attitudinal and physical barriers identified throughout this book. Those individuals need our help as friends, employers, and professional colleagues to restore their confidence in their abilities or to discover their giftedness and ways of using it to mitigate the limiting disability and enhance personal satisfaction. There are at least four ways in which you can be responsive to the needs of gifted persons with specific disabilities.

Individual Search and Support

In your work in community activities, constantly be alert to the possibility of discovering a disabled person who is intellectually gifted. When you discover one, become a facilitator of the growth and opportunities possible for that individual. As you develop a relationship with the person, you will accumulate knowledge and understandings that you and the gifted person may wish to share with others. But, most importantly, reach out to that person and touch his or her life. If you are a researcher, apply your skills to the analysis of the case studies that you and others collect. Share your interest and knowledge about gifted persons with disabilities with colleagues who may address our concerns through their research activity. If you are employed as a human services professional (educator, counselor, school psychologist, medical or rehabilitation professional), critically examine your practices and consider how they may need to change: How quickly do you make judgments about an individual's potential? How apt are you to identify giftedness through your assessment procedures? How much do you encourage the disabled individual to engage in self-evaluation and to provide you with significant personal information that will guide your assistance in the educational or rehabilitation/medical treatment process?

Active Advocacy

Respond to the challenges in this book by becoming active at the local, state, and federal levels of government as an advocate of gifted persons with specific disabilities. By asking pertinent questions about policies and practices and raising awareness, you can make those people with undesirable attitudes, values, and beliefs uncomfortable. See that accurate information about the needs of this subpopulation is disseminated systematically through all available and appropriate channels of communication in your community. Work to increase knowledge and improve practices within your own professional and/or social settings. Seek support for funds to establish, continue, and expand the needed services of agencies intended to serve disabled persons in the community. Publicize projects and programs that are needed or are providing resources and assistance to gifted disabled persons.

Active Participation in Organizations

The most effective way to advocate for the needs of gifted persons who are disabled is through existing organizations, which can raise a louder collective voice, can exert greater pressure on agencies and legislators, and can enable more to happen because of greater resources. Associations that have been established to advocate either for gifted or for handicapped persons need to extend their efforts to benefit this subpopulation, which has similar but also different needs. The organization that affords greatest potential for effective advocacy in behalf of gifted disabled persons is the Council for Exceptional Children (CEC). Membership includes parents, concerned citizens, and professional educators and is open to advocates of any population of exceptional persons. Membership supports the unified efforts of the total organization to advocate for all exceptional persons; for example, CEC dues provide support for the organization's dissemination of information through literature and conferences and the ongoing advocacy efforts of three full-time lobbyists on Capitol Hill. In addition, members can join specific divisions whose additional dues support their more narrowly focused advocacy activities. All advocates of gifted disabled persons should actively support CEC!

It also is important for all of us to increase awareness, promote understanding, and improve opportunities for gifted disabled persons through community and professional organizations whose members may not be sensitive to this need. Through influencing the programs offered by church and community groups, as well as the conference offerings and agendas of professional associations, a relatively small number of advocates can significantly extend awareness beyond professionals who work with gifted and/or disabled populations. Particularly important organizations to be influenced are those that have communication with regular classroom teachers, school administrators, school psychologists, physicians, nurses, therapists, counselors, and education and psychology professors and researchers.

Building the Field

The expertise available from disabled persons, their parents and caretakers, and diverse professionals must be coalesced around shared concerns and responsibility for improving services and opportunities. All persons can contribute to the development of a knowledge base about this specific population. By disseminating information about the needs of gifted disabled persons, support can be generated for systematic research efforts and the development of resource materials and equipment. Advocacy efforts can create pressure within institutions of higher education to modify appropriately their professional preparation programs and to support academic inquiry into the problem. Community advocates can bring similar pressure to bear upon the medical and rehabilitation professionals to make desirable changes in institutional practices and training programs. Together these forces will establish the field of inquiry and special services pertinent to the needs of gifted persons with disabling conditions.

We are glad you read our book, met our gifted acquaintances who taught us so much, and are thinking about the problems and needs suggested by our findings. Don't stop now! Continue the dialogue we have begun—with your families, friends, colleagues, and community leaders. Sustain your motivation as an advocate by remembering the individual stories shared in this book and focusing on the possibility that your efforts may result in one or more similar persons being enabled to develop and share their giftedness more fully and with more enabling support.

References

American Association for Gifted Children. (1978). *On being gifted*. New York: Walker & Company.

American Foundation for the Blind. (1961). *A teacher education program for those who serve blind children and youth*. New York: Author.

Ames, L. (1968). Learning disabilities: The developmental point of view. In H. Myklebust (Ed.), *Progress in learning disabilities* (Vol. 1). New York: Grune & Stratton.

Ashcroft, S.C. (1963). Blind and partially seeing children. In L.M. Dunn (Ed.), *Exceptional children in the schools*. New York: Holt, Rinehart & Winston.

Ayres, A. (1968). Reading—A product of sensory integrative process. In H. Smith (Ed.), *Perception and reading*. Newark, DE: International Reading Association.

Baker, H. (1970). *Biographical sagas of willpower*. New York: Vantage Press.

Barraga, N.C. (1964). *Increased visual behavior in low vision children*. New York: American Foundation for the Blind.

Bateman, B. (1963). *Reading and psycholinguistic processes of partially seeing children* (CEC Research Monograph, Series A, No. 5). Arlington, VA: Council for Exceptional Children.

Bateman, B. (1974). Educational implications of minimal brain dysfunction. *Reading Teacher, 27*, 662–668.

Bauer, R. (1982). Information processing as a way of understanding and diagnosing learning disabilities. *Topics in Learning and Learning Disabilities, 2*(2), 46–53.

Berdine, W.H. (Ed.). (in press). *Educational assessment in special education*. Boston: Little, Brown.

Berger, K.W. (1972). *Speechreading: Principles and methods*. Baltimore: National Education Press.

Birch, J., Tisdall, W.J., Peabody, R., & Sterrett, R. (1966). *School achievement and effect of type size on reading in visually handicapped children* (Cooperative Research Project No. 1766). Pittsburgh: University of Pittsburgh.

Bischoff, R.W. (1979). Listening: A teachable skill for visually impaired persons. *Journal of Visual Impairment and Blindness, 73,* 59–67.

Bleck, E.E. (1975). Myelomeningocele, meningocele, spina bifida. In E.E. Bleck & D.A. Nagel (Eds.), *Physically handicapped children: A medical atlas for teachers.* New York: Grune & Stratton.

Bleck, E.E., & Nagel, D.A. (Eds.). (1975). *Physically handicapped children: A medical atlas for teachers.* New York: Grune & Stratton.

Brannon, J.B. (1968). Linguistic word classes in the spoken language of normal, hard-of-hearing, and deaf children. *Journal of Speech and Hearing Research, 11,* 279–287.

Brannon, J.B., & Murray, T. (1966). The spoken syntax of normal, hard-of-hearing, and deaf children. *Journal of Speech and Hearing Research, 9,* 604–610.

Brasel, K., & Quigley, S. (1975). *The influence of early language and communication environments in the development of language in deaf children.* Urbana, IL: University of Illinois Institute for Research on Exceptional Children.

Bruininks, R., Glaman, G., & Clark, C. (1973). Issues in determining prevalence of reading retardation. *The Reading Teacher, 27,* 177–185.

Bryan, T., & Bryan, J. (1978). *Understanding learning disabilities* (2nd ed.). Sherman Oaks, Calif.: Alfred Publishing Company.

Carhart, R. (1970). Development and conservation of speech. In H. Davis & S.R. Silverman (Eds.), *Hearing and deafness.* New York: Holt, Rinehart & Winston.

Caton, H.R. (1981). Visual impairments. In A.E. Blackhurst & W.H. Berdine (Eds.), *An introduction to special education.* Boston: Little, Brown.

Chalfant, J.C., & Scheffelin, M.A. (1969). *Central processing dysfunctions in children: A review of research* (NINDS Monograph, No. 9). Bethesda, MD: United States Department of Health, Education, and Welfare.

Cohen, L., Reid, I., & Boothroyd, K. (1973). Validation of the Mehrabian need for achievement scale with college of education students. *British Journal of Educational Psychology, 43,* 269–278.

Cone, T., & Wilson, L. (1981). Quantifying a severe discrepancy: A critical analysis. *Learning Disability Quarterly, 4*(4), 359–371.

Cruickshank, W. (1963). *Psychology of exceptional children and youth.* Englewood Cliffs, NJ: Prentice-Hall.

Cruickshank, W. (1976). William M. Cruickshank. In J. Kauffman & D. Hallahan (Eds.), *Teaching children with learning disabilities: Personal perspectives.* Columbus, OH: Merrill.

Cutsforth, T.D. (1951). *The blind in school and society: A psychological study.* New York: American Foundation for the Blind.

Delacato, N. (1966). *Neurological organization and reading.* Springfield, IL: Charles C Thomas.

Duffy, J.K. (1967). Hearing problems of school age children. In I.S. Fusfeld (Ed.), *A handbook of readings in education of the deaf and postschool implications.* Springfield, IL: Charles C Thomas.

Dunkin, M.J., & Biddle, B.J. (1974). *The study of teaching.* New York: Holt, Rinehart & Winston.

Felker, D.W. (1973). *Building positive self-concepts.* Minneapolis: Burgess Publishing.

Flanagan, J.C. (1962). *Measuring human performance.* Pittsburgh: American Institute for Research.

Fox, L. (1984). The learning-disabled gifted child. *Learning Disabilities: An Interdisciplinary Journal, 8*(10), 117–128.

Frieze, I.H. (1976). Causal attributions and information-seeking to explain success and failure. *Journal of Research in Personality, 10,* 293–305.

Frostig, M. (1968). Education for children with learning disabilities. In H. Myklebust (Ed.), *Progress in learning disabilities.* New York: Grune & Stratton.

Frybus, R.J., & Karchmer, M.A. (1977). School achievement scores of hearing impaired children: National data on achievement status and growth patterns. *American Annals of the Deaf, 122,* 62–69.

Gage, N.L., & Berliner, D.C. (1979). *Educational psychology.* Chicago: Rand McNally.

Gallagher, J.J. (1966). *Research summary on gifted child education.* Springfield, IL: Office of the Illinois Superintendent of Public Instruction.

Gallagher, J.J. (1975). *Teaching the gifted child* (2nd ed.). Boston: Allyn & Bacon.

Gearheart, B.R., & Weishahn, M.W. (1976). *The handicapped child in the regular classroom.* St. Louis, MO: C.V. Mosby.

Getman, G. (1965). The visuomotor complex in the acquisition of learning skills. In J. Hellmuth (Ed.), *Learning disorders* (Vol. 1). Seattle, WA: Special Child Publications.

Gillingham, A., & Stillman, B. (1966). *Remedial training for children with specific disability in reading, spelling, and penmanship.* Cambridge, MA: Educators Publishing Service.

Goertzel, V.H., & Goertzel, M.G. (1962). *Cradles of eminence.* Boston: Little, Brown.

Goodman, L., & Mann, L. (1976). *Learning disabilities in the secondary school: Issues and practices*. New York: Grune & Stratton.

Gottesman, M.A. (1971). A comparative study of Piaget's developmental schema of sighted children with that of a group of blind children. *Child Development, 42*, 573–580.

Gottesman, M.A. (1973). Conservation development in blind children. *Child Development, 44*, 824–827.

Gottesman, M.A. (1976). Stage development of blind children: A Piagetian view. *New Outlook for the Blind, 70*, 94–100.

Green, W.W. (1981). Hearing disorders. In A.E. Blackhurst & W.H. Berdine (Eds.), *An introduction to special education*. Boston: Little, Brown.

Guilford, J.P. (1959). Three faces of intellect. *American Psychologist, 14*, 469–479.

Guilford, J.P. (1967). *The nature of human intelligence*. New York: McGraw-Hill.

Hamachek, D.E. (Ed.). (1965). *The self in growth, teaching, and learning*. Englewood Cliffs, NJ: Prentice-Hall.

Hammill, D., Leigh, J., McNutt, G., & Larsen, S. (1981). A new definition of learning disabilities. *Learning Disabilities Quarterly, 4*(4), 336–342.

Hayes, S.P. (1941). *Contributions to a psychology of blindness*. New York: American Foundation for the Blind.

Hickok, L.A. (1958). *The story of Helen Keller*. New York: Grosset.

Higgins, L.C. (1973). *Classification in congenitally blind children*. New York: American Foundation for the Blind.

Hobbs, N. (1975). *The futures of children: Categories, labels and their consequences* (Report of the Project on Classification of Exceptional Children). San Francisco: Jossey-Bass.

Hoffman, H.H. (undated). *The price of being born disabled*. Unpublished manuscript.

Hokanson, D.T., & Jospe, M. (1976). *The search for cognitive giftedness in exceptional children*. Hartford, Conn.: Connecticut State Department of Education.

Hollingworth, L. (1942). *Children above 180 IQ, Stanford-Binet*. New York: World Book Company.

Holm, V.A., & Kunze, L.H. (1969). Effect of chronic otitis media on language and speech development. *Pediatrics, 43*, 833.

Horney, K. (1945). *Our inner conflicts*. New York: W.W. Norton.

Houck, C. (1984). *Learning disabilities: Understanding concepts, characteristics, and issues*. Englewood Cliffs, NJ: Prentice-Hall.

Jensema, C. (1975). *The relationship between academic achievement and the demographic characteristics of hearing impaired children and youth*. Washington, DC: Gallaudet College, Office of Demographic Studies.

Jordan, I.K., Gustason, G., & Rosen, R. (1970). An update on communication trends in programs for the deaf. *American Annals of the Deaf, 124,* 350–357.

Karnes, M.B. (1979). Young handicapped children can be gifted and talented. *Journal for the Education of the Gifted, 1*(3), 157–171.

Karnes, M.B., & Bertschi, J.D. (1978). Identifying and educating gifted/talented nonhandicapped and handicapped preschoolers. *Teaching Exceptional Children, 10,* 114–119.

Keough, B. (1977). Working together: A new direction. *Journal of Learning Disabilities, 10,* 478–482.

Kephart, N. (1963). *The brain-injured child in the classroom*. Chicago: National Society for Crippled Children and Adults.

Kephart, J., Kephart, C., & Schwartz, G. (1974). A journey into the world of the blind child. *Exceptional Children, 40,* 421–429.

Kirk, S. (1967). Amelioration of mental abilities through psychodiagnostic and remedial procedures. In G. Jervis (Ed.), *Mental retardation*. Springfield, IL: Charles C Thomas.

Kirk, S. (1976). Samuel A. Kirk. In J. Kauffman & D. Hallahan (Eds.), *Teaching children with learning disabilities: Personal perspectives*. Columbus, OH: Merrill.

Kirk, S.A., & Gallagher, J.J. (1983). *Educating exceptional children* (4th ed.). Boston: Houghton Mifflin.

Kirk, S.A., & Kirk, W.D. (1971). *Psycholinguistic learning disabilities: Diagnosis and remediation*. Chicago: University of Illinois Press.

Knott, G. (1979). Nonverbal communication during early childhood. *Theory into Practice, 18*(4), 226–233.

Knott, G. (1980). Language assessment-intervention with special children. In J. Murray (Ed.), *Developing assessment programs for the multihandicapped child*. Springfield, IL: Charles C Thomas.

Knott, G. (1981). Secondary learning disabilities: Beyond phonics, punctuation and popularity. In W. Cruickshank (Ed.), *The best of ACLD* (Vol. 2). Syracuse, NY: Syracuse University Press.

Knott, G. (1983). Receptive and productive language processes in adolescents. In B. Hutson (Ed.), *Advances in reading/language research* (Vol. 2). Greenwich, CT: JAI Press.

Koppitz, E. (1972–1973). Special class pupils with learning disabilities: A five-year follow-up study. *Academic Therapy, 8,* 133–139.

Kroll, L.G. (1984). LD's—what happens when they are no longer children? *Academic Therapy, 20*(2), 133–148.

LaBenne, W.W., & Green, B.I. (1969). *Educational implications of self-concept theory.* Pacific Palisades, CA: Goodyear Publishing Company.

Larson, A.D., & Miller, J.B. (1978). The hearing impaired. In E.L. Meyen (Ed.), *Exceptional children and youth: An introduction.* Denver, CO: Love Publishing Company.

Lenneberg, E.H. (1967). *Biological foundations of language.* New York: John Wiley.

Lenneberg, E.H. (1970). What is meant by a biological approach to language? *American Annals of the Deaf, 115,* 67–72.

Leonard, J. (1978). *Chapel Hill services to the gifted/handicapped: Program description of a demonstration project for preschool children.* Chapel Hill, NC: The Seeman Printery.

Lerman, A., & Guilfoyle, G. (1970). *The development of pre-vocational behavior in deaf adolescents.* New York: Teachers College Press.

Lerner, J. (1981). *Learning disabilities: Theories, diagnosis, and teaching strategies* (3rd ed.). Boston: Houghton Mifflin.

Lovitt, T. (1978). The learning disabled. In N. Haring (Ed.), *Behavior of exceptional children* (2nd ed.) Columbus, OH: Merrill.

Lowenfeld, B., Abel, G., & Hatlen, P. (1969). *Blind children learn to read.* Springfield, IL: Charles C Thomas.

Macy, D., Baker, J., & Kosinski, S. (1979). An empirical study of the Myklebust learning quotient. *Journal of Learning Disabilities, 12,* 93–96.

Maker, C.J. (1976). Searching for giftedness and talent in children with handicaps. *The School Psychology Digest, 5*(3), 24–36.

Maker, C.J. (1977). *Providing programs for the gifted handicapped.* Reston, VA: Council for Exceptional Children.

Maker, C.J. (1979). Developing multiple talents in exceptional children. *Teaching Exceptional Children, 11,* 120–124.

Maker, C.J. (1982a). *Curriculum development for the gifted.* Rockville, MD: Aspen Systems Corporation.

Maker, C.J. (1982b). *Teaching models in education of the gifted.* Rockville, MD: Aspen Systems Corporation.

Maker, C.J., Morris, E., & James, J. (1981). The Eugene Field Project: A program for potentially gifted young children. In *Balancing the scale for the disadvantaged gifted.* Los Angeles, CA: National/State Leadership Training Institute on the Gifted and the Talented.

Maker, C.J., Redden, M.R., Tonelson, S., & Howell, R.M. (1978). *The self-perceptions of successful handicapped scientists*. Albuquerque, NM: University of New Mexico, The Department of Special Education.

Mann, L., Goodman, L., & Wiederholt, J. (Eds.). (1978). *Teaching the learning disabled adolescent*. Boston: Houghton Mifflin.

Marland, S.P., Jr. (1972). *Education of the gifted and talented* (Report to the Congress of the United States by the U.S. Commissioner of Education). Washington, DC: U.S. Government Printing Office.

Maslow, A. (1962). *Toward a psychology of being*. Princeton, NJ: Van Nostrand.

McClelland, D.C. (1958). *Talent and society*. Princeton, NJ: Van Nostrand.

McConnell, F. (1973). Children with hearing disabilities. In L.M. Dunn (Ed.), *Exceptional children in the schools: Special education in transition* (2nd ed.). New York: Holt, Rinehart & Winston.

McGrady, J. (1968). Language pathology and learning disabilities. In H.R. Myklebust (Ed.), *Progress in learning disabilities* (Vol. 1). New York: Grune & Stratton.

Meadow, K.P. (1968). Early communication in relation to the deaf child's intellectual, social, and communicative functioning. *American Annals of the Deaf, 113,* 29–41.

Meadow, K.P. (1980). *Deafness and child development*. Berkeley: University of California Press.

Meeker, M. (1973). *SOI abilities workbooks and manuals: Memory, cognition, evaluation, convergent production, divergent production*. El Segundo, CA: SOI Institute.

Melichar, J.F. (1977). *ISARE* (Vols. 1–7). San Mateo, CA: Adaptive Systems Corporation.

Melichar, J.F. (1978). ISARE, a description. *AAESPH Review, 3,* 259–268.

Minner, S., & Prater, G. (1984). College teachers' expectations of LD students. *Academic Therapy, 20*(2), 225–229.

Mitchell, M.M. (1976). Teacher attitudes. *High School Journal, 59,* 302–312.

Montgomery, G.W. (1966). Relationship of oral skills to manual communication in profoundly deaf children. *American Annals of the Deaf, 111,* 557–565.

Moore, D.F. (1976). A review of education of the deaf. In L. Mann & D.A. Sabatino (Eds.), *The third review of special education*. New York: Grune & Stratton.

Moores, D. (1982). *Educating the deaf: Psychology, principles, and practices* (2nd ed.). Boston: Houghton Mifflin.

Myerson, L. (1971). Somatopsychology of physical disability. In W.M. Cruickshank (Ed.), *Psychology of exceptional children and youth* (3rd ed.). Englewood Cliffs, NJ: Prentice-Hall.

Myklebust, H.R. (1964). *The psychology of deafness* (2nd ed.). New York: Grune & Stratton.

Myklebust, H. (1968). Learning disabilities: Definition and overview. In H.R. Myklebust (Ed.), *Progress in learning disabilities* (Vol. 1). New York: Grune & Stratton.

Myklebust, H., & Johnson, D. (1967). *Learning disabilities: Educational principles and practices.* New York: Grune & Stratton.

Newby, H.A. (1972). *Audiology.* New York: Appleton-Century-Crofts.

Newland, T.E. (1979). *The gifted in socio-educational perspective.* Englewood Cliffs, NJ: Prentice-Hall.

Northern, J.L., & Downs, M.P. (1974). *Hearing in children.* Baltimore: Williams & Wilkins.

Parnes, S.J. (1966). *Programming creative behavior.* Buffalo: State University of New York at Buffalo.

Parnes, S.J. (1975). *Aha! Insights into creative behavior.* Buffalo: D.O.K. Publishers.

Pless, J.B., & Douglas, J.W.B. (1971). Chronic illness in childhood: Part I. Epidemiological and clinical characteristics. *Pediatrics, 47,* 405–414.

Pless, J.B., & Roghmann, K.G. (1971). Chronic illness and its consequences: Observations based on three epidemiological surveys. *Journal of Pediatrics, 79,* 351–359.

Purkey, W.W. (1970). *Self-concept and school achievement.* Englewood Cliffs, NJ: Prentice-Hall.

Purkey, W.W. (1978). *Inviting school success.* Belmont, CA: Wadsworth Publishing.

Quigley, S.P. (1970). *Some effects of hearing impairment upon school performance.* Manuscript prepared for Office of the Illinois Superintendent of Public Instruction, Division of Special Education Services.

Quigley, S., & Kretschmer, R. (1982). *The education of deaf children.* Baltimore: University Park Press.

Redden, M.R. (1978). What is the state of the art? In H. Hoffman (Ed.), *Science education for handicapped students.* Washington, DC: National Science Teachers Association.

Reid, D., & Hresko, W. (1981). *A cognitive approach to learning disabilities.* New York: McGraw-Hill.

Renzulli, J.S., Smith, L.H., White, A.J., Callahan, C.M., & Hartman, R.K. (1976). *Scales for rating the behavioral characteristics of superior students (SRBCSS).* Wethersfield, CT: Creative Learning Press.

Report of the Ad Hoc Committee to Define Deaf and Hard of Hearing. (1975). *American Annals of the Deaf, 120,* 509–512.

Reynolds, M., & Birch, J. (1977). *Teaching exceptional children in all America's schools.* Reston, VA: Council for Exceptional Children.

Roedell, W.C. (1984). Vulnerabilities of highly gifted children. *Roeper Review, 6*(3), 127–130.

Salvia, J., & Clark, J. (1973). Use of deficits to identify the learning disabled. *Exceptional Children, 39,* 305–308.

Sartain, H. (1976). Instruction of disabled learners: A reading perspective. *Journal of Learning Disabilities, 9,* 489–497.

Schein, J.D., & Delk, M.T., Jr. (1974). *The deaf population of the United States.* Silver Spring, MD: National Association of the Deaf.

Schnur, J.O., & Stefanich, G.P. (1979). Science for the handicapped-gifted child. *Roeper Review, 2*(2), 26–28.

Schultz, C.B., & Pomerantz, M. (1976). Achievement motivation, locus of control, and academic achievement behavior. *Journal of Personality, 44,* 38–51.

Sears, P.S., & Sherman, V.S. (1964). *In pursuit of self-esteem.* Belmont, CA: Wadsworth Publishing.

Simpkins, K., & Stephens, B. (1974). Cognitive development of blind subjects. *Proceedings of the 52nd Biennial Conference of the Association for the Education of the Visually Handicapped,* 26–28.

Stevenson, E.A. (1964). *A study of the educational achievement of deaf children of deaf parents.* Berkeley: California School for the Deaf.

Suppes, P. (1975). A survey of cognition in handicapped children. In S. Chess & A. Thomas (Eds.), *Annual progress in child psychiatry and child development* (pp. 95–129). New York: Brunner/Mazel.

Tannenbaum, A. (1983). *Gifted children.* New York: Macmillan.

Terman, L.M. (1925). The mental and physical traits of a thousand gifted children. In L.M. Terman (Ed.), *Genetic Studies of Genius* (Vol. I). Stanford University Press.

Terman, L.M., & Oden, M.H. (1947). The gifted child grows up. In L.M. Terman (Ed.), *Genetic Studies of Genius* (Vol. IV). Stanford University Press.

Tillman, M.H., & Osborne, R.T. (1969). The performance of blind and sighted children on the Wechsler Intelligence Scale for Children: Interaction effects. *Education of the Visually Handicapped, 1,* 1–4.

Torrance, E.P. (1974). Differences are not deficits. *Teachers College Record, 75,* 471–487.

Towne, C.C. (1979). Disorders of hearing, speech, and language. In V.C. Vaughan, R.J. McKay, & R.E. Behrman (Eds.), *Textbook of pediatrics* (pp. 154–159). Philadelphia: W.B. Saunders.

Vernon, M., & Brown, D. (1964). A guide to psychological tests and testing procedures in the evaluation of deaf and hard of hearing children. *Journal of Speech and Hearing Disorders, 29,* 414–423.

Vernon, M., & Koh, S.D. (1970). Early manual communication and deaf children's achievement. *American Annals of the Deaf, 115,* 527–536.

Vernon, M., & Koh, S.D. (1971). Effects of oral preschool compared to early manual communication on education and communication in deaf children. *American Annals of the Deaf, 116,* 569–574.

Wallace, G., & McLoughlin, J. (1979). *Learning disabilities: Concepts and characteristics* (2nd ed.). Columbus, OH: Merrill.

Wallat, G., & Butler, K. (Eds.). (1984). *Language learning disabilities in school age children.* Baltimore: Williams & Wilkins.

Webb, J.T., Meckstroth, E.A., & Tolan, S.S. (1982). *Guiding the gifted child.* Columbus, OH: Ohio Psychology Publishing Company.

Weiner, B. (1972). *Theories of motivation: From mechanism to cognition.* Chicago: Rand McNally.

Weiner, B. (1974). *Cognitive views of human motivation.* New York: Academic Press.

Weiner, B., Frieze, I., Kukla, A., Reed, L., Rest, S., & Rosenbaum, R.M. (1972). Perceiving the causes of success and failure. In E. Jones, D. Kanouse, H. Kelley, R. Nisbett, S. Valines, & B. Weiner (Eds.), *Attribution: Perceiving the causes of behavior.* Morristown, NJ: General Learning Press.

Weiner, B., Heckhausen, H., Meyer, W.U., & Cook, R.C. (1972). Causal ascriptions and achievement behavior: The conceptual analysis of effort. *Journal of Personality and Social Psychology, 21,* 239–248.

Weiner, B., & Kukla, A. (1970). An attributional analysis of achievement motivation. *Journal of Personality and Social Psychology, 15,* 1–20.

Weiner, B., Nierenberg, R., & Goldstein, M. (1976). Social learning (locus of control) versus attributional (causal stability) interpretations of expectancy of success. *Journal of Personality, 44,* 52–68.

Weiner, B., & Potepan, P.A. (1970). Personality characteristics and affective reactions toward exams of superior and failing college students. *Journal of Educational Psychology, 61,* 144–151.

Wepman, J. (1968). The modality concept. In H. Smith (Ed.), *Perception and reading.* Newark, DE: International Reading Association.

White, A. (undated). *Music/sound assessment.* Unpublished paper (working copy).

Whitmore, J.R. (1980). *Giftedness, conflict, and underachievement.* Boston: Allyn & Bacon.

Whitmore, J.R. (1981). Gifted children with handicapping conditions: A new frontier. *Exceptional Children, 48*(2), 106–114.

Whitmore, J.R. (1983). Changes in teacher education: The key to survival for gifted education. *Roeper Review, 6*(1), 8–13.

Wiig, E., & Semel, E. (1976). *Language disabilities in children and adolescents.* Columbus, OH: Merrill.

Williams, B.R., & Vernon, M. (1970). Vocational guidance for the deaf. In H. Davis & S.R. Silverman (Eds.), *Hearing and deafness* (3rd ed.). New York: Holt, Rinehart & Winston.

Wrightstone, J.W., Aranow, M.S., & Moskowitz, S. (1963). Developing reading test norms for deaf children. *American Annals of the Deaf, 108,* 311–316.

Zehrbach, R.R. (1975). *CIP—Comprehensive Identification Process* (screening test for 2½–5½-year-old handicapped children). Bensenville, IL: Scholastic Testing Service.

Index

About the Authors

JOANNE RAND WHITMORE was trained as an early childhood educator at San Jose State University and completed her master's and doctoral degrees at Stanford University. After several years of teaching, she became involved with the issues of gifted education when assigned to teach primary-age gifted students in cluster classes of the Extended Learning Program in Cupertino, California. It was there that her interest in underachievers evolved and she designed and implemented the successful intervention program for highly gifted underachievers described in *Giftedness, Conflict, and Underachievement* (Allyn & Bacon, 1980).

Upon receiving her Ph.D. degree, Dr. Whitmore joined the faculty of George Peabody College for Teachers in Nashville, Tennessee as coordinator of the educational psychology programs. During her tenure there she directed the programs in early childhood, elementary, and special education and became extensively involved in efforts to better prepare teachers to work with exceptional students in regular classrooms. She is now Assistant Dean for Teacher Education at Kent State University where she also teaches courses and advises doctoral students in gifted education.

Since 1980 Dr. Whitmore has been a representative of teacher educators to the National Council for the Accreditation of Teacher Education. In 1982 she was elected to the presidency of The Association for the Gifted, a division of the Council for Exceptional Children. Recent publications of note include *EEPIGS: Evaluating Educational Programs for Intellectually Gifted Students* (United Educational Services, 1984), an evaluation instrument and process; and "New Challenges to Common Identification Practices," a chapter of J. Freeman (Ed.), *The Psychology of Gifted Children* (John Wiley, 1985).

C. JUNE MAKER is Associate Professor of Special Education at The University of Arizona in Tucson, Arizona. In this capacity, she is responsible for the development and coordination of graduate degree concentrations in education of the gifted both at the master's and doctoral levels. She has been active in several national, state, and local organizations for the gifted and for the handicapped. She has served on the Board of Directors for The National Association for Gifted Children (NAGC) since 1972, and has served as an officer and committee member or committee chairperson for The Association for the Gifted (TAG), the Association for Children with Learning Disabilities (ACLD), and the Arizona Association for the Gifted and Talented (AAGT).

Her publications are related to the topic areas of gifted handicapped, teacher training, the development of talents in exceptional children, teaching learning disabled students, curriculum development for the gifted, and teaching models in education of the gifted. Two major books are *Curriculum Development for the Gifted* and *Teaching Models in Education of the Gifted*. Both are published by Aspen Systems Corporation. She also serves on four editorial boards for journals in education of the gifted and special education. These include *The Gifted Child Quarterly* and *Topics in Early Childhood Special Education*. She is editor of a yearbook series entitled *Critical Issues in Gifted Education*, also published by Aspen.

In the past, she has been a teacher, a regional supervisor for a state department of education, an administrative intern in the federal office for the gifted, and an assistant professor at the University of New Mexico. She has consulted with numerous local school districts, state departments of education, and other public and private agencies both in the United States and in other countries. Her educational background consists of degrees in education of the gifted, and learning disabled, educational psychology, and elementary education from the University of Virginia (Ph.D.), Southern Illinois University (M.S.), and Western Kentucky University (B.S.).